NUTRITION
94/95

Sixth Edition

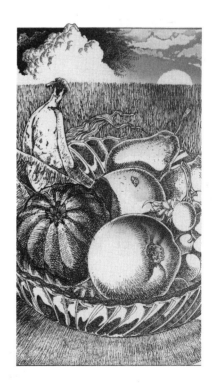

Annual Editions
A Library of Information from the Public Press

Editor

Charlotte C. Cook-Fuller
Towson State University

Charlotte Cook-Fuller has a Ph.D. in community health education and graduate and undergraduate degrees in nutrition. She has worked for several years in public health services and has also been involved with the federally funded WIC (Women, Infants, and Children) program. Now as a professor, she teaches nutrition within both professional and consumer contexts, as well as courses for health education students. She has co-authored a nutrition curriculum for grades K-12 and is currently involved in a multidisciplinary effort to provide strategies to public school teachers for teaching about global issues such as hunger.

Editorial Consultant

Stephen Barrett, M.D.
Editor, *Nutrition Forum*

Cover illustration by Mike Eagle

The Dushkin Publishing Group, Inc.
Sluice Dock, Guilford, Connecticut 06437

The Annual Editions Series

Annual Editions is a series of over 60 volumes designed to provide the reader with convenient, low-cost access to a wide range of current, carefully selected articles from some of the most important magazines, newspapers, and journals published today. Annual Editions are updated on an annual basis through a continuous monitoring of over 300 periodical sources. All Annual Editions have a number of features designed to make them particularly useful, including topic guides, annotated tables of contents, unit overviews, and indexes. For the teacher using Annual Editions in the classroom, an Instructor's Resource Guide with test questions is available for each volume.

VOLUMES AVAILABLE

Africa
Aging
American Foreign Policy
American Government
American History, Pre-Civil War
American History, Post-Civil War
Anthropology
Biology
Business Ethics
Canadian Politics
Child Growth and Development
China
Commonwealth of Independent States
Comparative Politics
Computers in Education
Computers in Business
Computers in Society
Criminal Justice
Drugs, Society, and Behavior
Dying, Death, and Bereavement
Early Childhood Education
Economics
Educating Exceptional Children
Education
Educational Psychology
Environment
Geography
Global Issues
Health
Human Development
Human Resources
Human Sexuality
India and South Asia

International Business
Japan and the Pacific Rim
Latin America
Life Management
Macroeconomics
Management
Marketing
Marriage and Family
Mass Media
Microeconomics
Middle East and the Islamic World
Money and Banking
Multicultural Education
Nutrition
Personal Growth and Behavior
Physical Anthropology
Psychology
Public Administration
Race and Ethnic Relations
Social Problems
Sociology
State and Local Government
Third World
Urban Society
Violence and Terrorism
Western Civilization, Pre-Reformation
Western Civilization, Post-Reformation
Western Europe
World History, Pre-Modern
World History, Modern
World Politics

Library of Congress Cataloging in Publication Data
Main entry under title: Annual editions: Nutrition. 1994/95.
1. Nutrition—Periodicals. 2. Diet—Periodicals. I. Cook-Fuller, Charlotte C., *comp.*
II. Title: Nutrition.
ISBN 1–56134–256–4   613.2′05

© 1994 by The Dushkin Publishing Group, Inc., Guilford, CT 06437

Sixth Edition

Printed in the United States of America

Printed on Recycled Paper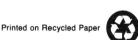

Editors/ Advisory Board

EDITORS

Charlotte C. Cook-Fuller
Towson State University

with Stephen Barrett, M.D.
Editor, *Nutrition Forum*

ADVISORY BOARD

Georgia Crews
South Dakota State University

Patricia Erickson
Skyline College

Sarah T. Hawkins
Indiana State University

Suzanne Hendrich
Iowa State University

David H. Hyde
University of Maryland
College Park

Dorothy Klimis-Tauantzis
University of Maine
Orono

Manfred Kroger
Pennsylvania State University
University Park

William M. London
Kent State University

Aden C. Magee
University of North Carolina

Sudma W. Mehta
Northern Illinois University

Gretchen Myers-Hill
Michigan State University

M. Zafar Nomani
West Virginia University

Thomas M. Richard
Keene State College

Diana M. Spillman
Miami University

Anna J. Svacha
Auburn University

Diane Witte
University of Wisconsin
Stevens Point

Members of the Advisory Board are instrumental in the final selection of articles for each edition of Annual Editions. Their review of articles for content, level, currentness, and appropriateness provides critical direction to the editor and staff. We think you'll find their careful consideration well reflected in this volume.

STAFF

Ian A. Nielsen, Publisher
Brenda S. Filley, Production Manager
Roberta Monaco, Editor
Addie Raucci, Administrative Editor
Cheryl Greenleaf, Permissions Editor
Diane Barker, Editorial Assistant
Lisa Holmes-Doebrick, Administrative Coordinator
Charles Vitelli, Designer
Shawn Callahan, Graphics
Meredith Scheld, Graphics
Steve Shumaker, Graphics
Lara M. Johnson, Graphics
Libra A. Cusack, Typesetting Supervisor
Juliana Arbo, Typesetter

To the Reader

In publishing ANNUAL EDITIONS we recognize the enormous role played by the magazines, newspapers, and journals of the *public press* in providing current, first-rate educational information in a broad spectrum of interest areas. Within the articles, the best scientists, practitioners, researchers, and commentators draw issues into new perspective as accepted theories and viewpoints are called into account by new events, recent discoveries change old facts, and fresh debate breaks out over important controversies.

Many of the articles resulting from this enormous editorial effort are appropriate for students, researchers, and professionals seeking accurate, current material to help bridge the gap between principles and theories and the real world. These articles, however, become more useful for study when those of lasting value are carefully *collected, organized, indexed,* and *reproduced* in a *low-cost format,* which provides easy and permanent access when the material is needed. That is the role played by *Annual Editions.* Under the direction of each volume's *Editor,* who is an expert in the subject area, and with the guidance of an *Advisory Board,* we seek each year to provide in each *ANNUAL EDITION* a current, well-balanced, carefully selected collection of the best of the public press for your study and enjoyment. We think you'll find this volume useful, and we hope you'll take a moment to let us know what you think.

Perhaps you may agree with Pudd'nhead Wilson (a character created by Mark Twain) who said, "The only way to keep your health is to eat what you don't want, drink what you don't like, and do what you'd rather not." Nutritionists would argue that you cannot achieve or maintain good health on a diet of soft drinks and vending machine foods. But you might be surprised to learn that many of your favorite foods can fit into a good diet. In making food choices, variety and moderation are two key words that will assist you in achieving positive health outcomes and avoiding the negative results of excesses or deficiencies.

An array of resources is available to help you make decisions, including popular publications, the news media, scientific journals, and people from many educational backgrounds. Your dilemma is to select reliable sources that will supply factual information without exaggeration or bias. An additional problem you have is to avoid overreacting to nutrition- and food-related news items or promotional materials, especially if they are sensational or have shock value. The exaggeration and the myth are what much of the public grasps and, in large measure, follows. My challenge to the reader is to use this volume, preferably with a standard nutrition text, as an invitation to learning. Become a discriminating learner. Compare what you hear and read to the accepted body of knowledge. If this volume provides you with useful information, challenges your thinking, broadens your understanding, or motivates you to take some useful action, it will have fulfilled its purpose.

While this entire volume is essentially one of current events, the first unit focuses on characteristics of today's food consumer, changes in the food industry, particularly the new labeling regulations, and a preview of the future. The next three units are devoted to nutrients, diet and disease, and weight control. All are topics directly related to health, and the dynamic state of knowledge requires each of us to be constantly learning and adjusting. Units on food safety and health claims follow, areas in which consumers are especially vulnerable to media and promotional hype and misinformation. Finally, unit 7 addresses hunger and malnutrition as a social and political issue as well as one requiring scientific knowledge for solution. Originally this was intended as a forum for global concerns, but it has become abundantly clear that hunger is also a national issue. Although the units in this book are distinct, many of the articles have broader significance. The *topic guide* will help you to find other articles on a given subject. You will also find that many of the articles contain at least some element of controversy, the origin of which may be incomplete knowledge, questionable policy, pseudoscience, or competing needs. Sometimes these are difficult issues to resolve, and frequently any resolution creates other dilemmas. But creatively solving problems is our challenge. We take the world as it is and use it as a foundation for tomorrow's discoveries and solutions.

This book is an anthology, and any anthology can be improved, including this one. You can influence the content of future editions by returning the article rating form on the last page of the book with your comments and suggestions.

Charlotte C. Cook-Fuller

Charlotte C. Cook-Fuller
Editor

Contents

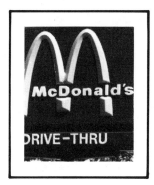

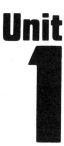

Unit 1

Trends Today and Tomorrow

Thirteen articles examine the eating patterns of people today. Some of the topics considered include nutrients in our diet, eating trends, food labeling, self-service outlets, and the latest in infant feeding.

The concepts in bold italics are developed in the article. For further expansion please refer to the Topic Guide, the Index, and the Glossary.

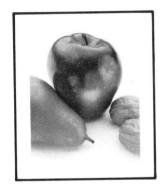
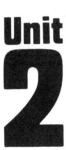

Unit 2

Nutrients

Eleven articles discuss the importance of nutrients and
fiber in our diet. Topics include dietary standards,
carbohydrates, fiber, vitamins, supplements, and
minerals.

The concepts in bold italics are developed in the article. For further expansion please refer to the Topic Guide, the Index, and the Glossary.

20. **Can Megadoses of Vitamin C Help Against Colds?** 69
Charles W. Marshall, *Nutrition Forum,* September/October 1992.

While many consumers continue to rely on **supplemental vitamin C** to prevent or cure colds, **scientific evidence** does not support this practice. This article summarizes the evidence and discusses **how scientific facts are determined.**

21. **Folic Acid: New Findings Renew Old Debate,** *Food Insight,* January/February 1993. 73

Neural tube defects (NTDs), which account for about five percent of **birth defects** in the United States, frequently may be linked to an insufficient amount of **folacin.** While **supplements** may seem like an easy answer, there are associated **risks.**

22. **Fluoride: Cavity-Fighter on Tap,** Dodi Schultz, *FDA Consumer,* January/February 1992. 74

Truly, the values of **fluoride** have been made clear by a dramatic reduction in **dental caries.** While excesses of **fluoride** can cause damage to teeth, the amounts put into **public water supplies** are carefully controlled to maximize the benefits. A **guide** for supplementing fluoride and tips for parents are included in this article.

23. **Might Americans Be Taking in Too Much Iron?** *Tufts University Diet & Nutrition Letter,* January 1993. 78

Recent research questions if there is a **connection between high iron levels and heart attack risk.** However, in the United States, **iron deficiency** is common among females and children. The degree of iron absorption depends on its form and the food eaten at the same time. Ironically, a few genetically predisposed people absorb too much iron even if they do not need it.

24. **The Importance of Fiber,** *University of California at Berkeley Wellness Letter,* April 1992. 83

Fiber, although not a nutrient, nevertheless performs significant **physiological functions** in the body. To meet the **recommendations** for fiber consumption, most Americans will have to eat more plant products.

Overview 86
25. **Eating Disorders Require Medical Attention,** Dixie Farley, *FDA Consumer,* March 1992. 88

Both **bulimia** and **anorexia** are fairly common disorders, especially among young women. The causes are unknown, but the consequences can be severe. Because both **eating disorders** are difficult to stop without assistance and because early treatment is necessary, professional help should be sought quickly.

26. **Nutrition and the Elderly,** Alexandra Greeley, *FDA Consumer,* October 1990. 90

Problems of social isolation, deteriorating health, and other factors often lead to **poor nutrition** habits among the **elderly.** In turn, health declines even further. **Ways to stimulate the appetite** are suggested in this article.

27. **Breakfast: Waking Up to a Healthy Start,** *Food Insight,* March/April 1992. 92

Those of us who are confirmed **breakfast-skippers** should review the performance and nutrient benefits to be gained from eating **breakfast.** Before you voice your reasons why you cannot (or will not) eat breakfast, check the tips in this article. These benefits apply to both **children** and adults.

28. **Benefits and Risks of Vegetarian Diets,** Susan Dingott and Johanna Dwyer, *Nutrition Forum,* November/December 1991. 95

Vegetarian diets must be planned well if they are to meet nutritional needs. Both **benefits and risks** are explored in this article. A chart also provides a key to **protein** complementation.

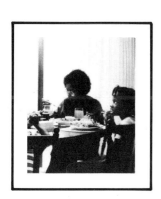 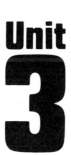

Unit 3

Through the Life Span: Diet and Disease

Eight articles examine our health as it is affected by diet throughout our lives. Some topics include the importance of childhood nutrition, the links between diet and disease, cholesterol levels, and the latest on high blood pressure.

The concepts in bold italics are developed in the article. For further expansion please refer to the Topic Guide, the Index, and the Glossary.

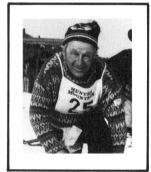

Unit 4

Fat and Weight Control

Nine articles examine weight management. Topics include the relationship between dieting and exercise, the genetic connection in weight control, the effects of various diet plans, and the relationship between being overweight and fit.

The concepts in bold italics are developed in the article. For further expansion please refer to the Topic Guide, the Index, and the Glossary.

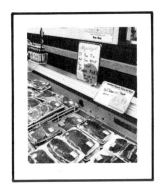
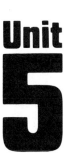

Unit 5

Food Safety

Nine articles discuss the safety of food. Topics include
the danger of poisons that can enter the foods in our
everyday diet.

47. **The Canning Process: Old Preservation Technique Goes Modern,** Dale Blumenthal, *FDA Consumer,* September 1990.   **164**

For nearly 200 years, food has been canned to prevent spoilage. Today's canning methods include not only cans and jars but paperboard and plastic formed into pouches and bowls as well. *Canning techniques* carefully destroy *hazardous bacteria* and retain food quality.

48. **The Unwelcome Dinner Guest: Preventing Food-Borne Illness,** Annabel Hecht, *FDA Consumer,* January/February 1991.   **167**

Consumers are frequently responsible for their own *food-borne illnesses.* Learning how to safely handle food could reduce the *risk* considerably. Information about the major food-borne organisms and symptoms of the diseases they cause are included.

49. **Burgers: Never Say "Rare,"** *University of California at Berkeley Wellness Letter,* June 1993.   **174**

A serious outbreak of *food-borne illness* in late 1992 in Washington State has made *undercooked hamburger* one of the hot news items of the year. While the disease is not usually fatal, it is serious. The lesson to be learned—no more steak tartare or pink hamburgers.

50. **Salmonella Enteritidis: From the Chicken to the Egg,** Dale Blumenthal, *FDA Consumer,* April 1990.   **175**

Continuing *salmonella* outbreaks both in the United States and abroad strengthen the data connecting it with uncracked, sanitized eggs. Public health issues and regulatory actions are discussed in this article, and *safety* tips are included.

Overview   **178**

51. **How Quackery Sells,** William T. Jarvis and Stephen Barrett, *Nutrition Forum,* March/April 1991.   **180**

Quacks are masters of the art of influencing people. As super manipulators, they sell *false hope* through products that cannot possibly produce the desired magical effects. This article exposes the tricks they use.

52. **The Multilevel Mirage,** Stephen Barrett, *Priorities,* Summer 1991.   **185**

Being an independent distributor who sells *health-related products* is a popular money-making scheme. It pays, however, to be wary of the products and *health claims.* Usually expensive, they are often unnecessary, unproven, or outright *fraudulent.*

53. **Food News Blues,** Anthony Schmitz, *Health,* November 1991.   **188**

How can the ordinary consumer separate *sense from nonsense* in the *latest news*? Start with understanding the motivations of a newspaper editor. Then apply some basic questions, healthy skepticism, and common sense.

54. **Vitamin Pushers and Food Quacks,** Victor Herbert, *Nutrition Forum,* March/April 1993.   **192**

Since the discovery of *vitamins,* we have been both blessed by the knowledge of the true miracles they produce and plagued by their excessive and dangerous use. In fact, promoting *megadose usage of vitamins* is, at the same time, both a major industry and outright *quackery.* Some of the selling strategies are presented in this article.

55. **Chiropractors and Nutrition: The "Supplement Underground,"** Stephen Barrett, *Nutrition Forum,* July/August 1992.   **199**

Whatever one's position concerning the value of *chiropractic,* it is useful to know that many *chiropractors* rely heavily on the *inappropriate use of supplements.* Evidence presented here shows that supplements can be a major source of the chiropractor's income.

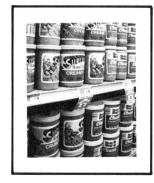

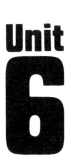

Unit

6

Health Claims

Nine articles examine some of the health claims made by today's "specialists." Topics include quacks, fad diets, and nutrition myths and misinformation.

The concepts in bold italics are developed in the article. For further expansion please refer to the Topic Guide, the Index, and the Glossary.

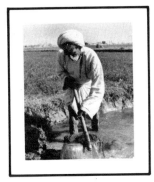
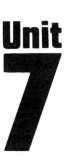

Unit 7

Hunger and Global Issues

Five articles discuss the world's food supply. Topics include global malnutrition, famine, and wasteful food production in the United States.

The concepts in bold italics are developed in the article. For further expansion please refer to the Topic Guide, the Index, and the Glossary.

Topic Guide

This topic guide suggests how the selections in this book relate to topics of traditional concern to students and professionals involved with the study of nutrition. It is useful for locating articles that relate to each other for reading and research. The guide is arranged alphabetically according to topic. Articles may, of course, treat topics that do not appear in the topic guide. In turn, entries in the topic guide do not necessarily constitute a comprehensive listing of all the contents of each selection.

TOPIC AREA	TREATED IN:	TOPIC AREA	TREATED IN:
Additives	9. Ingredient Labeling: What's in a Food? 44. Is the Artificially Sweetened Stuff the Right Stuff? 45. Low-Calorie Sweeteners: Aspartame	**Fat/Fat Substitutes**	6. Fat Replacers Now and in Your Future 15. Basic Primer on Fats in the Diet 16. Fat for the Fit
Antioxidants	18. Supplement Story	**Fiber**	24. Importance of Fiber 32. Diet/Cancer Connection
Biotechnology	7. Biotechnology—The Designer Genes 43. Hot Potato	**Food Safety**	42. Scientists Urge Skepticism of Reports About an Unsafe Food Supply 43. Hot Potato 46. Good Food You Can't Get 47. Canning Process 49. Burgers: Never Say "Rare" 50. Salmonella Enteritidis
Breakfast	27. Breakfast: Waking Up to a Healthy Start		
Children	22. Fluoride: Cavity-Fighter on Tap 27. Breakfast: Waking Up to a Healthy Start 60. Nutrition/World Hunger 62. Hunger and Undernutrition in America	**Food-Borne Illness**	46. Good Food You Can't Get 47. Canning Process 48. Unwelcome Dinner Guest 49. Burgers: Never Say "Rare" 50. Salmonella Enteritidis
Cholesterol	29. Cholesterol		
Controversial Issues	7. Biotechnology—The Designer Genes 11. Look for 'Legit' Health Claims on Foods 12. ADA Timely Statement on Proposed Revision of U.S. RDAs 23. Might Americans Be Taking in Too Much Iron? 43. Hot Potato 44. Is the Artificially Sweetened Stuff the Right Stuff? 45. Low-Calorie Sweeteners: Aspartame 46. Good Food You Can't Get	**Guidelines/ Recommendations**	4. Dietary Guidelines Revised 5. Food Pyramid—Food Label Connection 11. Look for 'Legit' Health Claims on Foods 14. Things Nobody Ever Told Rocky Balboa About Protein 15. Basic Primer on Fats in the Diet 16. Fat for the Fit 22. Fluoride: Cavity-Fighter on Tap 23. Might Americans Be Taking in Too Much Iron? 24. Importance of Fiber 29. Cholesterol 30. Lifelong Program to Build Strong Bones 31. Hypertension 36. Quit Watching the Scales? 40. Rating the Diets 48. Unwelcome Dinner Guest 49. Burgers: Never Say "Rare" 50. Salmonella Enteritidis 59. Nutritional Supplements for Athletes?
Diet and Disease	11. Look for 'Legit' Health Claims on Foods 16. Fat for the Fit 19. What Can E Do for You? 24. Importance of Fiber 29. Cholesterol 30. Lifelong Program to Build Strong Bones 31. Hypertension 32. Diet/Cancer Connection 57. Nutrition Myths and Misinformation		
Diet Methods/ Programs	40. Rating the Diets 58. FDA Bans Diet Pill Ingredients	**Hunger/Malnutrition**	14. Things Nobody Ever Told Rocky Balboa About Protein 60. Nutrition/World Hunger 61. Hunger and Undernutrition in America 63. Hunger in the United States: Policy Implications 64. Effects of Human Starvation
Eating Disorders	25. Eating Disorders 37. Nondiet Movement Gains Strength		
Eating Patterns/ Preferences	1. Food Americans Buy 2. Changing American Diet 3. War and Peas: How Wars Have Shaped America's Diet	**Infants**	21. Folic Acid: New Findings Renew Old Debate 41. Causes of Obesity in Infants 60. Nutrition/World Hunger 62. Hunger and Undernutrition in America
Elderly	26. Nutrition and the Elderly 30. Lifelong Program to Build Strong Bones		

Trends Today and Tomorrow

Today is not yesterday./We ourselves change./How then, can our works and thoughts, if they are always to be the fittest, continue always the same. / Change indeed is painful, yet ever needful. . . .

—Carlyle

Indeed, the average consumer is almost a phantom, constantly reshaping under the influences of the food industry, the media, activist organizations, and whatever health messages are currently most persuasive. Some trends, such as decreased consumption of certain higher fat products, do emerge over time (see "The Food Americans Buy" and "The Changing American Diet"), and at least one major grocery chain has laid off meat cutters as a result. Conversely, consumption of fresh fruits and vegetables has risen (increasing two- and ten-fold respectively for cauliflower and broccoli, 300 percent for squash). To supply this increased demand, the produce import business has greatly increased to 13 billion pounds yearly. Mexico is a major supplier of limes and vegetables. Canada supplies 18 percent of the vegetables we consume, and other supplies come from South and Central America as well as Europe. Still, Americans spend less of their incomes for food than do citizens of any other country.

Evidence of contradictory trends is common. Some pollsters say we are becoming less concerned about fat and reverting to a greater interest in taste, that we are more willing to indulge ourselves and to forgive ourselves for doing it. Ample support for this contention exists. Seventy-six percent of Americans told the *Washington Post* that they are reducing dietary fat, but the USDA says we consume 45 percent more lard and shortening than 5 years ago. According to a study by the American Dietetics Association, 78 percent of women carefully select foods for a healthy diet, but a North Carolina study determined that women also eat twice as much pizza and pasta with rich cheese sauces, 24 percent more desserts, and nearly 60 percent more fatty snacks than they did in 1977. The number of restaurant diners who carefully watch what they eat is said to be declining also, and Mega Mac, McDonald's newest, biggest burger is said to be doing much better than the McLean DeLuxe, which may be phased out. Analysts argue over whether we are simply treating ourselves through these behaviors, perhaps compensating emotionally for the hardships of an economic depression, or we are establishing a genuine disregard for healthy behavior. In contradiction, new low-fat, low-cholesterol food products are being introduced in grocery stores at the rate of 30 to 35 per month, and they are doing well in the marketplace (see "Fat Replacers Now and in Your Future").

Today's sophisticated consumer wants information, and much has been done to fill that desire. Dietary Guidelines for Americans, the third edition ("Dietary Guidelines Revised"), was published earlier, and more recently the Food Guide Pyramid (see "The Food Pyramid—Food Label Connection") has replaced the Basic Four to show daily recommended amounts from five food groups. So far, only about half of the population say the pyramid is even somewhat familiar. And, of course, knowledge does not indicate practice. In a Gallup survey, a mere 5 percent of those responding admitted to currently following the new recommendations, and no more than 15 percent indicated willingness to comply with the recommended grain consumption of at least 6 servings daily.

Over half of the population, 52 percent according to a Roper poll, turn to packaging labels for information. Yet many consumers found the old labeling system to be confusing and impractical. New label specifications are ready for implementation (articles 8–11), and big changes are on the way. Perhaps the most obvious changes are the expanded information on fats and how the product fits into the overall daily diet. For this purpose, new reference values, Reference Daily Intakes (RDIs), will replace the U.S. Recommended Daily Allowances (U.S. RDAs), but this will be only a name change until a review process takes place. Additionally, health claims considered to be scientifically valid will be allowed, and there will be standard definitions for descriptive terms such as "light" and "reduced." The cost of these labeling changes, ultimately to be borne by the consumer, is estimated at between $1.6–$2 billion. Some critics assert that the label changes are not in the consumer's best interests, and one is tempted to speculate if a pocket guidebook will be needed. Still, there is general agreement that changes are necessary, and the really interested consumer should be able to make more sense of the new labels. A supporting position is taken in the article "ADA Timely Statement on Proposed Revision of U.S. RDAs for Use on Food Labels."

The Food and Drug Administration (FDA) promotes other sources of nutrition information as well. In grocery stores, food shoppers are already helping themselves to pamphlets, leaflets, and recipes. Point-of-purchase information is required for at least the 20 most frequently eaten raw vegetables, fruits, and fish. While technically a voluntary program, it will remain so only if 60 percent or more of a representative sample of grocery stores nationwide are in compliance. In a newer ruling, the FDA will require

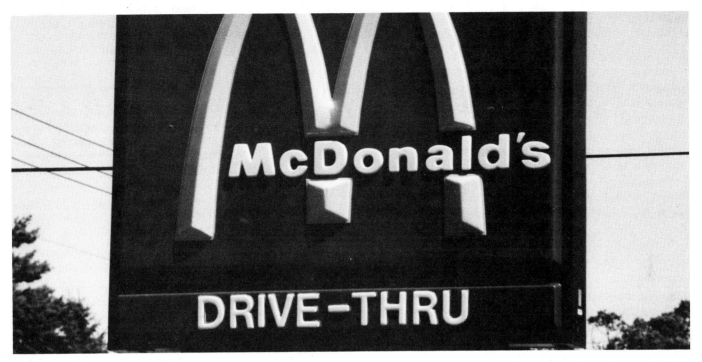

restaurants to support nutrition claims made in menus. Although the menus need not contain the information, chefs must be able to justify claims such as "healthy" or "low fat" to inspectors. Additional consumer information, for those willing to make the effort, can be secured from the FDA itself or other agencies (see article 13).

Trends in biotechnology enable foods to be designed for special health needs, plants and animals for disease resistance, and produce for better flavor and longer shelf life. These trends are addressed in "Biotechnology—The New Designer Genes," and in the article "Hot Potato" in unit 5. Irradiation, a trend in food preservation, though a controversial one, is also addressed in unit 5.

From time to time historical events effect a lasting impact on eating habits. Both the tomato and the potato originated in the Andes Mountains and reached Europe only after the age of exploration began. But, can you imagine Italian food now without tomatoes? Wars have been equally important. The canning process was developed in response to Napoleon's request for better food preservation methods to feed his troops. "An army marches on its stomach," he said. Article 3 describes how other wars have shaped today's food styles. More recently, the Persian Gulf War has speeded up the technology to provide shelf-stable pizzas, carbonated beverages in compressed tablets, and chocolate that withstands high heat.

Cultural change is occurring in our lifetimes. An orange was a treat in the toe of my mother's Christmas stocking. As a child, I had fresh oranges and orange juice in cans. For my daughters frozen orange juice was commonplace, and my grandchildren enjoy drinking it from sealed cartons, although all of the previous options remain. By the year 2001, eating is expected to be "grazing style" and combined with other activities rather than an event in itself. Breakfast will be eaten in the car, where there will be a microwave in the glove compartment. What other possibilities will there be for the next generation?

Looking Ahead: Challenge Questions

Explain contradictory trend results from surveys.

Do you feel that the packaging label changes are appropriate and useful? Will it have a good return for the costs involved?

Which trends in the food industry will or will not support healthier life-styles?

Discuss the implications of biotechnology as they relate to health and ethical issues.

Does change always equal progress? Why or why not?

The Food Americans Buy: An Economic Perspective

Fast Scan: Americans spend a smaller portion of their income for food than any other country. The budget share for food was only 11.8% in 1990. An economic perspective explains many factors affecting the food Americans buy. In 1960, 37.7% of women were in the labor force; in 1989, 57.4% were. This change has had a major impact on the food we buy. Time-pressured consumers want convenience. Food products are increasingly thought of as composed of attributes which can be altered in response to consumer demands. Packaging and advertising are now important product attributes.

Ben Senauer, Ph.D.

Professor
Department of Agricultural and
Applied Economics
University of Minnesota
St. Paul, Minnesota 55108

O ur food system in the United States has become consumer driven. New food products are developed to respond to consumer wants and needs, and the most successful food companies have acquired a consumer-oriented marketing focus. A knowledge of consumer food trends and their implications is vital. Moreover, the food Americans buy is changing dramatically, and the underlying factors behind these changes are increasingly complex (1). An economic perspective can enrich our understanding of the food-buying behavior of American consumers.

[1]This article draws on the author's new book *Food Trends and the Changing Consumer*, written with Elaine Asp and Jean Kinsey. It is published by Eagan Press, 3340 Pilot Knob Road, St. Paul, MN 55121-2097.

Share of Budget Spent for Food Still Declining in U.S.

The share of the budget spent for food is a basic yet informative statistic. Engel's law says that as income increases, the proportion spent for food will decrease. The basic factor behind this law is the limited capacity of the human stomach, and the many other goods and services people wish to purchase (1).

In Table 1, an average of only 11.8% of disposable (after taxes) income was spent for food in 1990: 7.3% for food at home and 4.5% for food away from home. The share of income spent for food consumed at home and for total food has steadily declined, whereas the portion going to food away from home has risen. Engel's law holds for food at home and total food, even though Americans are buying food with more value added (i.e., more processing and convenience). It is important to look beyond the overall averages though.

Higher income households (with incomes over $50,000) spent 9.9% of their income on food, whereas lower income households (with incomes less than $10,000) spent over 30.0% in 1989 (2). This pattern also reflects Engel's law.

As shown in Table 2, Americans spend a smaller share of their budget on food at home than any other country. Only 8.4% of total personal consumption expenditures were for food consumed at home in the United States. The share is also the lowest for any country when total food, beverage and tobacco expenditures are compared to disposable income per person (3). This achievement reflects not only our high average income level and the operation of Engel's law, but also results from the efficiency of the U.S. food system in providing reasonably priced food.

People in poor Third World countries, such as the Philippines and India, must devote over half their budgets to food. Although Switzerland actually has a higher

TABLE 1. Food Expenditures by Families and Individuals as a Share of Disposable Personal Income[1]			
	Percent of Income Spent for Food		
Year	At Home	Away from Home	Total
1929	20.7	3.2	23.9
1939	18.6	3.3	21.9
1949	18.0	4.1	22.1
1959	14.3	3.5	17.8
1970	10.4	3.7	14.1
1980	9.3	4.5	13.8
1990	7.3	4.5	11.8

[1] Data from (10, p. 50)

From *Food & Nutrition News*, Vol. 64, No. 2, March/April 1992, pp. 11-12. Copyright © 1992 by the National Live Stock and Meat Board. Reprinted by permission.

> "Because it is limited, time has an economic value. As incomes have risen and the pressures on available time increased, life seems to become more hectic."

> "Over $11 billion was spent on food-related advertising in 1988." (8)

total expenditure and income level per person than the United States, their budget share for food is much higher. This reflects the high price the Swiss pay for food.

Increasing Number of Working Women Increases Demand for Convenience

Greatly increased participation of women in the labor force is one of the major economic and social trends of our time. The labor force participation rate for women has gone from 37.7% in 1960 to 57.4% in 1989 (4). The rate for married women went from 31.9% to 57.8% during the same period.

Three out of four women 35 to 44 years old are now in the labor force. Even for married women with a child less than 6 years old, the participation rate reached 58.4% in 1989 (4).

Given this trend, it should not be surprising that convenience has become such an important attribute in food products. Surveys have found that women still do over 90% of the cooking in American families (5). Time-pressured consumers do not want to buy ingredients used to prepare a meal; they want to buy a meal that is ready to heat and serve. Some 75 to 80% of American households now have microwave ovens. The demand for convenience is also behind the rapid growth in home meal delivery and take-out-to-eat (TOTE) food.

The economic concepts of Gary Becker stress the importance of productive activity in the household and the scarcity of time (6). People confront not only a limited budget, but also a time constraint. Everyone faces the limitation that there are just 24 hours in a day. Because it is limited, time has an economic value. As incomes have risen and the pressures on the available time increased, life seems to become more hectic.

Women who are in the labor force and have families have the greatest demands on their time, since they continue to do most of the work in the home (1). Furthermore, Becker suggests that work activity occurs not just in the labor force, but in the home where many things are produced, such as home-cooked meals.

This household work of cooking meals resembles in a basic economic sense the production process that occurs in a factory: Preparation of a meal requires inputs purchased at the supermarket, household capital such as stoves and refrigerators, and labor. Efficiency of household production can vary. A skilled cook can create a more appetizing meal with the same ingredients than someone with little training or experience in cooking. A technical innovation like the microwave oven increases efficiency by reducing the time, and perhaps energy, necessary to cook many foods.

The full price of a home-cooked meal includes not just the purchased ingredients, but the value of the time spent in its preparation. As labor force participation by women rises, the value of their time increases, the cost of home-cooked meals goes up, and the demand for convenience increases.

Food Product Attributes Influence Consumer Demand

According to Kevin Lancaster, consumers buy goods for the characteristics or attributes which they embody (7). Demand for food products is determined by the characteristics they contain. Food scientists are now asked to develop products that contain specific attributes that consumers want. Many line extensions alter only a few, and perhaps even just one, attribute. This allows products to be targeted at particular market "niches," but also contributes to product proliferation. Some 9,200 new food products were introduced in 1989 (8).

In response to the demand for convenience, almost 1,000 new microwave products were introduced in 1989 (9). Companies are also scrambling to develop low-fat or nonfat products. Some fast-food chains have introduced reduced-fat hamburgers. Fat-free ingredients with the functional properties of fat are now available for some uses. However, consumers want products that do not sacrifice taste and quality characteristics.

Attributes that compose a food product encompass its advertising and packaging. Over $11 billion was spent on food-related advertising in 1988 (8). Advertising tries to influence consumer perceptions of a product's characteristics. Companies use advertising to attempt to create a specific impression of their product among consumers. They want to differentiate their product from competing ones and generate brand loyalty. Much of the takeover activity in the food industry in the 1980's was motivated by a desire to acquire highly profitable, market-leading brand name products (1).

Packaging costs now account for 8% of total food expenditures and totaled $36 billion in 1990 (10). Packaging contributes to storability, appearance, convenience and quality attributes. The package's appearance can be very important. If consumers do not find it attractive, they may never buy the product. Increasingly though, packaging affects other product characteristics. For example, with microwave products, the package may actually be the cooking utensil and contain features such as susceptors that affect the heating of the food.

TABLE 2. Expenditures for Food Consumed at Home as a Share of Total Personal Consumption Expenditures for Selected Countries, 1986[1]

Country	Percent of Total Consumption Expenditures	Total Personal Consumption
		Dollars per person
United States	8.4	11,673
Canada	12.1	8,280
United Kingdom	14.3	5,830
Australia	15.8	6,479
Hong Kong	17.3	4,190
France	17.3	7,904
West Germany	17.4	8,042
Sweden	18.3	7,989
Japan	19.4	9,235
Switzerland	21.4	12,341
Italy	21.8	6,361
USSR	28.0	NA[2]
Israel	28.6	4,081
Mexico	33.1	1,340
Greece	36.0	2,649
Thailand	38.1	513
Jamaica	40.3	663
China	47.8	NA
Philippines	52.3	389
India	54.2	198

[1] Data from (2, p. 142)
[2] Not available

1. TRENDS TODAY AND TOMORROW

Food packaging adds to the trash disposal problem, however, and pressures are increasing to reduce food packaging or make it recyclable or degradable.

The Environmental Protection Agency considers *source reduction* to be the best method for decreasing solid waste and *recycling* to be the second most desirable approach (11). Reduced packaging may require some difficult choices, however, which may necessitate trade-offs with other attributes such as convenience or appearance. Recyclable materials are already replacing materials that are difficult to recycle in food packaging (11). Some fast food companies have switched to paper packaging from plastic foam containers (12).

Speculation

The budget share for food at home will probably continue to decline, but more gradually, since it is already so low. On the other hand, the steady increase in the share of food consumed away from home is expected to continue. The greatest time pressures fall on women in the labor force, who still do most of the work within the home. This time crunch will continue to fuel the demand for convenience, especially for microwave products and take-out food. The ability of food scientists to design particular attributes into food products will undoubtedly expand even more. Environmental concerns will have an increasing impact on food packaging. ◆

References

1. Senauer, B.; Asp, E.; Kinsey, J. Food trends and the changing consumer. St. Paul, Minn.: Eagan Press; 1991.
2. Putnam, J.; Allshouse, J.E. Food consumption, prices, and expenditures, 1968-89. Econ. Res. Serv., U.S. Dept. Agric., Stat. Bull. 825; Washington, D.C.; May 1991.
3. Dunham, D. Food spending and income. Econ. Res. Serv., U.S. Dept. Agric. Natl. Food Rev. 37:24-33; 1987.
4. U.S. Department of Commerce, Bureau of the Census. Statistical Abstract of the United States, 1991; Washington, D.C.; 1991.
5. Burros, M. Women: out of the house but not out of the kitchen. New York Times. 1988 Feb. 24.
6. Becker, G.S. A theory of the allocation of time. Econ. J. 75:493-517; 1965.
7. Lancaster, K.J. A new approach to consumer theory. J. Polit. Econ. 74:132-157; 1966.
8. U.S. Department of Agriculture, Economic Research Service. Food marketing review, 1989-90. Agric. Econ. Rep. 639; Washington, D.C.; Nov. 1990.
9. Dornblaser, L. Take the "F" train. Prep. Foods New Prod. Annu. 159:70-74;1990.
10. Dunham, D. Food cost review, 1990. Econ. Res. Serv., U.S. Dept. Agric., Agric. Econ. Rep. 651; Washington, D.C.; June 1991.
11. Dziezak, J.D. Packaging waste management. Food Technol. 44:98-101; 1990.
12. Holusha, J. McDonald's announces end to foam packaging. Minneapolis Star Tribune, 1990 Nov. 2.

The Changing American Diet

BONNIE LIEBMAN

f the United States got a Food Report Card, it would barely be pulling a C+ average. The Surgeon General and our other "teachers" have told us to eat:

■ fewer fatty foods like red meat, cheese, whole milk, butter, and margarine,

■ more complex carbohydrates like fruits, vegetables, whole grains, and beans, and

■ fewer sugary foods like soft drinks, candy, and ice cream.

New figures from the U.S. Department of Agriculture show that we're following *some* of this advice. We're eating fewer eggs, less whole milk, and less beef than we did a decade ago. And avoiding the saturated fat and cholesterol in these foods has paid off. Since 1978, the number of Americans dying of heart disease has dropped by 29 percent.

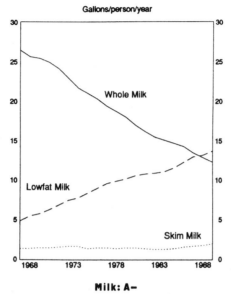

Milk: A−

Is the national milk glass half-full or half-empty? In 1960, lowfat milk was virtually non-existent. Now it has surpassed whole milk (terrific). But most of that "lowfat" is not-so-low two-percent milk, rather than truly-low one-percent (oops).

But other changes show that we're not quite ready for the Honor Roll. Instead of replacing saturated fats with complex carbohydrates, we've replaced them with unsaturated fats.

"It's clear we haven't made much progress in getting people to eat less [total] fat, but we have been successful in changing the composition of fat," says Mark Hegsted, of Harvard University.

In other words, we're eating more chicken instead of beef, but it's fried chicken; more baked goods, but they're fatty baked goods; and more salads, but they're smothered in oily dressings.

It's not just our fat tooth that's insatiable. Despite the popularity of artificial sweeteners, we're consuming more sugars than ever before. And we now down more soft drinks than milk.

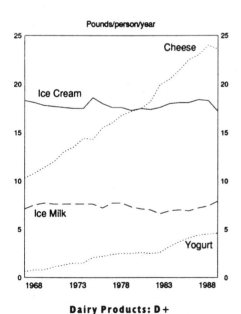

Dairy Products: D+

Since 1968, consumption of high-fat hard cheese has more than doubled. The reason? Fast-food pizzas and cheeseburgers. Yogurt's popularity continues to grow, in part because of its healthy reputation (which is well-deserved if it's low- or nonfat).

What's remarkable about our consumption of ice milk and ice cream is how little they've budged —either up or down.

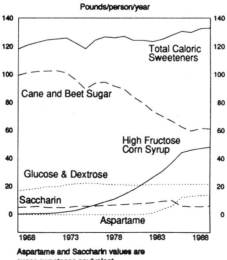

Aspartame and Saccharin values are sugar-sweetness equivalent.

Sweeteners: F

You might expect us to use less calorie-containing sweeteners like sugar or corn syrup as we eat more artificial ones. Wrong. Far from curbing the American sweet tooth, the switch has actually fed it. Apparently, the more we get, the more we want.

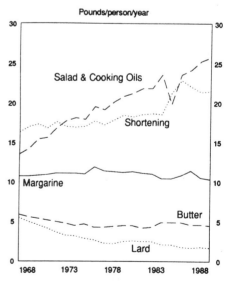

Fats & Oils: C−

We're now eating twice as much margarine as butter and 15 times more vegetable oil than lard. By substituting "good" (unsaturated) fats for "bad" (saturated) ones, we're doing our hearts a favor.

But we're not eating less fat. It's all those fried foods, fatty baked goods, and salad dressings that are doing us in. And we wonder why so many American bellies are bulging.

1. TRENDS TODAY AND TOMORROW

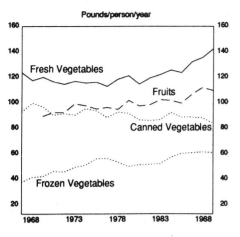

Pounds/person/year

Fruits & Vegetables: A−

Potatoes, which account for about 37 percent of all fresh vegetables, and lettuce, which makes up about 17 percent, are both on the upswing, as are less-popular vegetables like broccoli, tomatoes, carrots, and cauliflower. We should probably thank fast-food baked potatoes and salad bars for both trends.

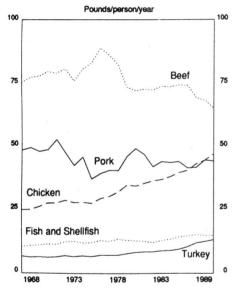

Pounds/person/year

Meat, Poultry & Fish: B

No wonder the beef industry is running scared. Whether it's price or concern about clogged arteries, something seems to be curbing our taste for burgers, roasts, and steaks. All told, we ate 10 pounds less per person per year in the 1980s than the 1970s. Nevertheless, we still eat more beef than any other food in this group.

Why did we eat as much pork in the 1980s as in the 70s? Perhaps the industry's misleading ads,

---

The influence of fast-food restaurants on our eating habits continues to grow. Chicken, soft drinks, salad, American and pizza cheese—just about all the foods we're eating more of are prominent on fast-food menus.

These grades rate not *what* we eat, but *how we've changed* what we eat over the last decade. For example, even though we still eat too many eggs (yolks), they get an "A," because we're eating fewer of them.

which call pork "The Other White Meat," have tricked us into thinking that pork is as low in fat as chicken, turkey, or fish (it isn't).

Chicken's rise isn't as promising as it seems. Most of the increase probably ends up as greasy nuggets, entrees, and McChicken sandwiches.

Turkey is finally breaking its Thanksgiving-Day stereotype, probably because it's being sold ground-up and in parts. Fish and shellfish consumption is only inching upwards, perhaps because prices have risen sharply. But much of the additional fish is fried fast-food, which is a far cry from broiled flounder.

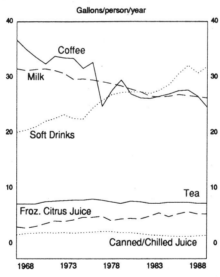

Gallons/person/year

Beverages: D+

Soft drinks have now surpassed milk as the nation's most popular beverage. And with milk consumption falling, the only reason Beverages didn't get an F is coffee's continuing 26-year decline. That's probably due to competition from soft drinks, concern about caffeine, quicker breakfasts, and central heating.

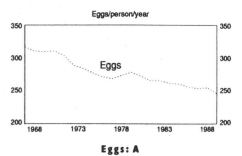

Eggs/person/year

Eggs: A

Egg-eating continues its 45-year decline, hitting a low of 234 per person in 1989. The cholesterol in the yolks is largely responsible, but it's only fair to acknowledge another reason: Moms who once had time to poach, boil, fry, or scramble are now scrambling to get to work.

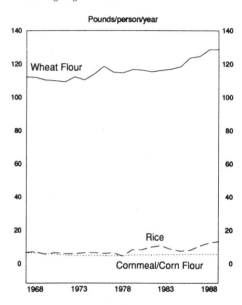

Pounds/person/year

Flour & Cereal Products: B−

We're eating 17 percent more complex carbohydrates than we did a decade ago (Yay!). That's largely due to a rise in wheat flour and rice. But we still eat less than half as much bread, cereal, pasta, and rice as our grandparents did in 1910.

The trick is to eat the bun without the burger, the pasta without the pesto, and the rice without the "roni."

> *The charts overestimate what people actually eat, because they don't account for the food that gets thrown away . . . before or after it reaches our plates. Nevertheless, the figures are computed the same way for each food and for each year, so comparisons and changes are reliable.*
>
> *Lorraine Jones and Bill Dugan helped compile information for this article.*

WAR AND PEAS

How Wars Have Shaped America's Diet

Susan Stiger
Albuquerque Journal Food Editor

The landscape of the American table—shaped by history, altered by battle—owes some of its favorite dishes, its most appreciated conveniences and its tried-and-true dietary knowledge to times of war.

Apple pie, sweet potato pie and pepper pot soup. Coffee, condensed milk and doughnuts. RDAs frozen foods and Betty Crocker herself. By legend or fact, history ties each of these dishes and developments to times of battle. In some cases war was the mother of invention; in others, merely the teacher that took an existing item and proved its worth.

Apple pie, the culinary symbol of America, may owe its lofty status to the Revolutionary War. In "American Food, the Gastronomic Story," author Evan Jones notes that the Pennsylvania Dutch probably invented the dish. In southeastern counties of the state, potters were already making pie plates and cooks were known to wrap crisp crusts around all of the regional fruits. Pennsylvania historian Frederic Klees suggests that men from other colonies may have enjoyed the dish in Pennsylvania and fostered that love at home when the war ended.

PHILADELPHIA PEPPER POT SOUP, A mélange of tripe, veal knuckle, potatoes, carrots and herbs, is the stuff of legend: The setting was Valley Forge, a brutal winter. General Washington grew desperate, his men in ragged uniforms, their shoes worn thin. Food supplies dwindled in the face of great hunger, and the desertion rate was alarming.

Washington summoned the chef of the Revolutionary armed forces and demanded a great dish to sustain his weary men. The chef protested, his larder full of nothing but a few hundred pounds of tripe (the gift of a nearby butcher), peppercorns (from a Germantown patriot), and scraps, scraps, scraps. But the relentless Washington ordered his chef to prepare something from nothing. So the tripe was scrubbed and simmered, the peppercorns were ground and added, the scraps were tossed into the pot.

At the call of the bugle, the men ate their fill of the fragrant, hearty dish and, with spirits renewed, called, "Bring on the Redcoats!"

Washington proclaimed it the stuff of heroes and asked its name. The chef suggested pepper pot, but Washington countered with an amendment: "Call it Philadelphia Pepper Pot, in honor of your hometown."

DURING THE CIVIL WAR, INSPIRATION came with the challenge to stretch short supplies. Southerners boiled the dirt under their smokehouses to get salt, and took soda from burnt corncobs. The sweet potato, long a major player in the Southern diet, lent its flavor to an even greater variety of dishes—among them, Sweet Potato Pie, destined to become a classic dessert.

The Union Army bought large quantities of Gail Borden's 1856 invention, sweetened condensed milk, the first product of the Borden Co. However, it seldom found its way to troops on the march, who might have used it to sweeten their coffee. Many men had never seen coffee until the war, but they embraced it with enthusiasm. Since the caffeine helped keep them going, coffee was commonly considered their most important ration.

In "Hard Tack and Coffee," John Billings quotes from the writings of one soldier: "How often, after being completely jaded by a night march . . . have I had a wash, if there was water to be had, made and drunk my pint or so of coffee, and felt as fresh and invigorated as if just arisen from a night's sound sleep."

When the war ended, coffee became America's national drink.

AT SUCH A MOMENT IN HISTORY, could the doughnut be far behind? Hardly. The doughnut took its place in American culinary history during World War I. One theory holds that it was invented in 1847, when Captain Hanson Crockett Gregory of Rockport, Maine, solved his mother's baking problem with the poke of a fork. Her fried cakes were always soggy in the center, so he poked out the middles. By the first world war, doughnuts had become part of the American mainstream, a symbol of comfort to start the day.

During the war, the doughnut made history of the sentimental sort. A Salvation Army worker in France made a batch for the boys "over there," triggering a wave of national sentiment that led the American Expeditionary Force to be called "doughboys."

The troops were far less thrilled with corned beef, which had been invented in 1872. It wasn't until the war that quality corned beef came into general use. Along with canned salmon, it became standard rations for the doughboys, who disdainfully referred to the pair as goldfish and corned willie.

Back home, Americans answered food shortages with big backyard gardens, baked goods made without butter and eggs, meals concocted without meat or wheat. Margarine took the place of butter, and honey, corn syrup or molasses stood in for sugar. Ingenious cooks learned to do without everything but flavor as rationing was part of the war-time lifestyle.

In Washington, D.C., the wives of Cabinet members pledged "to reduce living to its simplest form and deny ourselves luxuries in order to free those who produce them for the cultivation of necessities."

They drastically cut back their usual entertaining and social activities to allow time "for constructive preparedness and relief work." They bought simple clothing and food and did without the luxury of out-of-season items. "To hasten the end of the struggle and win the war," they appealed to women across America to follow suit.

WORLD WAR II BROUGHT TWO DEVEL-opments that often seem at odds today: nutrition guidelines and convenience foods.

The science of nutrition—at least a general understanding of calories, vitamins and other nutrients—was part of the public psyche by 1940, thanks in part to Margaret Mead and her colleagues at the National Research Council's Committee on Food Habits, who had been conducting nutritional research since the 1930s. The Food and Nutrition Board began preparing RDAs (Recommended Dietary Allowances) in 1941, but the first edition of the RDAs wasn't published until

1943 to help deal with wartime nutrition problems at home and to ensure a proper diet for the troops.

At the same time, the war moved so many women out of the home and into the work force that the usual lengthy meal preparation no longer fit the American lifestyle. Manufacturers assumed part of the homemaker's role, developing food products that cut cooking times and offering canned and frozen foods.

Mixes for baked goods were one of the most popular innovations of the time. By 1944, mixes for muffins, gingerbread, biscuits, pudding, pastry and pancakes were available. By 1949, women were buying butter cake, corn bread, brownie, hot roll and angel food mixes, according to "Better Homes and Gardens Heritage Cookbook."

It was during the war, too, that America began the transition from canned to frozen foods. When the Japanese invaded Southeast Asia, capturing a large portion of the world's tin resources, manufacturers were forced to look for alternatives to canning.

Frozen food had been around for some time, most notably through the work of Clarence Birdseye in 1923, but it had a bad image from early, unsuccessful ventures. In addition, few retailers had adequate display cases and consumers had no home freezers. But as the supply of canned goods diminished, the sale of frozen items took off.

By the end of the war, the quality of frozen foods still hadn't won over the American consumer. Had it not been for the development of frozen concentrated orange juice, which would become the industry's top-volume item, the nation probably would have gone back to canned goods to answer its need for convenience.

The trend away from the kitchen as a woman's place continued after the war, as restaurant dining went into full swing. And the All-American "all-you-can-eat" concept was born.

IN 1942, DURING THE WORST OF THE war shortages, M. F. K. Fisher wrote one of her more famous books, "How to Cook a Wolf" (the wolf being, as it were, at the door).

It was both serious and whimsical, practical and inspiring, a how-to for

shopping and cooking and stocking a blackout shelf. And it was wrapped in the poetic prose that was to make Fisher America's pre-eminent food writer—the doyenne of American cuisine.

Cook ahead, she said, and use every square inch of your oven to avoid wasting the heat.

Save the broth from cooking rice and macaroni to make soup. Save the water from cooking vegetables. Put it in an old gin bottle in the ice box, next to the old gin bottle filled with the juices from canned fruit. Use it to make soup, or drink it as a tonic.

If you can get your hands on 50 cents, she said, you can dine for at least three days, maybe a week, depending how luxurious your tastes are. And she gave specific instructions for doing so.

In the chapter "How to Be Cheerful Though Starving," she honored the practice of sharing a meal: "No matter what your hunger nor how fiercely your fingers itch for the warmness of the food, the fact that you are not alone makes flavors clearer and a certain philosophic slowness possible."

In "How To Be a Wise Man," she supported man's right to pleasure, even, or perhaps especially, in times of suffering: "All men are hungry. They have always been. They must eat, and when they deny themselves the pleasures of carrying out that need, they are cutting off part of their possible fullness, their natural realization of life, whether they are poor or rich."

In the chapter "How To Drink the Wolf," she paired the virtues of preparedness and faith: "Use as many fresh things as you can, always, and then trust to luck and your blackout cupboard and what you have decided, inside yourself, about the dignity of man."

And in the chapter "How To Practice True Economy," she wrote with compassion of the need to escape the limits and challenges of wartime: "And if by chance you can indeed find some anchovies or a thick slice of rare beef and some brandy, or a bowl of pink curled shrimps, you are doubly blessed, to possess in this troubled life both the capacity and the wherewithal to forget (the war) for a time."

DIETARY GUIDELINES REVISED

The third (1990) edition of *Nutrition and Your Health: Dietary Guidelines for Americans* has been published. The document presents dietary advice for healthy Americans and constitutes the central statement of federal nutrition policy. Issued jointly by the U.S. Departments of Agriculture and Health and Human Services, the guidelines were released originally in 1980 and updated in 1985. The two Departments distributed more than five million copies of the 1985 edition, and millions more were printed and distributed by others.

The new edition is based on recommendations of a nine-member advisory committee: Malden C. Nesheim, Ph.D. (chairman); Lewis A. Barness, M.D.; Peggy R. Borum, Ph.D.; C. Wayne Callaway, M.D.; John C. LaRosa, M.D.; Charles S. Lieber, M.D.; John A. Milner, Ph.D.; Rebecca M. Mullis, Ph.D.; and Barbara O. Schneeman, Ph.D. This committee and departmental reviewers concluded that the central messages of the 1985 guidelines remain sound and of major importance in choosing food for a healthful diet. The new edition is more specific and quantitative than previous versions, and is written in a more positive tone. The changes reflect new scientific evidence on the relationships between diet and health, information on the usefulness of the earlier editions, and formal comments from individuals and groups outside the government.

Seven Guidelines

The new report states that food alone cannot make people healthy. Smoking, alcohol abuse, other lifestyle factors, and heredity are also important. The American food supply is varied, plentiful, and safe to eat. But many Americans eat diets with too many calories, too much fat (especially saturated fat), cholesterol and sodium, and low in complex carbohydrates and fiber. The revised guidelines are:

- *Eat a variety of foods.* To assure variety and a well-balanced diet, choose foods each day from five major food groups: vegetables (3–5 servings); fruits (2–4 servings); breads, cereals, rice, and pasta (6–11 servings); milk, yogurt, and cheese (2–3 servings); and meats, poultry, fish, eggs, and dry beans and peas (2–3 servings). Vitamin or mineral supplements at or below the RDAs are safe, but are rarely needed except by women who are menstruating, pregnant, or breastfeeding. Many women and adolescent girls need to eat more calcium, and children, teenage girls, and women of childbearing age should take care to consume enough iron-rich foods.

- *Maintain healthy weight.* Obesity is associated with many serious illnesses. Being too thin is linked to osteoporosis in women and early death in both men and women. The guidelines recommend ranges of weights for adults ages 19 to 34 and higher ranges for

COMPARISON OF 1985 AND 1990 DIETARY GUIDELINES

1985	1990	Reason for Change
Eat a variety of foods	Eat a variety of foods	(No change)
Maintain desirable weight	Maintain healthy weight	Focus on total diet in more positive way
Avoid too much fat, saturated fat, and cholesterol	Choose a diet low in fat, saturated fat, and cholesterol	New interim health-based weight criteria
Eat foods with adequate starch and fiber	Choose a diet with plenty of vegetables, fruits, and grain products	Focus on foods, rather than food component, in total diet
Avoid too much sugar	Use sugars only in moderation	Focus on targeted food in a more positive way
Avoid too much sodium	Use salt and sodium in moderation	Focus on both in a more positive way
If you drink alcoholic beverages, do so in moderation	If you drink alcoholic beverages, do so in moderation	(No change)

From *Nutrition Forum*, Vol. 8, No. 1, January/February 1991, pp. 5-6. Reprinted with permission from *Nutrition Forum Newsletter*, now published by Stephen Barrett, M.D., P. O. Box 1747, Allentown, PA 18105.

those 35 and over. Waist measure should be smaller than hip measure. For those who are overweight, the recommended loss of 1/2 to 1 pound a week should be accomplished by increasing physical activity and eating less fat and fatty foods, more fruits, vegetables, and cereals, less sugar and other sweets, and little or no alcohol.

- *Choose a diet low in fat, saturated fat, and cholesterol.* This advice is tied to the goal of maintaining blood cholesterol level below 200 mg/dl. It recommends a fat intake of 30% or less of calories, with less than 10% of calories as saturated fat. Have your blood cholesterol level checked. If it is within a desirable range, help keep it that way with a diet low in saturated fat and cholesterol. If it is high, follow the doctor's advice about diet and medication.
- *Choose a diet with plenty of vegetables, fruits, and grain products.* This guideline recommends that adults eat at least three servings of vegetables and two servings of fruit daily. It also recommends at least six servings of grain products, with an emphasis on whole grains. Because foods differ in the kinds of fiber they contain, it is best to include a variety of fiber-rich foods. Fiber should be obtained from foods, not supplements.
- *Use sugars only in moderation.* The major health concern with excess sugar consumption is tooth decay. The risk does not depend simply on the amount of sugar consumed but on the frequency of consumption of sugars and starches and how long they remain in contact with the teeth. Eating such foods as frequent between-meal snacks may be more harmful to teeth than having them at meals. Teeth should be brushed (with a fluoride toothpaste) and flossed regularly. Fluoridated water or another fluo-

ride source is especially important for children while their teeth are forming.
- *Use salt and sodium in moderation.* Noting that high sodium intake can be a factor in high blood pressure, the guidelines suggest that sodium intake be moderated. This can be accomplished by learning to enjoy the flavors of unsalted foods; adding little or no salt during cooking or at the table; flavoring foods with herbs, spices, or lemon juice; and limiting intake of foods that are obviously salty or contain significant amount of hidden salt. A blood pressure check is also recommended.
- *If you drink alcoholic beverages, do so in moderation.* Alcoholic beverages supply calories but few or no nutrients. Drinking them has no proven health benefit and is linked with many health problems, is the cause of many accidents, and can lead to addiction. Since birth defects have been attributed to drinking during pregnancy, women who are pregnant or trying to conceive are advised to abstain completely from alcohol. People planning to drive a car or engage in another activity that requires attention or skill are also advised to abstain.

In October 1990, Congress enacted the National Nutritional Monitoring and Related Research Act of 1990 (Public Law 101–445), a bill intended to ensure more complete information while reducing duplication of efforts among government agencies studying the eating habits of Americans. The bill calls for the establishment of a National Nutrition Monitoring Advisory Council and an Interagency Board for Nutrition Monitoring and Related Research. It also states that *Dietary Guidelines* for Americans will be updated and published every five years.

The Food Pyramid—Food Label Connection

Etta Saltos, Ph.D., R.D.

Etta Saltos is a nutritionist with USDA's Human Nutrition Information Service.

What foods fit in a healthy diet? How can you compare the nutritional values of food? Can the new food label help you answer these questions?

It can, if you use the label information to follow the Dietary Guidelines for Americans.

Food Pyramid

The Food Guide Pyramid can help you put the Dietary Guidelines into action. The pyramid illustrates the research-based food guidance developed by the U.S. Department of Agriculture and supported by the Department of Health and Human Services. It is based on USDA's research on what foods Americans eat, what nutrients are in these foods, and how to make the best food choices to promote good health. It outlines what to eat each day, but it is not a rigid prescription. You can use it as a general guide in choosing a healthful diet that is right for you. The pyramid calls for eating a variety of foods to get the nutrients you need, and, at the same time, the right amount of calories to maintain a healthy weight. It also focuses on fat because most American diets are too high in fat, especially saturated fat.

You don't have to avoid foods that are high in fat, saturated fat, cholesterol, and sodium completely. It's your average intake over a few days, not in a single food or even a single meal, that's important. If you eat a high-fat food or meal, balance your intake by choosing low-fat foods the rest of the day or the next day. The new food label can help you "budget" your intake of fat, saturated fat, cholesterol, and sodium over several days.

The new food label also can help you identify good sources of fiber and vitamins and minerals.

Look to the Label

How does it do this? First, descriptors such as "free," "low" or "reduced" on the front of the package can signal that a food is low in a certain dietary component, such as calories, fat, saturated fat, or sodium. Eating those foods can then help you moderate your intake of these and other nutrients.

Descriptors such as "good source" and "high" can help you identify foods that contain significant amounts of dietary fiber, vitamins, and minerals.

Claims about the relationship between a nutrient or a food and the risk of a disease or health-related condition also may show up on the front of the package of FDA-regulated products. These are called health claims, and FDA has authorized seven of them. They can help you identify foods with certain nutritional qualities that are of interest to you. (See "Starting This Month: Look for 'Legit' Health Claims on Foods" in the May 1993 *FDA Consumer*.)

However, you don't have to select only foods with descriptors or health claims on the label to follow the Dietary Guidelines. In moderation, all foods can fit into a healthy diet.

Second, look at the nutrition panel, now titled "Nutrition Facts." With a few exceptions, the nutrition panel will list calories, calories from fat, and the amount of nutrients of greatest public health concern contained per serving of the food. (See " 'Nutrition Facts' to Help Consumers Eat Smart" in the May 1993 *FDA Consumer*.) Similar information also will be available voluntarily for some raw foods. (See "Nutrition Info Available for Raw Fruits, Vegetables, Fish" in the January–February 1993 *FDA Consumer*.)

On the nutrition panel, nutrient content will be expressed not only as an amount by weight but also as a percent of the Daily Value, or DV—a new label reference value. (See " 'Daily Values' Encourage Healthy Diet" in the May 1993 *FDA Consumer*.)

These percentages can help you decide whether a food contributes a lot or a little of a particular nutrient. Lower percentages indicate the food contributes less of the nutrient, and higher percentages indicate that it contributes more of the nutrient.

Look to see whether the nutrients you would like to get more of (such as carbohydrate, dietary fiber, and vitamins and minerals) have high percentages and the nutrients you may need to limit (such as fat, cholesterol and sodium) have low per-

Food Guide Pyramid
A Guide to Daily Food Choices

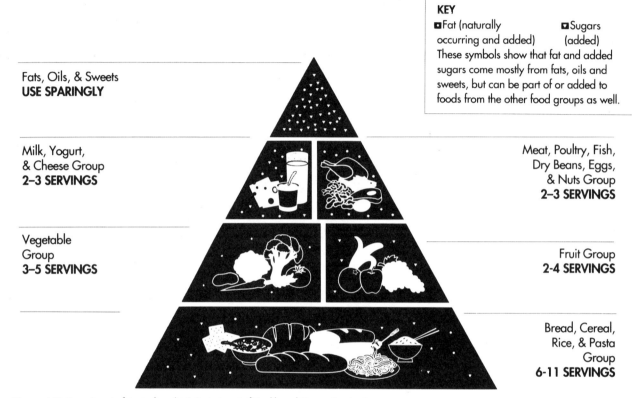

KEY
■ Fat (naturally occurring and added)   ▲ Sugars (added)
These symbols show that fat and added sugars come mostly from fats, oils and sweets, but can be part of or added to foods from the other food groups as well.

Fats, Oils, & Sweets
USE SPARINGLY

Milk, Yogurt, & Cheese Group
2–3 SERVINGS

Meat, Poultry, Fish, Dry Beans, Eggs, & Nuts Group
2–3 SERVINGS

Vegetable Group
3–5 SERVINGS

Fruit Group
2-4 SERVINGS

Bread, Cereal, Rice, & Pasta Group
6-11 SERVINGS

(Source: U.S. Department of Agriculture/U.S. Department of Health and Human Services)

How to Use the Daily Food Guide

What Counts as One Serving?

Breads, Cereals, Rice, and Pasta
1 slice of bread
1/2 cup of cooked rice or pasta
1/2 cup of cooked cereal
1 ounce of ready-to-eat cereal

Vegetables
1/2 cup of chopped raw or cooked vegetables
1 cup of leafy raw vegetables

Fruits
1 piece of fruit or melon wedge
3/4 cup of juice
1/2 cup of canned fruit
1/4 cup of dried fruit

Milk, Yogurt, and Cheese
1 cup of milk or yogurt
1 1/2 to 2 ounces of cheese

Meat, Poultry, Fish, Dry Beans, Eggs, and Nuts
2 1/2 to 3 ounces of cooked lean meat, poultry or fish
Count 1/2 cup of cooked beans, or 1 egg, or 2 tablespoons of peanut butter as 1 ounce of lean meat (about 1/3 serving)

Source: *FDA Consumer,* June 1993

Fats, Oils, and Sweets
Limit calories from these, especially if you need to lose weight

The amount you eat may be more than one serving. For example, a dinner portion of spaghetti would count as two or three servings of pasta.

Descriptors such as "free," "low" or "reduced" on the front of the package can signal that a food is low in a certain dietary component, such as calories, fat, saturated fat, or sodium.

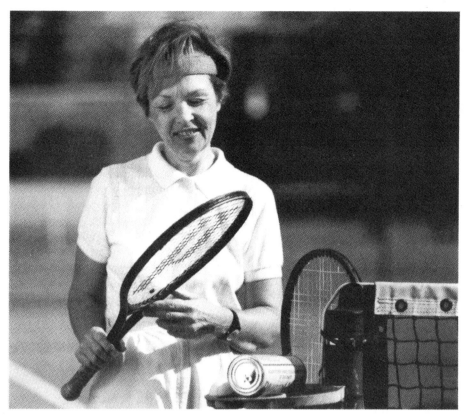

A daily diet of 2,000 calories—the basis for the "% Daily Value" on food labels—is about right for women who engage in moderate activity, such as an occasional tennis game. It is also the target calorie level for teenage girls and sedentary men.

centages. The percent Daily Values, while based on a 2,000-calorie diet, will indicate in a relative way the nutritional contributions of a food to your diet regardless of your calorie intake.

Also, because serving sizes are now more uniform across product lines, comparing the nutritional content of foods is easier.

However, the amount of food you eat may be different from the stated serving size. For example, the serving size for ice cream is a half cup, so if you usually eat one cup of ice cream, you would have to double the number of calories and the percentages of the Daily Values listed to learn the nutrient content of the portion you eat.

Figuring Fat

While the food label provides a reliable general guide for most people, you may want to use the information on it to make more personal choices.

You may be concerned about fat, for example. The Dietary Guidelines suggest that you eat a diet that provides 30 percent or less of calories from fat and less than 10 percent of calories from saturated fat. Thus, the recommended upper limit on the grams of fat and saturated fat in your diet depends on the calories you need (see chart on this page). The percent DVs for fat and saturated fat are based on a 2,000-calorie diet, which is about right for moderately active women, teenage girls, and sedentary men.

Some people keep a running total of the amount of fat and saturated fat they eat in

Find Your Fat Limit

Recommended upper limits of total fat and saturated fat intake at different calorie levels:

	Calories			
	1,600	2,000	2,500	2,800
Total Fat (grams)	53	65	80	93
Saturated Fat (grams)	18	20	25	31

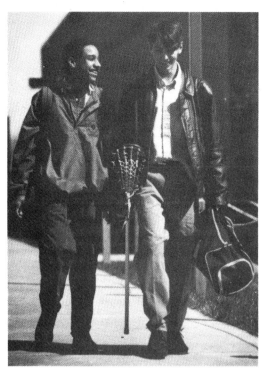

Teenage boys are among those who may need 2,500 calories a day. Daily values for that calorie level are required on the labels of larger food packages.

a day and compare this to their target level. If you eat about 2,000 calories a day, you can simply monitor the percent DV information from the foods you eat so that the total is close to or less than 100 percent over the day.

If you eat fewer than or more than 2,000 calories a day, you can keep a total of the actual amount of fat and saturated fat contained in the foods you eat. This information is listed immediately after the nutrient name (for example, "Total Fat 13 g").

Daily values based on an intake of 2,500 calories a day are listed in a footnote, at least on the nutrition panels of larger packages. These values can be used as a target level for many men, teenage boys, and active women.

The chart on page 17 lists recommended upper limits of fat and saturated fat intakes for other calorie levels. Many older adults, children, and sedentary women need fewer than 2,000 calories a day and may want to select target levels based on 1,600 calories a day. Some active men and teen-

age boys and very active women may want to select target levels based on 2,800 calories per day.

Sugars and Others

The percent DV column also can be used to help you moderate your intake of sodium and cholesterol. The Daily Values for sodium and cholesterol are the same for everyone, regardless of total calories consumed, so you do not have to make adjustments based on your caloric needs.

Food labels also can be helpful if you're trying to moderate your sugar intake. The nutrition panel lists the amount of sugars in grams (4 grams is equivalent to 1 teaspoon) in a serving of the food.

Note that this amount includes sugars that are present *naturally* in the food (such as lactose in milk and fructose in fruit), as well as sugars *added* to the food during processing. If you're interested in finding out whether a sweetener has been added to a food, check the ingredient listing. Terms such as "sugar (sucrose)," "fructose," "maltose," "lactose," "honey," "syrup," "corn syrup," "high-fructose corn syrup," "molasses," and "fruit juice concentrate" are used to describe sweeteners added to foods.

If one of these terms appears first or second in the list of ingredients, or if several of them appear, the food is likely to be high in added sugars. A percent DV is not given for sugars because there is no target quantity of sugars to aim for each day.

Labeling of the alcohol content of beverages is regulated by the Bureau of Alcohol, Tobacco, and Firearms. Alcohol content (in percentage by volume) appears on the front panel of some alcoholic beverage labels. Alcohol content of foods and beverages is not required to be listed on the nutrition panel. However, some alcoholic beverages, such as light beers and wine coolers, provide information about the amount of calories, carbohydrate, protein, and fat they contain. You may find this information useful if you're counting calories because alcoholic beverages are generally rich in calories and poor in nutrients.

You'll find lots of information on food labels. So take the time to read them. The information can help you plan a healthful diet that meets the recommendations of the Dietary Guidelines.

Dietary Guidelines

The Dietary Guidelines, developed by the Department of Health and Human Services and the U.S. Department of Agriculture, represent the best, most current advice for healthy Americans 2 years and older. They reflect recommendations of health and nutrition experts, who agree that enough is known about the effect of diet on health to encourage certain eating practices. The seven Dietary Guidelines are:

• *Eat a variety of foods* to get the energy (calories), protein, vitamins, minerals, and fiber you need for good health.

• *Maintain a healthy weight* to reduce your chances of having high blood pressure, heart disease, a stroke, certain cancers, and the most common kind of diabetes.

• *Choose a diet low in fat, saturated fat, and cholesterol* to reduce your risk of heart disease and certain types of cancer. Because fat contains more than twice the calories of an equal amount of carbohydrates or protein, a diet low in fat can help you maintain a healthy weight.

• *Choose a diet with plenty of vegetables, fruits, and grain products* that provide needed vitamins, minerals, fiber, and complex carbohydrates. They are generally lower in fat.

• *Use sugars only in moderation.* A diet with lots of sugars has too many calories and too few nutrients for most people and can contribute to tooth decay.

• *Use salt and other forms of sodium only in moderation* to help reduce your risk of high blood pressure.

• *If you drink alcoholic beverages, do so in moderation.* Alcoholic beverages supply calories, but little or no nutrients. Drinking alcohol is also the cause of many health problems and accidents and can lead to addiction.

FAT Replacers
Now and in Your Future

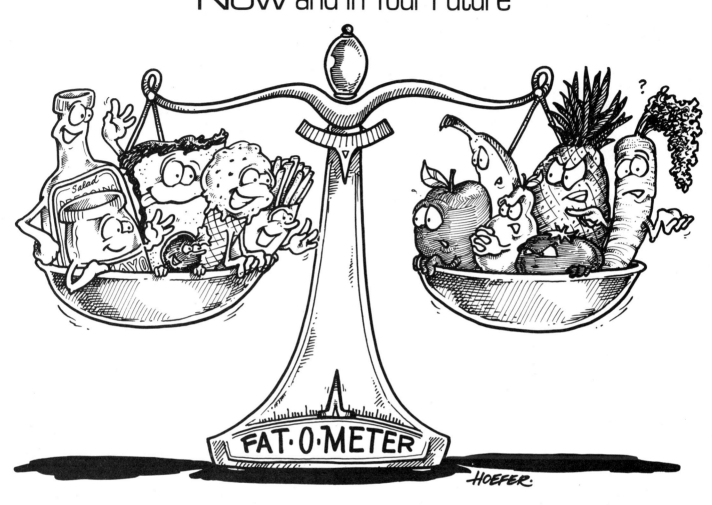

HOEFER.

Mary Carole McMann

Mary Carole McMann, M.P.H., R.D./ L.D., is a freelance writer living in Houston, TX.

If the 1970s were the decade of sugar substitutes, the 1990s are shaping up as the decade of fat replacers. Fat replacer is the term used to describe a substance (or combination of substances) that gives reduced-fat or fat-free foods the texture and "mouthfeel" of higher-fat foods.

Many people enjoy the "richness" of high-fat foods. However, they don't like the results of overindulgence — excess weight and adverse health consequences. While it is estimated that Americans consume 36 to 37

> Fat replacers are one way food technology has responded to this tug-of-war between rich food cravings and the desire to avoid high-fat eating habits.

percent of calories from fat, health experts recommend that fat not exceed 30 percent of daily calorie intake. Fat replacers are one way food technology has responded to this tug-of-war between rich food cravings and the desire to avoid high-fat eating habits.

Fat replacers can be categorized in several ways. Some substances already exist in nature while others are synthesized in the laboratory. Naturally occurring substances, which do not undergo chemical changes but may be physically processed, require less rigorous testing before being allowed into the food supply. Manufacturers of these naturally occurring fat replacers petition the Food and Drug Administration (FDA) to categorize their products as "generally recognized as safe" — the coveted GRAS sta-

From *Priorities*, Spring 1992, pp. 11-13. Reprinted with permission from *Priorities*, a publication of the American Council on Science and Health, New York, NY.

19

tus. To date, the FDA has not approved the use of any synthetic fat replacers, which are categorized as food additives.

Perhaps the most useful way of looking at fat replacers is to consider their source. Some of the following are already on the market; others await FDA approval or are still in the process of development.

Protein-Based Fat Replacers

Simplesse™ (The NutraSweet Company), the fat replacer most familiar to the American public, is produced by heating and then blending protein from milk and/or eggs in a patented process called microparticulation that forms very tiny round particles. The tongue perceives the particles as having a creamy texture and the "mouthfeel" of fat. Simplesse contains less than 2 calories per gram, compared to 9 calories per gram from fat.

Simplesse is currently being marketed in a frozen dairy dessert called Simple Pleasures™, which the manufacturer describes as having the texture of premium ice cream. This fat replacer is suitable for use in other dairy products, such as yogurt, cream cheese and sour cream, and in a number of fat-based foods, including margarine, mayonnaise and salad dressing. Because heat coagulates protein, Simplesse cannot be used in foods that are exposed to high temperatures, as in baking or frying.

Trailblazer™ (Kraft General Foods) is another protein-based fat replacer manufactured from protein in egg white and skim milk using a process other than microparticulation.

Carbohydrate-Based Fat Replacers

Carbohydrate-based fat replacers have been used for years to replace all or part of the fat in a wide variety of foods.

Carrageenan, which is extracted from a type of seaweed, has been used for centuries to thicken foods. Its superior gel-forming properties have long made carrageenan useful in foods such as frozen desserts, pie filling, yogurt, relishes and chocolate milk. More recently, carrageenan has been added to ground beef containing less than ten percent fat to yield moist, juicy cooked meat with the texture of higher-fat beef. McDonald's

McLean™ burger is a combination of very lean ground beef and carrageenan.

LeanMaker is a brand of very lean ground beef containing a fat replacer based on oat bran.

ConAgra is marketing a very lean ground beef combined with a fat substitute called LEANesse™ under the Healthy Choice label. LEANesse is based on oatrim, an ex-

> **Use of fat replacers allows food manufacturers to offer appetizing foods that taste sinfully rich but contain little or no fat.**

tract of oat bran, and provides one calorie per gram. Four ounces (raw) of Healthy Choice Extra Lean Ground Beef™ provide 4 grams of fat compared to 19 grams of fat in the same amount of extra lean ground beef.

Although gums are not fat replacers in the accepted meaning of the term, food manufacturers have used their thickening and gelling properties since the early 1980s to produce reduced-fat or fat-free foods, such as salad dressings.

Polydextrose (Pfizer Chemical Division), which provides one calorie per gram, is commonly used as a bulking agent. However, it may be partially substituted for fat in certain foods, such as candy and candy coatings; frozen dairy desserts; pudding, cake and cookie mixes; chewing gum; meal replacement bars; and cake frosting.

Cornstarch maltodextrin (Grain Processing Corporation), which is marketed under the name Maltrin™ M040, forms a bland-tasting gel with the smooth "mouthfeel" of fat. The manufacturer is testing its acceptability as partial fat replacement in margarine, table spread, salad dressing, frozen dessert and imitation sour cream.

Stellar™ (A.E. Staley Manufacturing Company) is a cornstarch-based fat replacer, providing one calorie per gram. It can replace part of the fat in baked goods, cheese, puddings, soups and sauces. The same company also manufactures Sta-Slim 143™ from modified potato starch. This fat replacer, which provides four calories per gram, can be used for partial fat replacement in cheesecakes, soups, imitation cream cheese, and both pourable and spoonable salad dressings.

N-Oil™, Instant N-Oil™, and Instant N-Oil II™ (National Starch and Chemical Corporation) are made from tapioca dextrins and maltodextrin and provide one calorie per gram. They are used in fat-free frozen desserts and reduced-fat puddings, imitation sour cream, salad dressings, table spreads, and microwaveable cheese sauces.

Paselli SA2 (Avebe America, Inc.) is the brand name used to market potato starch maltodextrin, which provides one calorie per gram. It can be used to replace fat in bakery products, pourable and spoonable salad dressings, frozen desserts, table spreads, dips, meat products, candies and cake frosting.

Synthetic Fat Replacers

Fat replacers which are synthesized in the laboratory and are not digested in the human body do not qualify for GRAS status. Before the FDA allows the addition of synthetic fat replacers to foods, the manufacturers must conduct extensive testing to prove that these new products do not have harmful side effects.

Sucrose polyester, better known as olestra, is a synthetic fat replacer developed by Proctor & Gamble a number of years ago. Olestra consists of a sugar molecule to which fatty acids have been attached. Since the resulting substance does not appear in nature, it must be treated as a food additive. Olestra resembles standard fats and oils in many ways, including its ability to withstand frying and baking at high temperatures. Suggested uses for olestra include partial replacement of fat in cooking fats and oils and partial or complete replacement of fat in cheese, salad dressings, table spreads and frozen desserts. Since it does not break down in the human digestive system, olestra has no caloric value.

In the spring of 1987, Proctor & Gamble filed a food additive petition asking FDA approval of olestra in replacing up to 35 percent of the fat in shortenings and cooking oils designed for home use and up to 75 percent of the fat in shortenings used for commercial deep-fat frying and in the production of fried snack foods (*e.g.*, potato chips and corn chips). The FDA has yet to approve the petition.

Esterified propoxylated glycerols, EPG, (ARCO Chemical Company) is formed by changing the chemical structure of fat. Since EPG is not broken down in the body, it provides no calories. EPG is being testing as a replacement for fats and oils in bakery products, frozen desserts, table spreads and salad dressings. Several more years of testing will be necessary before petitioning FDA for approval of EPG as a food additive.

Dialkyl dihexadecymalonate, DDM, (Frito-Lay, Inc.) is being developed to partially replace the fat used to fry chips. Chips fried in a combination of vegetable oil and DDM have been judged as good as or superior to the original. This fat replacer is also being evaluated for use in lower-fat versions of mayonnaise and margarine. Unlike olestra and EPG, a small amount of DDM is digested and absorbed in the body.

Trialkoxytricarballate, TATCA, (Best Foods) is being evaluated for use in reduced-fat mayonnaise and margarine-like products and may also be used to replace other types of fats and oils. TATCA evidently is not broken down in the digestive tract and so will not be a source of calories.

Combination Fat Replacers

Some companies have combined certain of the fat replacers described above with other substances.

Reach Associates Inc. markets a number of combination fat replacers. Prolestra™ (su-

> Before the FDA allows the addition of synthetic fat replacers to foods, the manufacturers must conduct extensive testing to prove that these new products do not have harmful side effects.

crose polyester and protein) is suitable for use in salad oil, mayonnaise and table spread, frozen desserts, baked products, snacks and sauces. The NutriFat brand is used on several products that replace varying amounts of fat in foods. The manufacturer describes these products as blends of several hydrolyzed starches, some of which have proteins and/or polysaccharides added. Finesse is a protein-based fat replacer containing specially treated proteins.

Colestra™ (Food Ingredients and Innovations) is a low-calorie polyester sucrose.

Answer to a Fat-Fighter's Prayer?

Introduction of substances like fat replacers into the food supply always raises important questions and concerns. Is the public being misled into thinking that all low-fat and fat-free foods are also automatically low in calories? Many reduced-fat foods contain increased amounts of other ingredients, such as sugar, and the resulting product may not actually be low in calories. Will people using reduced-fat foods feel free to increase their intake of other fats, thereby not decreasing their overall fat intake? Surveys show that sugar intake has not decreased in spite of the wide use of sugar substitutes. Will increased use of reduced-fat non-essential foods result in less emphasis on eating a balanced diet? And, do we really know the long-term effects of consuming appreciable amounts of fat replacers?

Although the total story on fat replacers has yet to be told, their introduction into foods has the potential for changing consumers' eating habits. Use of fat replacers allows food manufacturers to offer appetizing foods that taste sinfully rich but contain little or no fat. Now consumers can continue to eat "low fat" while still enjoying their favorite foods. As long as the public understands that "fat-free" does not mean "calorie-free" these lower-fat foods can play a nutritious, delicious part in a balanced diet.

Biotechnology — The New Designer Genes

Mary Carole McMann

MARY CAROLE MCMANN, M.P.H., R.D./L.D., IS A FREELANCE WRITER LIVING IN HOUSTON, TX.

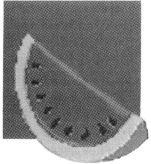

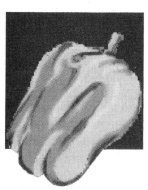

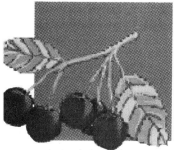

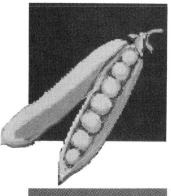

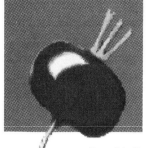

IT'S EVERY SALAD LOVER'S DREAM — TO garnish a bowl of crisp greens with wedges of red, ripe, firm, juicy tomato that doesn't have to be home grown to be delicious. Take heart, the answer to the tomato-lover's prayer may be just around the corner, thanks to advances in biotechnology.

Building on the Old Technology

For centuries man has employed cross-breeding to improve fruits, vegetables and grains by combining the best characteristics of different plants. However, traditional methods can take several generations to produce results, and there is always the chance of unfavorable traits being transmitted along with the desired ones.

The first step in the development of biotechnology was the discovery of the basis of heredity in plants and in animals. Simply put, the nucleus of each living cell contains identical pairs of chromosomes, which are made up of deoxyribonucleic acid (DNA), containing hereditary information in the form of genes. When a cell divides, each new cell usually contains the entire heredity of the original cell. On the other hand, sex cells contain one chromosome from each pair. When a new organism is formed, the offspring receives chromosomes from both parents, giving it inherited characteristics from each.

This knowledge found practical application in agriculture. Different plants are cross-bred to try to produce offspring with the best traits of both parents. For example, wheat cross-bred with wild grasses has a greater yield; increased resistance to fungal and bacterial diseases; and a higher tolerance for salt and unfavorable weather conditions. However, conventional cross-breeding is time consuming, often requiring many generations to achieve the desired combination. The process is also somewhat of a gamble since the offspring may receive undesirable traits on the same chromosome with desirable ones.

Moving into the New Technology

Biotechnology took a giant step forward when, in 1974, American scientists first isolated and duplicated specific genes (cloning). This discovery made recombinant-DNA technology — the deliberate formation of new gene combinations not present in the chromosomes of either "parent" — possible. The gene carrying a desirable trait is identified in the DNA of a donor, duplicated and inserted directly into the DNA of the host. This technology allows genes to be transferred without regard to the usual barriers to cross-breeding, making it feasible to produce gene combinations not possible by conventional methods. Also, desirable traits can be transferred without simultaneously transferring other less desirable traits. Thus, new plants with the most desirable characteristics can be developed in just one generation.

Applying Biotechnology

Several varieties of genetically engineered plants should reach consumers by the mid-1990s. At present, recombinant-DNA techniques are being used to develop more than 70 food crops that contain new proteins, enzymes and other substances that make them superior in quality. The main applications of biotechnology in agriculture are in developing fruits, vegetables and grains that have improved characteristics for nutrient content and processing and that are resistant

From *Priorities*, Spring 1993, pp. 24-26. Reprinted with permission from *Priorities*, a publication of the American Council on Science and Health, New York, NY.

Biotechnology helps to provide larger quantities of more nutritious food than ever before and for a more reasonable price.

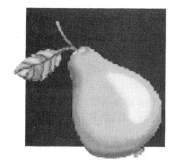

to adverse weather conditions (cold, heat, frost and drought), pests, diseases, herbicides and salt.

Crops that are being genetically altered to improve their resistance to herbicides include corn, potatoes, rice, soybeans, lettuce and cole (a cross between broccoli and cauliflower). Herbicides produced in recent years usually work by inactivating an enzyme needed for some vital plant system (*e.g.*, photosynthesis). Through genetic engineering, plants can be developed that produce greater quantities of the enzyme or that produce an enzyme either less sensitive to the herbicide or capable of inactivating it. These improved crop plants will allow farmers to use broad-spectrum herbicides that are less toxic, have low soil mobility and degrade more quickly. These effects ultimately decrease the amount of herbicide required and minimize harmful effects on the environment.

Through biotechnology, scientists are now able to breed plants with an increased resistance to pests. They have identified the gene in a particular type of bacterium that controls the production of a protein, called delta endotoxin, which is lethal to some insect larvae. Transfer of this gene into the DNA of a host plant results in subsequent generations capable of producing delta endotoxin, and therefore, defending themselves against certain pests. At present, delta endotoxin is lethal to the larvae of moth, butterfly, beetle and certain fly species but has no apparent toxic effects in animals, fish, birds, most plants or beneficial insects. A modified form of endotoxin is being developed that will affect a larger variety of pests.

Crop plants resistant to viruses that can destroy entire harvests are in development. They include tomatoes, potatoes, alfalfa, melons, soybeans, strawberries, sugar beets and cole. Host plants are made more resistant to viral infections by inserting a gene that retards subsequent infection with the virus and/or delays its reproduction and spread. Increased resistance to viruses not only improves crop quality and increases

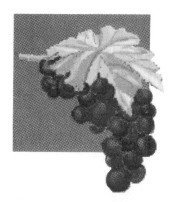

yield but also decreases the need for insecticides targeted to insects known to spread the virus.

Bioengineering has also been used to change the nutrient content of certain plant foods. The rapeseed plant, the source of canola oil, has been genetically changed to increase its content of unsaturated fatty acids. A new strawberry strain is being developed that has an increased level of ellagic acid, a cancer-protective agent normally present in strawberries at low levels.

In some cases the goal of biotechnology may not be the improvement of an existing foodstuff, but the creation of an altogether different food. For example, the tangelo (the result of cross-breeding a grapefruit and tangerine by traditional methods) is entirely different from either "parent."

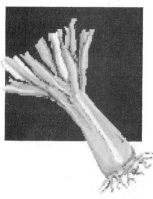

Tomorrow's Tomato — Terrific!

The first genetically engineered plant food that should reach consumers is the Flavr Savr™ tomato, which should be available by late 1993. At present tomatoes are picked green and treated with ethylene to ripen them before shipping. Shoppers need skill and luck to find a ripe and full-flavored tomato that has not yet become mushy and begun to spoil. The ripening process can be slowed and shelf life increased by inserting a gene that retards the rapid ripening and spoiling of tomatoes. The resulting genetically engineered tomato is not only identical nutritionally to an ordinary tomato but looks, smells, feels and tastes the same.

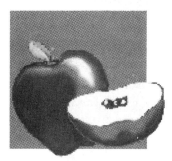

"Anti" Activities

People who are hesitant to accept new scientific discoveries, alarmed at terms like "gene splicing" and "cloning," have already begun to fight the new technology. One such anti-science group, the Foundation on Economic Trends, has petitioned the Food and Drug Administration (FDA) to demand more regulatory action against genetically engineered foods. In one instance, activists

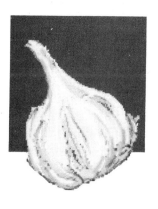

1. TRENDS TODAY AND TOMORROW

in Maryland delayed the field testing of genetically engineered corn which was designed to resist a caterpillar that normally requires heavy pesticide treatment. Unchecked, this caterpillar causes crop losses of $400 million per year. In a similar case in Wisconsin, researchers had difficulty getting approval for field tests on green beans genetically altered to resist the devastating brown spot disease.

The All-Important Issue of Safety

The safety of genetically altered plant foods has been evaluated by many individuals and groups both in the United States and around the world. The basic concerns focus on the possible effects of gene splicing in plant foods on the people and animals consuming them and on the environment.

In May 1992 the FDA announced a policy to improve the variety of food available to consumers by promoting the development of safe new foods through biotechnology. The policy allows the sale of genetically engineered fruits, vegetables and grains without government testing if their new properties can be found in plant foods already being safely consumed.

Companies interested in developing new plant varieties have a number of questions to resolve. For example, many common foods naturally contain toxicants (poisonous substances) in amounts so tiny that they present no danger. Other foods, such as the potato and the rapeseed plant, must be screened routinely to ensure that toxicant levels are within an acceptable range. One legitimate question is whether the level of these toxicants has been increased in a genetically engineered food crop.

Other questions include:

- Has an allergen (substance causing an allergic reaction) not commonly found in the plant been introduced?

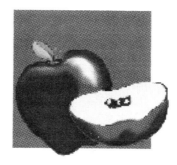

Increased resistance to viruses not only improves crop quality and increases yield but also decreases the need for insecticides targeted to insects known to spread the virus.

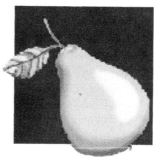

At present, recombinant-DNA techniques are being used to develop more than 70 food crops that contain new proteins, enzymes and other substances that make them superior in quality.

- Have levels of important nutrients been changed?

- Have any new substances that raise questions of safety been introduced into the food?

- What are the effects of the new food crop on the environment?

- Have both the genetic material and its "expression product" been well characterized?

- Have developers of the new food crop followed accepted, established scientific practices?

The FDA policy is consistent with recommendations of expert panels on biotechnology convened by the National Academy of Sciences of the National Research Council (NRC) and jointly by the World Health Organization and the Food and Agriculture Organization of the United Nations. In 1989, the NRC stated that, "Crops modified by molecular and cellular methods (biotechnology) pose risks no different from those modified by classical genetic methods for similar traits."

Why Biotechnology?

World population continues to grow, intensifying the need for increased food production. Meanwhile, we in America continue to expect fresh, varied, delicious produce throughout the year. We demand healthier food products with less fat, more vitamins and great taste. Biotechnology helps to provide larger quantities of more nutritious food than ever before and for a more reasonable price. It increases crop yields and minimizes losses through disease, pests and inclement weather while decreasing the need for pesticides and herbicides. The application of genetic engineering brings agricultural practices into the twenty-first century. A safer, healthier, less expensive and more varied food supply is on the way.

'NUTRITION FACTS'

To Help Consumers Eat Smart

Paula Kurtzweil

Paula Kurtzweil is a member of FDA's public affairs staff.

Susan Thom, of Parma, Ohio, knows how important it is for people to know the number of calories from fat they eat each day.

As a registered dietitian, she counsels patients on the need to limit fat consumption to 30 percent or less of total daily calories. As a person with diabetes, and thus at increased risk for heart disease, she strives to do the same for herself.

But, in the past, obtaining that information from the food label has required some mathematical skill—namely, multiplying the total grams (g) of fat in a serving by 9, since 1 g of fat contains 9 calories.

"It does take time," Thom said. "But if you want to feed yourself well, you have to look at the label."

Help is on the way. For Thom and millions of other Americans who seek to restrict their fat intake to recommended levels, a new dietary component is being added to the food label—"calories from fat."

It's just one of many new items of diet-related information manufacturers are required to offer on their food products by 1994. There also will be information on saturated fat, cholesterol, dietary fiber, and other nutrients that relate to today's health concerns, such as heart disease, cancer, and other diseases linked, at least in part, to diet.

There will be more complete nutrient content information because almost all the required nutrients will have to be listed as a percent of the Daily Value. There will be more uniform serving sizes, too, which will make nutritional comparisons between foods easier. And, because nutrition labeling is now mandatory for almost all processed foods, there will be a lot more products with this important information.

"The new information is going to be very helpful for consumers," said Virginia Wilkening, a registered dietitian in FDA's Office of Food Labeling.

"Some of the nutrients—saturated fat and cholesterol—have been allowed on the label before but on a voluntary basis," she said. "Dietary fiber and sugars were not allowed in the nutrition label. With the new label, consumers will soon have information about these and other nutrients, which can help them choose their foods more wisely."

The new requirements for nutrition labeling are spelled out in regulations issued in January 1993 by FDA and the U.S. Department of Agriculture's Food Safety and Inspection Service (FSIS). FDA's regulations meet the provisions of the Nutrition Labeling and Education Act of 1990 (NLEA), which, among other things, requires FDA to make nutrition labeling mandatory for almost all processed foods. FSIS' regulations, which cover meat and poultry products, largely parallel FDA's. (Meat and poultry products were not covered by NLEA.)

Old Label

NUTRITION INFORMATION	PER SERVING	PERCENTAGE OF U.S. RECOMMENDED DAILY ALLOWANCES (U.S. RDA)	
SERVING SIZE	5 OZ.	PROTEIN	10
SERVINGS PER CONTAINER	4	VITAMIN A	*
		VITAMIN C	*
CALORIES	250	THIAMINE	8
PROTEIN	9g	RIBOFLAVIN	15
CARBOHYDRATE	19g	NIACIN	2
FAT	11g	CALCIUM	20
SODIUM	530mg	IRON	4

*CONTAINS LESS THAN 2% OF THE U.S. RDA OF THIS NUTRIENT

Starting this year, the 'old' nutrition label format above will be replaced by the one on the next page. Both labels are for a frozen macaroni and cheese product.

Reprinted from *FDA Consumer,* May 1993, pp. 22-27.

Key Aspects of the New Nutrition Label

A number of consumer studies conducted by FDA, as well as outside groups, enabled FDA and the Food Safety and Inspection Service of the U.S. Department of Agriculture to agree on a new nutrition label. The new label is seen as offering the best opportunity to help consumers make informed food choices and to understand how a particular food fits into the total daily diet.

New heading signals a new label.

More consistent serving sizes, in both household and metric measures, replace those that used to be set by manufacturers.

Nutrients required on nutrition panel are those most important to the health of today's consumers, most of whom need to worry about → getting too much of certain items (fat, for example), rather than too few vitamins or minerals, as in the past.

Conversion guide helps consumers learn caloric value of the energy-producing nutrients.

New mandatory component helps consumers meet dietary guidelines recommending no more than 30 percent of calories from fat.

%Daily Value shows how a food fits into the overall daily diet.

Reference values help consumers learn good diet basics. They can be adjusted, depending on a person's calorie needs.

Nutrition Facts

Serving Size 1 cup (228g)
Servings Per Container 2

Amount Per Serving

Calories 260   Calories from Fat 120

	% Daily Value*
Total Fat 13g	**20**%
Saturated Fat 5g	**25**%
Cholesterol 30mg	**10**%
Sodium 660mg	**28**%
Total Carbohydrate 31g	**10**%
Dietary Fiber 0g	**0**%
Sugars 5g	
Protein 5g	

Vitamin A 4%	•	Vitamin C 2%
Calcium 15%	•	Iron 4%

* Percent Daily Values are based on a 2,000 calorie diet. Your daily values may be higher or lower depending on your calorie needs:

	Calories:	2,000	2,500
Total Fat	Less than	65g	80g
Sat Fat	Less than	20g	25g
Cholesterol	Less than	300mg	300mg
Sodium	Less than	2,400mg	2,400mg
Total Carbohydrate		300g	375g
Dietary Fiber		25g	30g

Calories per gram:
Fat 9 • Carbohydrate 4 • Protein 4

FDA has set May 8, 1994, as the date by which food manufacturers must comply with the new nutrition labeling regulations. FSIS requires meat and poultry processors to relabel their products by July 6, 1994. However, some newly labeled products may begin appearing in grocery stores much sooner than the deadlines.

Dietary Components

What can consumers expect? First, they will see a new name for the nutrition panel. It used to go by "Nutrition Information Per Serving." Now, it will be called "Nutrition Facts." That title will signal to consumers that the product is newly labeled according to FDA and FSIS' new regulations.

The new panel will be built around a new set of dietary components. (See graphic, page 26.) The mandatory (underlined) and voluntary dietary components and order in which they must appear are:

- total calories
- calories from fat
- calories from saturated fat
- total fat
- saturated fat
- stearic acid (on meat and poultry products only)
- polyunsaturated fat
- monounsaturated fat
- cholesterol
- sodium
- potassium
- total carbohydrate
- dietary fiber
- soluble fiber
- insoluble fiber
- sugars
- sugar alcohol (for example, the sugar substitutes xylitol, mannitol and sorbitol)
- other carbohydrate (the difference between total carbohydrate and the sum of dietary fiber, sugars, and sugar alcohol, if declared)
- protein
- vitamin A
- percent of vitamin A present as beta-carotene
- vitamin C
- calcium
- iron
- other essential vitamins and minerals.

If a food is fortified or enriched with any of the optional components, or if a claim is made about any of them, the pertinent nutrition information then becomes mandatory.

These mandatory and voluntary components are the only ones allowed on the nutrition panel. The listing of single amino acids, maltodextrin, calories from polyunsaturated fat, and calories from carbohydrate, for example, may not appear on the label.

The reason, according to Wilkening, is to help consumers focus on nutrients of public health significance. "Too much additional information could clutter the label or mislead or confuse the consumer," she said.

Nutrients required on the label, she pointed out, reflect current public health concerns and coincide with current public health recommendations. She noted that the order in which the food components and nutrients are required to appear reflects their public health significance and the order in which they were specified in NLEA.

On the new food label, the listing of thiamin, riboflavin and niacin will not be mandatory. Under the old nutrition labeling program, these vitamins were required to be listed. But because deficiencies of these are no longer a public health problem in this country, listing them is now optional.

New Format

Consumers also will see a new format, one that calls for many of the macronutrients (such as fat, cholesterol, sodium, carbohydrate, and protein) to be declared as a percent of the Daily Value—a new label reference value. The amount, in grams or milligrams per serving, of these nutrients still must be listed to their immediate right. But, for the first time, a column headed "%Daily Value" will appear.

According to Wilkening, the percent declaration of the Daily Value offers an advantage over amount declaration: The percent Daily Values put the nutrients on an equal footing in the context of a total daily diet.

For example, she said, a food is low in sodium if it has less than 140 mg of sodium. "But people look at that number, 140, and think it's a tremendous amount, when it actually is less than 6 percent of the Daily Value."

On the other hand, she said, a food with 5 g of saturated fat could be construed as being low in that nutrient just because 5 is a small number. Actually, that food would provide one-fourth the total Daily Value of 20 g of saturated fat for a 2,000-calorie diet.

"People are affected by the size of numbers," she said. "That's why percentages are helpful. They put all of the nutrients on a level playing field."

The percent Daily Value listing will carry a footnote stating that the percentages are based on a 2,000-calorie diet and that a person's individual dietary goal is based on his or her calorie needs. Some nutrition labels—at least those on larger packages—will list daily values for selected nutrients for a 2,000- and a 2,500-calorie diet and the number of calories per gram of fat, carbohydrate and protein. The calorie conversion information is required as a general guide about the caloric contributions of fat, carbohydrate and protein.

The content of micronutrients—that is, vitamins and minerals—will continue to be expressed as a percent, although the term "Daily Value" will replace "U.S. Recommended Daily Allowance."

Modifications

Some foods will carry a variation of this format. For example, the label of foods for children under 2 (except infant formula, which is exempt from nutrition labeling under NLEA) will not carry information about calories from fat, calories from saturated fat, saturated fat, polyunsaturated fat, monounsaturated fat, and cholesterol.

The reason, according to Wilkening, is to prevent parents from inadvertently assuming that infants and toddlers should restrict their fat intake, when in fact, they should not. Fat is important during this life stage, she said, to ensure adequate growth and development.

The labels of food for children under 4 cannot include percentages of Daily Values for macronutrients, except protein, nor any footnote information, including the lists of Daily Values for selected nutrients. The reason: Other than protein, FDA has not established Daily Values for macronutrients for this age group. The percent Daily Values for vitamins and minerals is allowed, however. The content of the other nutrients must be expressed as an amount by weight in a separate column to the right of the macronutrients.

Other foods may qualify for a simplified label format. This format is allowed when the food contains insignificant amounts of seven or more of the mandatory dietary components, including total calories. "Insignificant" means that a declaration of "zero" could be made in nutrition labeling or, for total carbohydrate, dietary fiber, and protein, a declaration of "less than 1 g."

For foods for children under 2, the simplified format may be used if the product contains insignificant amounts of six or more of the following: calories, total fat, sodium, total carbohydrate, dietary fiber, sugars, protein, vitamins A and C, calcium, and iron.

When the simplified format is used, information on total calories, total fat, total carbohydrate, protein, and sodium—even if they are present in insignificant amounts—must be listed. Calories from fat and other nutrients must be listed if they are present in more than insignificant amounts. Nutrients added to the food must be listed, too.

Serving Sizes

Whatever the format, the serving size remains the basis for reporting each nutrient's amount. However, unlike in the past, serving sizes now will be more uniform and closer to the amounts that many people actually eat. They also must be expressed in both common household and metric measures. (See accompanying table.)

Before, the serving size was up to the discretion of the food manufacturer. As a result, said Youngmee Park, Ph.D., a nutritionist in FDA's Office of Special Nutritionals, serving sizes often varied widely, making it difficult for consumers to compare nutritional qualities of similar products or to determine the nutrient content of the amount of food they normally ate.

The uniformity also is important, she said, for giving consistency to health claims and words describing nutrient content, such as "high fiber" and "reduced fat."

FDA and FSIS define serving size as the amount of food customarily eaten at one time. It is based on FDA- and USDA-established lists of "Reference Amounts Customarily Consumed Per Eating Occasion."

These reference amounts, which are part of the new regulations, are broken down into 139 FDA-regulated food product categories, including 11 groups of foods for children under 4, and 23 USDA meat and poultry product categories. They list the amounts of food customarily consumed per eating occasion for each food category, based primarily on national food consumption surveys. FDA's list also gives the suggested label statement for serving size declaration.

For example, the category "breads (excluding sweet quick type), rolls" has a reference amount of 50 g, and the appropriate label statement for sliced bread is "__ piece(s) __ (g)" or, for unsliced bread, "2 oz (56 g/__ inch slice)."

The serving size of products that come in discrete units, such as cookies, candy bars, and sliced products, is the number of whole units that most closely approximates the reference amount. For example, cookies have a reference amount of 30 g. The household measure closest to that amount is the number of cookies that comes closest to weighing 30 g. Thus, the serving size on the label of a cookie package in which each cookie weighs 13 g would read "2 cookies (26 g)."

If one unit weighs more than 50 percent but less than 200 percent of the reference amount, the serving size is one unit. For example, the reference amount for bread is 50 g; therefore, the label of a loaf of bread in which each slice weighs more than 25 g would state that a serving size is one slice.

For food products packaged and sold individually, if an individual package is less than 200 percent of the applicable reference amount, the item qualifies as one serving. Thus, a 360-milliliter (mL) (12 fluid-ounce) can of soda is one serving because the reference amount for carbonated beverages is 240 mL (8 fluid ounces).

However, if the product has a reference amount of 100 g or 100 mL or more and the package contains more than 150 percent but less than 200 percent of the reference amount, manufacturers have the option of deciding whether the product is one or two servings.

For example, the serving size reference amount for soup is 245 g. So a 15-ounce (420 g) can can be listed as either one or two servings.

Metric Conversion Chart

Units as they will appear for serving sizes on label

Household Measure	Metric Measure
1 tsp	5 mL
1 tbsp	15 mL
1 cup	240 mL
1 fl oz	30 mL
1 oz	28 g

tsp = teaspoon

tbsp = tablespoon

fl oz = fluid ounce

oz = ounce

mL = milliliter

g = gram

Presentation

There also are rules governing how the nutrition information is displayed. Under existing FDA regulations, nutrition information must appear on the information panel to the immediate right of the principal panel. Thus, on boxed foods, for example, in which the principal panel is on the front of the box, the nutrition information appears on the right side of the box. Packages whose area to the immediate right is too small or not suited for such labeling may provide information on the next panel to the right.

FSIS allows nutrition information to be listed on the principal or information panels.

The new food labeling rules call for one additional variation: For packages that are 40 square inches or less, the nutrition information may be placed on any label panel.

The rules also address size and prominence of the typeface. For example, the

28

heading "Nutrition Facts" must be set in the largest type on the nutrition panel and be highlighted in some manner, such as boldface, all capital letters, or another graphic to distinguish it from the other information. Such highlighting also is required for headings such as "Amount per serving" and "%Daily Value" and for the names of dietary components that are not subcomponents—that is, calories, total fat, cholesterol, sodium, total carbohydrate, and protein.

Exceptions and Exemptions

In some instances, special provisions exist for providing nutrition information. For example:

• Nutrition information about game meat, such as deer, bison, rabbit, quail, wild turkey, and ostrich, may be provided on counter cards, signs, or other point-of-purchase materials. Because little nutrient data exists for these foods, FDA believes that allowing this option will enable game meat producers to give first priority to collecting appropriate data and make it easier for them to update the information as it becomes available.

• FDA-regulated food packages with less than 12 square inches available for nutrition labeling do not have to carry nutrition information. However, they must provide an address or telephone number for consumers to obtain the required nutrition information.

• Packages with less than 40 square inches for nutrition labeling may present nutrition information in a tabular format, abbreviate the names of dietary components, and omit the footnotes with the list of daily values and caloric conversion information but include a footnote stating that the percent Daily Values are based on a 2,000-calorie diet or place nutrition information on other panels.

Some foods are exempt from nutrition labeling. These include:

• food produced by small businesses. (As mandated by NLEA, FDA defines a small business as one with food sales of less than $50,000 a year or total sales of less than $500,000. FSIS defines a small business as one employing 500 or fewer employees and producing no more than a certain amount of product per year.)

• food served for immediate consumption, such as that served in restaurants and hospital cafeterias, on airplanes, and by food service vendors (such as mall cookie counters, sidewalk vendors, and vending machines)

• ready-to-eat foods that are not for immediate consumption, as long as the food is primarily prepared on site—for example, many bakery, deli, and candy store items

• food shipped in bulk, as long as it is not for sale in that form to consumers

• medical foods

• plain coffee and tea, flavor extracts, food colors, some spices, and other foods that contain no significant amounts of any nutrients

• donated foods

• products intended for export

• individually wrapped FSIS-regulated products weighing less than half an ounce and making no nutrient content claims.

Although these foods are exempt, they are free to carry nutrition information, when appropriate—as long as it complies with the new regulations.

But, there will be plenty of other foods carrying the new nutrition information. Dietitian Susan Thom sees that as a plus.

"We'll all know exactly what we're putting in our mouths," she said. "So there'll be little room for excuses."

Ingredient Labeling

WHAT'S IN A FOOD?

"Yankee Doodle went to town a ridin' on a pony,

Stuck a feather in his hat and called it

Macaroni."

Marian Segal

Marian Segal is a member of FDA's public affairs staff.

MR. DOODLE can call his hat whatever he likes. Pasta makers, however, have long had to be very specific about what they call "macaroni." That's because since shortly after the Federal Food, Drug, and Cosmetic Act was passed in 1938, macaroni, along with some other foods people commonly prepared at home in those days, was exempted from the law's requirement that food manufacturers list their products' ingredients on the food label. Instead, the new act provided for "standards of identity"—prescribed recipes—for these foods, which the manufacturers had to follow.

"The law resulted in standardized recipes for such foods as dairy products, mayonnaise, ketchup, jelly, and orange juice," says Elizabeth Campbell, director of the programs and enforcement policy division in the Office of Food Labeling of FDA's

Center for Food Safety and Applied Nutrition. "When a consumer bought a jar of jelly she knew it would have at least 45 percent fruit, as the standard provided, because that's what it takes to make jelly," she explained. "It's roughly half fruit and half sugar. People knew that because they used to make it themselves."

Well, maybe so, but we're in the '90s now, and with the fast pace of today's lifestyles, homemade breads and jellies mostly exist in Grandma's memories. It can hardly be taken for granted that people still know what's in those standardized foods. And yet, more and more, health-conscious consumers and people with dietary restrictions want and need to know what's in the foods they buy.

So, the law is changing to catch up with the times. FDA now requires that ingredients for all standardized foods be listed on the label, the same as for all other foods. This is one of several provisions of a final rule published in the Jan. 6, 1993, *Federal Register* concerning declaration of ingredients on food labels. (The U.S. Department of Agriculture requires full ingredient labeling on all meat and poultry products, including standardized products, such as chili or sausages.)

Two of the provisions of the rule on declaration of ingredients respond directly to the 1990 Nutrition Labeling and Education Act (NLEA). One is the requirement to list ingredients in standardized foods; the other requires the label to list FDA-certified color additives by name.

Before passage of the NLEA, the Food, Drug, and Cosmetic Act did not require flavorings, colorings or spices to be identified by their common or usual names. Instead, they could be declared collectively under the general terms "flavorings," "spices" or "colorings." Under the NLEA, however, color additives that FDA certifies for food use—FD&C colors Yellow No. 5, Red No. 40, Red No. 3, Yellow No. 6, Blue No. 1, Blue No. 2, and Green No. 3, and their lakes (specially formulated nonsoluble colors)—now must be declared on all foods except butter, cheese, and ice cream. Colors exempt from certification, such as caramel, paprika, and beet juice, do not have to be specifically identified; they can still be listed simply as "artificial colors."

People often look to the ingredient label for health reasons—perhaps to avoid substances they are allergic or sensitive to—or for religious or cultural reasons.

 Reprinted from *FDA Consumer,* April 1993, pp. 14-18.

When Is Peach Juice Apple Juice?

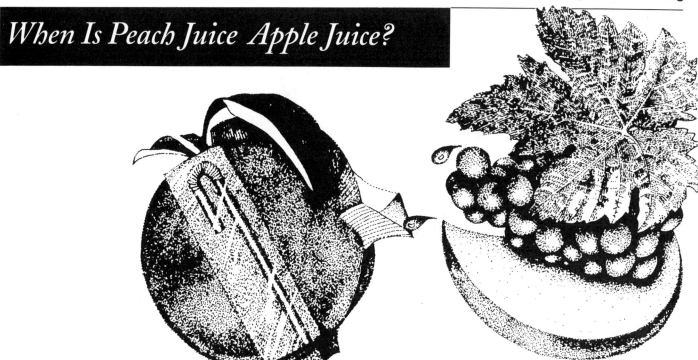

When it comes to juice labeling, there are those who would disagree with Shakespeare's sentiment that "a rose by any other name would smell as sweet." If the label implies that it's peach juice, they contend, it shouldn't consist mostly of apple and white grape juice—especially without saying so on the label.

The final rule on percentage juice declaration published in the Jan. 6, 1993, *Federal Register* will help remedy this problem. Beginning May 8, 1993, juice manufacturers will have to declare the total amount of juice in a beverage. (As this article goes to press, FDA is proposing to exempt from this requirement until May 8, 1994, foods that claim to be beverages containing vegetable or fruit juice.)

In addition, when the label of a multi-juice beverage names one or more, but not all, the juices in the beverage, and if the named juices are present in minor amounts, manufacturers must either:
• state the beverage is flavored by the named juice, such as "raspberry flavored juice drink," *or*
• declare the amount of the named juice in a 5 percent range, as "juice blend, 2 to 7 percent raspberry juice."

The rule-making process on declaration of percentages of juice goes back many years, beginning with debates over standards of identity for diluted juice beverages. In 1974, FDA proposed a regulation to establish common or usual names for juice drinks instead of developing standards.

After many objections, tie-ups, and reworkings—including a final regulation in 1980 that never had an effective date and two more proposals in 1984 and 1987—the Nutrition Labeling and Education Act came along in 1990 requiring that "a food that purports to be a beverage containing juice must declare the percent of total juice on the information panel."

But this alone would not solve the problem of misleading labels. Many manufacturers today use bland juices, like apple or white grape, as diluents instead of water and call the product a 100 percent juice blend.

"Some of these labels are just not informative," Campbell says. "The label says 100 percent juice blend or 100 percent natural juices, but only the expensive juices—the raspberry or strawberry, which are in smaller amounts—appear prominently on the principal display panel. You have to look for the grape and the apple in the fine print."

To correct this, FDA elaborated on the 1990 law, proposing that manufacturers be required to declare not only the total percent of juice, but the percent of each juice named or pictured on the label of a multi-juice beverage.

In responding to the proposal, however, manufacturers protested that this requirement would be impractical and difficult to comply with. They explained that juice, as an agricultural product, varies in strength, flavor, solids, and color. If they were required to state a percentage, they wouldn't have the flexibility necessary to adjust the amount of juice—using a little bit less or a little bit more or a little sweetening—to get the desired flavor. Nor would they be able to vary their formulas as driven by fluctuations in cost or availability of individual juices.

In addition, they said the amount of juice they use in their formulations is proprietary information, and requiring them to reveal this information in 1 percent increments would force them to divulge their secret formulas.

The final rule allowing a statement that the beverage is flavored, or declaring the amount of juice named in a 5 percent range, addresses manufacturers' concerns, while providing more accurate information for consumers.

—*M.S.*

FDA

now requires that ingredients for all standardized foods be

listed on the label, the same as for all other foods.

Manufacturers must comply with the requirements for ingredient listing of standardized foods and declaration of certified color additives by May 8, 1993. Other provisions of the final rule become effective May 8, 1994.

Caseinate

If it says "nondairy," does it mean no milk? Many people are not aware that certain products claiming to be nondairy, such as some coffee whiteners, contain a milk derivative called caseinate, in this case used to whiten effectively.

"People expect there to be no milk ingredients in products marketed as dairy substitutes," Campbell says, "but some states require the label 'nondairy.' This issue is particularly important for people with milk allergies. The nondairy label may lead consumers to think that caseinates are not milk derived. Furthermore, it guides people away from even checking the label for milk-derived ingredients."

Under the new rule, caseinate will have to be identified as a milk derivative in the ingredient statement when it's used in foods that claim to be nondairy. This requirement will help to flag it for casein-sensitive people.

Protein Hydrolysates

Consumers will get more information about protein hydrolysates in their food, too. Hydrolyzed proteins (proteins broken down by acid or enzymes into amino acids) are added to foods to serve various functions. They can be used as leavening agents, stabilizers (to impart body or improve consistency, for example), thickeners, flavorings, flavor enhancers, and as a nutrient (protein source), to name a few uses.

Since the law does not require flavors to be identified by their common or usual names, some in industry have made a practice of declaring protein hydrolysates as "flavorings" or "natural flavors" even when they are used as flavor enhancers—a use not exempt from declaration. After reviewing the data, FDA concluded that protein hydrolysates added to foods as flavorings always function as flavor enhancers as well and, as such, must be declared by their common or usual name.

The source of protein in hydrolysates used for flavor-related purposes also must be identified. Previously the general terms "hydrolyzed vegetable protein," "hydrolyzed animal protein," or simply "hydrolyzed protein" were permitted, but the new regulation requires identification of the specific protein source, such as "hydrolyzed corn protein" or "hydrolyzed casein." There are two reasons for this.

First, the law requires that the common or usual name of a food should adequately describe its basic nature or characterizing properties or ingredients. FDA reasoned that the more general terms "animal" and "vegetable" don't meet this requirement because protein hydrolysates from different sources best serve different functions. Manufacturers select protein hydrolysates from specific sources depending on how they will be used in a product. Hydrolyzed

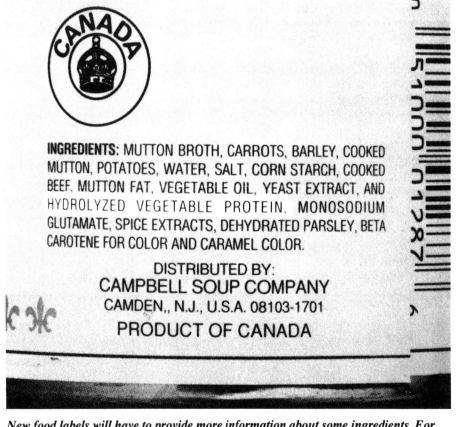

INGREDIENTS: MUTTON BROTH, CARROTS, BARLEY, COOKED MUTTON, POTATOES, WATER, SALT, CORN STARCH, COOKED BEEF, MUTTON FAT, VEGETABLE OIL, YEAST EXTRACT, AND HYDROLYZED VEGETABLE PROTEIN, MONOSODIUM GLUTAMATE, SPICE EXTRACTS, DEHYDRATED PARSLEY, BETA CAROTENE FOR COLOR AND CARAMEL COLOR.

DISTRIBUTED BY:
CAMPBELL SOUP COMPANY
CAMDEN,, N.J., U.S.A. 08103-1701
PRODUCT OF CANADA

New food labels will have to provide more information about some ingredients. For example, the terms "hydrolyzed vegetable protein," "hydrolyzed animal protein," or simply "hydrolyzed protein"—permitted in the past—will now have to identify the protein source, such as corn, casein or other.

Standardized Foods

To comply with the new food labeling laws, manufacturers now will have to list ingredients that are in standardized foods. The following product categories of standardized foods are:

- milk and cream
- cheeses and related products
- frozen desserts
- bakery products

- cereal flours and related products
- macaroni and noodle products
- canned fruits
- canned fruit juices
- fruit butters, jellies, and jams or preserves
- fruit pies
- canned vegetables
- vegetable juices
- frozen vegetables

- eggs and egg products
- fish and shellfish
- cacao products (for example, cocoa, chocolate)
- tree nut and peanut products
- margarine
- sweeteners and table syrups
- food dressings and flavorings (for example, mayonnaise, salad dressing, vanilla flavoring)

*P*eople often look to the ingredient label

for health reasons, or

for religious or cultural reasons.

casein is generally used in canned tuna, for example, whereas hydrolyzed wheat protein is used in meat flavors.

Second, the source of the additive is particularly important to consumers who have special dietary requirements, whether for religious, cultural or health reasons. If hydrolyzed casein is added to canned tuna, for example, it must be identified as such, rather than simply as "hydrolyzed protein" or "hydrolyzed milk protein."

Furthermore, after reviewing comments on the June 1991 proposal, the agency concluded that to minimize confusion, the source of protein in hydrolysates used for non-flavor-related purposes should also be identified. Thus, the source of all protein hydrolysates—regardless of use—will now have to be identified.

Other final provisions of the new rule will:

- Permit voluntary inclusion of the food

source in the names of sweeteners. For example, "corn sugar monohydrate" would be permitted in addition to names previously permitted, such as "dextrose" or "dextrose monohydrate."
- Provide a uniform format for voluntary declaration of percentage ingredient information. Manufacturers who choose to declare ingredients by percent of content would present them by weight rather than volume to avoid inconsistent calculations. Firms may use percentage declarations for as many or as few ingredients as they choose, as long as the information is not misleading. Manufacturers must still list ingredients in descending order, by weight, as required by law.
- Require label declaration of sulfiting agents in standardized foods. This is required because some people are sensitive to these preservatives. FDA has required listing of sulfiting agents in nonstandardized foods since 1986.

Dori Stehlin

Dori Stehlin is a member of FDA's public affairs staff.

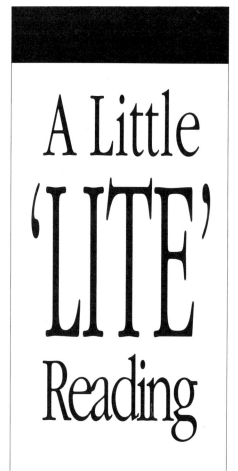

"Low fat." "No cholesterol." "High in oat bran." "Light." And don't forget "lite."

Until now, many of these claims have been nothing more than advertising hype. The public has been misled with products like the "light" vegetable oil that was just light in color and the "lite" cheesecake that was just light in texture.

But with the publication of new food labeling regulations in January 1993, the Food and Drug Administration and the U.S. Department of Agriculture's Food Safety and Inspection Service (FSIS) address the problem of misleading nutrition claims and help reestablish the credibility of the food label. The regulations spell out which nutrient content claims are allowed and under what circumstances they can be used.

There are 11 core terms:
* free
* low
* lean
* extra lean
* high
* good source
* reduced
* less
* light
* fewer
* more

Free

The new regulations allow manufacturers the option to use the following synonyms for the term "free":
* without
* trivial source of
* negligible source of
* dietarily insignificant source of
* no
* zero

Whatever term the manufacturer chooses, the product must either be absolutely free of the nutrient in question or, if the nutrient is in the food, the amount must be dietetically trivial or physiologically insignificant.

For example, zero fat cannot be required because it is impossible to measure below a certain amount. So, the regulation will allow a fat-free claim on foods with less than 0.5 grams (g) of fat per serving, an amount that is physiologically insignificant even if a person eats several servings.

Foods that don't contain a certain nutrient naturally must be labeled to indicate that all foods of that type meet the claim. For example, a fat-free claim on applesauce would have to read "applesauce, a fat-free food."

"Free" also can be used in reference to saturated fat, cholesterol, sodium, sugars, and calories.

Low

A food meets the definition for "low" if a person can eat a large amount of the food without exceeding the Daily Value for the nutrient. (See " 'Daily Values' Encourage Healthy Diet" in the May 1993 *FDA Consumer*.)

The synonyms allowed for "low" are:
* little
* few
* contains a small amount of
* low source of

"Low" claims can be made in reference to total fat, saturated fat, cholesterol, sodium, and calories.

A claim of "very low" can be made only about sodium.

Lean and Extra Lean

"Lean" and "extra lean" can be used to describe the fat content of meat, poultry, seafood, and game meats. (FSIS regulates meat and poultry products; FDA oversees seafood and game meats.)

"Lean" means the food has less than 10 g of fat, less than 4 g of saturated fat, and less than 95 milligrams (mg) of cholesterol per serving and per 100 g. An example of a serving is 55 g (2 oz.) for fish, shellfish or game meat. Some "lean" foods are Spanish mackerel, bluefin tuna, and domesticated rabbit.

"Extra lean" means the food has less than 5 g of fat, less than 2 g of saturated fat, and less than 95 mg of cholesterol per

Reprinted from *FDA Consumer*, June 1993, pp. 12-16.

serving and per 100 g. Examples of "extra lean" foods are haddock, swordfish, clams, and deer.

Percent Fat Free

FDA and FSIS believe that this claim implies, and consumers expect, that products bearing "percent fat free" claims contain relatively small amounts of fat and are useful in maintaining a low-fat diet. Therefore, products with these claims must meet the definitions for low fat.

In addition, the claim must accurately reflect the amount of fat present in 100 g of the food. For example, if a food contains 2.5 g of fat per 50 g, the claim must be "95 percent fat free."

Good Source and High

"High" and "good source" focus on nutrients for which higher levels are desirable. To qualify for the "high" claim, the food must contain 20 percent or more of the Daily Value for that nutrient in a serving. Approved synonyms for high are "rich in" or "excellent source."

"Good source" means a serving contains 10 to 19 percent of the Daily Value for the nutrient.

Comparison Claims

Manufacturers who want to compare a nutritionally altered product with the regular product may make a relative claim—that is, "reduced," "less," "fewer," "more," or "light." The regular products, or reference foods, may be either an individual food or a group of foods representative of the type of food—for example, an average of three market leaders.

Restrictions on these claims and the reference foods include:
• A relative claim must include the percent difference and the identity of the reference food.
• "Reduced," "less" and "light" claims can't be made on products whose nutrient level in the reference food already meets the requirement for a "low" claim.
• Reference foods for "light" and "reduced" claims must be similar to the product bearing the claim—for example, reduced fat potato chips compared with regular potato chips.
• Reference foods for "less" and, in the case of calories, "fewer" may use dissimilar products within a product category—

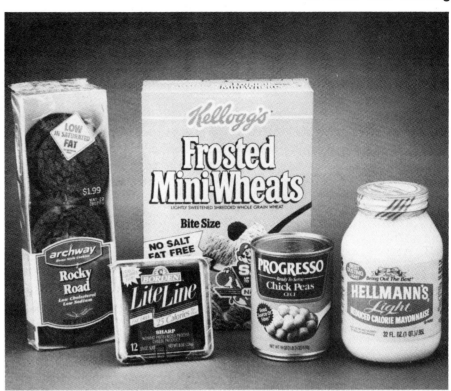

By 1994, claims about the nutrient content of a food, such as "low cholesterol," "light," and others on these food packages, will have to mean the same on every product on which they appear.

for example, pretzels with 25 percent less fat than potato chips.

At the other end of the spectrum, a serving of a food carrying a "more" claim (or claims of fortified, enriched or added) must have at least 10 percent more of the Daily Value for a particular nutrient (that is, dietary fiber, potassium, protein, or an essential vitamin or mineral) than the reference food that it resembles.

Light/Lite

"Light" or "lite" can mean one of two things:

First, that a nutritionally altered product contains one-third fewer calories or half the fat of the reference food. If the food derives 50 percent or more of its calories from fat, the reduction must be 50 percent of the fat.

Second, that the sodium content of a low-calorie, low-fat food has been reduced by 50 percent.

The term "light in sodium" is allowed if the food has at least 50 percent less sodium than a reference food. If the food

still does not meet the definition for "low sodium," the label must include the disclaimer "not a low-sodium food."

"Light" will be allowed to describe color or texture, provided qualifying information is included. However, names that have a long history of use, such as "light brown sugar," can still be used without qualifying information.

Meals and Main Dishes

Any product represented as or in a form commonly understood to be breakfast, lunch or dinner is subject to the special rules for meal products. Examples include frozen dinners, some pizzas, and shelf-stable items.

Under FDA rules, a main dish must weigh at least 6 ounces and contain at least two different foods from at least two of four specified food groups. (While FDA endorses the five food groups recommended in current dietary guidelines, the agency believes treating fruits and vegetables as separate groups in this situation would allow the inappropriate classi-

Special Situations

"Standards of identity" define a food's composition and specify the ingredients it must contain. The government originally developed these standards to protect consumers from economic deception.

But some standards of identity require high amounts of nutrients that many consumers would like to avoid. For example, the standard for sour cream requires that the food contain 18 percent fat and the standard for mozzarella cheese requires it to be 45 percent fat. Before the new regulations, "reduced-fat" sour cream or mozzarella cheese were required to have their own standards of identity or be called "imitation" or "substitute," names that consumers may perceive as negative.

The new regulations allow manufacturers to reduce the fat content of such products and call them "low fat" or "light," as appropriate, as long as the food is still nutritionally equivalent to the regular version. For example, sour cream can be called "light" as long as its fat content is reduced to 9 percent and it has vitamin A added to replace the amount lost when the fat was removed. If the company decides not to add the vitamin A, it must call the product "imitation light sour cream."

FDA is not allowing nutrient content claims on foods for infants and children under 2, unless explicit permission has been given.

FDA allows manufacturers to use the terms "unsweetened" and "unsalted" on these foods because these claims are considered to be about taste rather than nutrient content. However, current dietary guidelines do not call for limiting salt or sugar in the diets of children under 2. Therefore, FDA will not allow phrases that imply low or reduced amounts of sodium and calories, such as "no salt added" and "no sugar added," on these types of foods.

—D.S.

fication of a fruit and a vegetable product as a main dish.)

FDA requires a "meal" to weigh at least 10 ounces and have at least three different foods from at least two of the four specified food groups.

USDA defines a meal-type product as one weighing between 6 and 12 ounces per serving and containing ingredients from two or more of four specified food groups.

Claims that a meal or main dish is "free" of a nutrient, such as sodium or cholesterol, must meet the same requirements as those for individual foods.

"Low" claims can be made if the main dish or meal has:
• 120 calories or less per 100 g
• 140 mg sodium or less per 100 g
• 3 g fat or less and no more than 30 percent of calories from fat per 100 g
• 1 g saturated fat or less and no more than 10 percent calories from saturated fat per 100 g **or**
• 20 mg cholesterol or less per 100 g and no more than 2 g of saturated fat per 100 g.

Implied Claims

"Made with oat bran" and "no tropical oils" are examples of statements that may be implied nutrient content claims. Such claims are prohibited when they wrongfully imply that a food contains or does not contain a meaningful level of a nutrient. They are allowed if the food's nutrient content meets the definition for appropriate nutrient content descriptors that are implied by the claim.

For example, FDA considers statements about some types of oil as an ingredient, such as "made with canola oil" or "contains corn oil," to imply that the oil in the product is low in saturated fat. Therefore, to carry that claim, a food would have to meet the definition of "low saturated fat."

A serving of a food carrying a "more" claim (or claims of fortified, enriched or added) must have at least 10 percent more of the Daily Value for a particular nutrient (that is, dietary fiber, potassium, protein, or an essential vitamin or mineral) than the reference food that it resembles.

Getting Specific

Here are examples of the meanings of some descriptive words for specific nutrients:

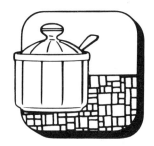

Sugar

Sugar free: less than 0.5 grams (g) per serving

No added sugar, Without added sugar, No sugar added:
• No sugars added during processing or packing, including ingredients that contain sugars (for example, fruit juices, applesauce, or dried fruit).
• Processing does not increase the sugar content above the amount naturally present in the ingredients. (A functionally insignificant increase in sugars is acceptable from processes used for purposes other than increasing sugar content.)
• The food that it resembles and for which it substitutes normally contains added sugars.
• If the food doesn't meet the requirements for a low- or reduced-calorie food, the product bears a statement that the food is not low-calorie or calorie-reduced and directs consumers' attention to the nutrition panel for further information on sugars and calorie content.

Reduced sugar: at least 25 percent less sugar per serving than reference food

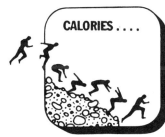

Calories

Calorie free: fewer than 5 calories per serving

Low calorie: 40 calories or less per serving and if the serving is 30 g or less or 2 tablespoons or less, per 50 g of the food

Reduced or Fewer calories: at least 25 percent fewer calories per serving than reference food

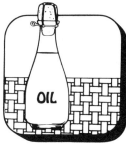

Fat

Fat free: less than 0.5 g of fat per serving

Saturated fat free: less than 0.5 g per serving and the level of trans fatty acids does not exceed 1 percent of total fat

Low fat: 3 g or less per serving, and if the serving is 30 g or less or 2 tablespoons or less, per 50 g of the food

Low saturated fat: 1 g or less per serving and not more than 15 percent of calories from saturated fatty acids

Reduced or Less fat: at least 25 percent less per serving than reference food

Reduced or Less saturated fat: at least 25 percent less per serving than reference food

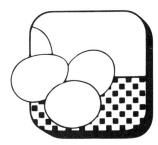

Cholesterol

Cholesterol free: less than 2 milligrams (mg) of cholesterol and 2 g or less of saturated fat per serving

Low cholesterol: 20 mg or less and 2 g or less of saturated fat per serving and, if the

serving is 30 g or less or 2 tablespoons or less, per 50 g of the food

Reduced or Less cholesterol: at least 25 percent less and 2 g or less of saturated fat per serving than reference food

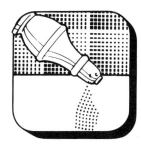

Sodium

Sodium free: less than 5 mg per serving

Low sodium: 140 mg or less per serving and, if the serving is 30 g or less or 2 tablespoons or less, per 50 g of the food

Very low sodium: 35 mg or less per serving and, if the serving is 30 g or less or 2 tablespoons or less, per 50 g of the food

Reduced or Less sodium: at least 25 percent less per serving than reference food

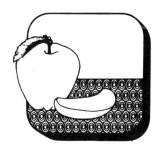

Fiber

High fiber: 5 g or more per serving. (Foods making high-fiber claims must meet the definition for low fat, or the level of total fat must appear next to the high-fiber claim.)

Good source of fiber: 2.5 g to 4.9 g per serving

More or Added fiber: at least 2.5 g more per serving than reference food

1. TRENDS TODAY AND TOMORROW

The statement "made only with vegetable oil" implies that because vegetable oil is used instead of animal fat, the oil component contributes no cholesterol and is low in saturated fat. In this case, the claim could be used only if the food meets the definition of "cholesterol free" and "low saturated fat."

And the statement "contains no oil" implies that the product contains no fat and thus is fat free. Such a claim on a product that contained another source of fat, such as animal fat, would be misleading. Therefore, this statement would be allowed only if the food is truly fat free.

Claims that imply a product contains a particular amount of fiber, such as "high in oat bran," can be made only if the food actually meets the definition for "high" fiber or "good source" of fiber, whichever is appropriate.

Statements that don't fall under the rules for nutrient content implied claims and therefore are still allowed are:

• those that help consumers avoid certain foods because of religious beliefs or dietary practices—for example, a "milk-free" claim
• those about nonnutritive ingredients, such as "no preservatives" or "no artificial colors"
• those about ingredients that provide added value, such as "contains real fruit"
• statements of identity, such as "Colombian coffee" and "100 percent corn oil"

Fresh

Although not mandated by the Nutrition Labeling and Education Act of 1990, as regulations for the other nutrient content claims are, FDA has issued a regulation for the term "fresh." Under this regulation, "fresh" can be used only on a food that is raw, has never been frozen or heated, and contains no preservatives. (Irradiation at low levels is allowed.) "Fresh frozen," "frozen fresh," and "freshly frozen" can be used for foods that are quickly frozen while still fresh. Blanching (brief scalding before freezing to prevent nutrient breakdown) is allowed.

Other uses of the term "fresh," such as in "fresh milk" or "freshly baked bread," are not affected.

Healthy

Along with the final rule on nutrient content claims published last January, FDA and FSIS published proposed rules that would allow manufacturers to make a "healthy" claim on the label. Under FDA's proposal, "healthy" could be used if the food is low in fat and saturated fat and a serving does not contain more than 480 mg of sodium or more than 60 mg of cholesterol. USDA's proposal would allow the term if the food meets the definition for "lean" and contains no more than 480 mg of sodium per serving.

Final rules are expected in 1993.

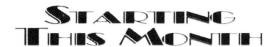

Look For 'LEGIT' Health Claims On Foods

Dixie Farley

Dixie Farley is a staff writer for FDA Consumer. *Ellen Anderson, Ph.D., a research chemist in FDA's Center for Food Safety and Applied Nutrition, also contributed to this article.*

Planning a healthy diet will soon be easier. Beginning this May 8, food labels may provide not only the nutrient content of products but also claims about certain relationships between diet and disease.

As mandated by the Nutrition Labeling and Education Act of 1990, the Food and Drug Administration has issued final food labeling rules for health claims. (See accompany summary.) The rules, published in the Jan. 6, 1993, *Federal Register,* allow claims about seven relationships:

• calcium and a reduced risk of osteoporosis (a condition of lowered bone mass)
• sodium and an increased risk of hypertension (high blood pressure)
• dietary saturated fat and cholesterol and an increased risk of coronary heart disease
• dietary fat and an increased risk of cancer
• fiber-containing grain products, fruits, and vegetables and a reduced risk of cancer
• fruits, vegetables, and grain products that contain fiber, particularly soluble fiber, and a reduced risk of coronary heart disease

• fruits and vegetables and a reduced risk of cancer.

"These rules allow information on food labels that can help to educate the public about recognized diet-disease relationships," says Elizabeth Yetley, Ph.D., acting director of FDA's Office of Special Nutritionals. "Authorized claims must meet requirements to pre-

> *Diets low in saturated fat and cholesterol and rich in fruits, vegetables, and grain products that contain some types of dietary fiber, particularly soluble fiber, may reduce the risk of heart disease, a disease associated with many factors.*

vent label information that would be false or misleading." Yetley coordinated the agency's health claims evaluation.

Health claims became a hot issue in the 1980s, when food marketing strategies began reflecting increased recognition of the role of nutrition in promoting health. A 1984 ad campaign by the Kellogg Company for All Bran cereal advised consumers to maintain proper weight and eat a well-balanced diet including low-fat, high-fiber foods, fresh fruits, and vegetables. Stating the National Cancer Institute "believes eating the right foods may reduce your risk of some kinds of cancer," the health message was both attributed to and approved by NCI.

According to an FDA survey by Alan Levy, Ph.D., and Raymond Stokes, Ph.D., sales of high-fiber cereals increased 37 percent within a year as consumers apparently discriminated between high- and low-fiber products.

Under the provisions of the Federal Food, Drug, and Cosmetic Act in effect at that time, FDA took the position that information about a disease on a food label implied that eating the food could beneficially affect the course of the disease. The agency considered such statements to be drug claims.

In 1987, however, in response to developing scientific data on the relationship between diet and disease, FDA proposed changing its policy to permit appropriate health messages on food labels. The agency noted that the rapid increase in in-

Reprinted from *FDA Consumer,* May 1993, pp. 15-21.

formation and of public interest in nutrition "argues for recognition and dissemination of such new knowledge, and food labels offer one appropriate vehicle for this dissemination."

Soon, many claims appeared on foods—often only partly meeting FDA's proposed criteria. For this reason and because of widely divergent comments on the proposal, FDA solicited additional comments and held a public hearing. The agency withdrew the 1987 proposal and reproposed regulations in February 1990 to more narrowly define health claims and more clearly state its criteria for claims.

Scientific support for diet-disease relationships and public interest in health continued to grow, encouraging Congress in the fall of 1990 to pass the Nutrition Labeling and Education Act. The new law confirmed FDA's authority to regulate health claims on food. Among other things, it required that the agency determine whether health claims were appropriate for 10 relationships:
• calcium and osteoporosis
• sodium and hypertension
• lipids (fats and fat-like substances) and cardiovascular (heart and blood vessel) disease
• lipids and cancer
• dietary fiber and cardiovascular disease
• dietary fiber and cancer
• folic acid and neural tube defects
• antioxidant vitamins and cancer (antioxidants inhibit or prevent oxidation—a chemical reaction whose effect in the body is not well-understood)
• zinc and immune function in the elderly
• omega-3 fatty acids and heart disease.

FDA evaluated the scientific evidence and published its tentative findings in the Nov. 27, 1991, *Federal Register* food labeling proposal. The health claims proposals garnered more than 6,000 letters. To reach its final decisions about health claims, FDA reviewed more than 1,400 scientific studies and authoritative reports.

Definitions, Restrictions

According to the final rule, a "health claim" is any claim on the package label or other labeling (such as an ad) of a food, including fish and game meats, that characterizes the relationship of any nutrient or other substance in the food to a disease or health-related condition.

An example of a health claim is, "Development of cancer depends on many factors. A diet low in total fat may reduce the risk of some cancers." This claim associates the two necessary components: a specific nutrient or food substance and a specific health problem.

Health claims include implied claims, which indirectly assert a relationship. Implied claims may appear as third-party references, such as "The National Cancer Institute recommends a high-fiber diet." Brand names (such as "Heart Smart"), symbols (such as heart-shaped logos), and vignettes (descriptions), when used with specific nutrient information, may within the context of the label result in a health claim.

In contrast, claims about general health or food classes are not health claims. Some examples: the Food Guide Pyramid logo (a pyramid-shaped depiction of the Dietary Guidelines for Americans), valentine candy in a heart-shaped box, and "Eat five servings of fruits and vegetables a day for good health." FDA would consider those examples health claims if a specific nutrient and disease were introduced—the term "low fat" and a heart logo, for instance. Context is the key.

The definition does not cover nutrient-deficiency diseases—such as scurvy, caused by lack of vitamin C. Such diseases, which are no longer of major public health significance in the United States, are adequately regulated under other portions of the FD&C Act. Thus, FDA believes it would be inappropriate to subject these relationships to the health claims rules.

Finally, health claims do not apply to:
• exempt infant formulas
• foods intended for children under 2 years
• medical foods, which are foods formulated for dietary management of diseases or other medical conditions
• foods regulated as drugs.

To qualify for labeling with a health claim, foods must contain:
• a nutrient (such as calcium) whose consumption at a specified level as part of an appropriate diet will have a positive effect on the risk of disease **or**
• a nutrient of concern (such as fat) below a specified level.

The foods must contribute nutrition to the diet by containing at least 10 percent of the Daily Value (DV) of one or more of the nutrients vitamin A, vitamin C, iron, calcium, protein, and fiber. These nutrients must occur naturally in the food at least at 10 percent of the DV.

The Nutrition Labeling and Education Act specifies that foods bearing health claims must not contain any nutrient or food substance in an amount that increases the risk of a disease or health condition. Because dietary guidance calls for people to limit intake of fat, saturated fat, cholesterol, and sodium, FDA identified these substances as risk nutrients and set disqualifying levels for them per serving and per reference amount and, when a food has a small reference amount (30 grams or two tablespoons or less), per 50 g of the food. (As stated in FDA's new rule, the "reference amount" is the amount customarily consumed on an eating occasion. The serving size will be close, but not necessarily identical, to the reference amount.) Foods bearing health claims, then, must contain 20 percent or less of the DV of: fat (13 g), saturated fat (4 g), cholesterol (60 milligrams), and sodium (480 mg).

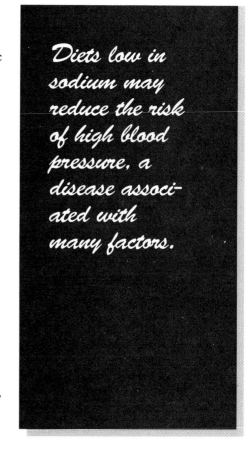

Diets low in sodium may reduce the risk of high blood pressure, a disease associated with many factors.

About Supplements. . .

The Dietary Supplement Act, Title II of the Prescription Drug User Fee Act of 1992, prohibits FDA until at least Dec. 15, 1993, from making final labeling rules for supplements and from taking action against supplements for unauthorized health claims. The legislation became law Oct. 30, 1992.

As with conventional food, however, a supplement component may qualify for a health claim under the Nutrition Labeling and Education Act of 1990 if it confers a health benefit due to its nutritive value and meets other FDA health claims criteria.

"If a nutrient is shown to provide the benefit, then it's the nutrient content that's important, not its source," says Elizabeth Yetley, Ph.D., of FDA's Center for Food Safety and Applied Nutrition, who coordinated the agency's review of health claims.

Dietary supplements include products providing nutrition, such as vitamins, minerals, amino acids, and fatty acids. They also include substances such as herbs and bee pollen.

Under the Nutrition Labeling and Education Act, even when a supplement contains a nutrient in an amount in excess of that found in conventional food, the rule doesn't necessarily prevent a health claim. For example, a calcium-osteoporosis health claim would be permitted in supplements containing calcium in higher potencies than those found naturally in foods such as dairy products, provided the supplement meets the claim's other criteria. If the potency exceeds 400 milligrams a day, however, the labeling must state there's no known benefit from taking more than 2,000 mg a day.

Meanwhile, the new supplements act requires that, during 1993, the General Accounting Office study FDA's management of dietary supplements, and the Office of Technology Assessment study the relationship between supplements regulation (in other countries as well as the United States) and health outcomes. Under the act, FDA is to publish proposed rules (by June 15) and final rules (by Dec. 31, but no earlier than Dec. 15) that are responsive to the Nutrition Labeling and Education Act regarding supplements.

Thus, whole milk, which is high in calcium, may not bear a calcium-osteoporosis claim because its fat content exceeds the disqualifying levels, and excess fat increases the risk of cancer and heart disease. Skim, 1 percent, and 2 percent milks and milk products generally qualify for calcium-osteoporosis health claims.

Main dish products (6 ounces or more with not less than 40 g of two foods from two or more of the four food groups) and meal products (10 ounces or more with not less than 40 g of three or more foods from two or more food groups) may not bear claims if they contain, respectively, 30 or 40 percent or more of the DV for a disqualifying nutrient. FDA may by regulation permit a claim on food that contains a nutrient in amounts that exceed the disqualifying level if the agency finds that the claim will help consumers maintain a healthy diet, and the labeling discloses the presence of the nutrient at that level. No such exceptions have yet been made.

Every statement, phrase or symbol on a food label (health claim or not) must be truthful and not misleading. Because many factors affect disease development, it would be misleading to overemphasize the role of the food substance in a claim, such as indicating it will prevent the disease. Claims that a substance will prevent a disease are drug claims. Thus, in discussing the diet-disease relationship, health claims may only say the substance "may" or "might" reduce the risk. Claims must indicate the disease depends on many factors and may be required to mention other factors that affect the benefit—such as regular exercise, in calcium-osteoporosis claims.

Health claims cannot substitute a disease risk indicator for the disease itself, unless authorized. Claims for fat and heart disease, for instance, may optionally include the link of lowering blood cholesterol—as in, "Development of heart disease depends upon many factors. A healthful diet low in saturated fat and cholesterol may lower blood cholesterol levels and may reduce the risk of heart disease."

Many claims will be consistent with certain recognized dietary guidelines and may state them. A sodium-hypertension health claim, for instance, may say it is consistent with dietary guidelines to "use salt and sodium in moderation." Some

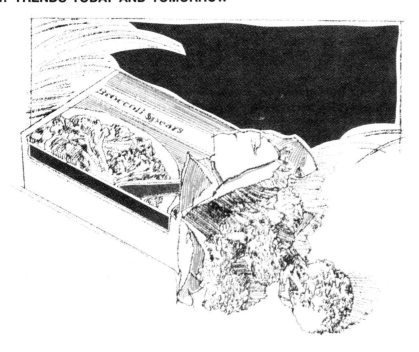

While many factors affect heart disease, diets low in saturated fat and cholesterol may reduce the risk of this disease.

Claim Specifics

Calcium and osteoporosis. Low calcium intake is one risk factor for osteoporosis, a condition of lowered bone mass, or density. Lifelong adequate calcium intake helps maintain bone health by increasing as much as genetically possible the amount of bone formed in the teens and early adult life and by helping to slow the rate of bone loss that occurs later in life. ***Typical foods.*** Low-fat and skim milks, yogurts, tofu, calcium-fortified citrus drinks, and some calcium supplements. ***Requirements.*** A food or supplement must be "high" in calcium (at least 200 milligrams of assimilable calcium per reference amount or per daily dose of a calcium supplement; a "reference amount" is the amount customarily consumed on an eating occasion). It must not contain more phosphorus than calcium. Claims must cite other risk factors, such as a person's gender, race and age; state the need for regular exercise and a healthful diet; explain that the way adequate calcium intake early in life helps reduce fracture risk later in life is by increasing as much as genetically possible a person's peak bone mass; and indicate that those at greatest risk of developing osteoporosis later in life are white and Asian teenage and young adult women, who are in their bone-forming

years. Claims for foods or supplements with more than 400 mg of calcium per reference amount or daily dose must state that a daily intake over 2,000 mg offers no added known benefit to bone health.

Sodium and hypertension (high blood pressure). Hypertension is a risk factor for coronary heart disease and stroke deaths. The most common source of sodium is table salt. Diets low in sodium may help lower blood pressure and related risks in many people. Guidelines recommend daily sodium intakes of not more than 2,400 mg. Typical U.S. intakes are 3,000 to 6,000 mg. ***Typical foods.*** Unsalted tuna, salmon, fruits and vegetables, and low-fat milks, low-fat yogurts, cottage cheeses, sherbets, ice milk, cereal, flour, and pastas (not egg pastas). ***Requirements.*** Foods must meet criteria for "low sodium" (140 mg or less of sodium per reference amount and, when a food has a small reference amount of 30 g or 2 tablespoons or less, per 50 g of the food). Claims must use "sodium" and "high blood pressure" in discussing the nutrient-disease link.

Dietary fat and cancer. Diets high in fat increase the risk of some types of cancer, such as cancers of the breast, colon and prostate. While scientists don't know how total fat intake affects cancer development, low-fat diets reduce the risk. Experts recommend that Americans consume 30 percent or less of daily calories as fat. Typical U.S. intakes are 37 percent. ***Typical foods.*** Fruits, vegetables, reduced-fat milk products, cereals, pastas, flours, and sherbets. ***Requirements.*** Foods must meet criteria for "low fat" (3 g or less of fat per reference amount and, when a food has a small reference amount, per 50 g of the food). Fish and game meats must meet criteria for "extra lean." Claims may not mention specific types of fats and must use "total fat" or "fat" and "some types of cancer" or "some cancers" in discussing the nutrient-disease link.

Dietary saturated fat and cholesterol and risk of coronary heart disease. Diets high in saturated fat and cholesterol increase total and low-density (bad) blood cholesterol levels and, thus, the risk of coronary heart disease. Diets low in saturated fat and cholesterol decrease the risk. Guidelines recommend that American diets contain less than 10 percent of calories from saturated

other optional information is allowed, such as the number of people affected by the disease.

New Claims

When petitioned, FDA will authorize new claims if specific requirements are met.

First, the nutrient or food substance must be related to a disease or health condition for which most people or a specific group of people, such as the elderly, are at risk.

Second, for a claim to be valid, the rules require significant agreement among qualified experts that the claim is supported by the "totality of publicly available scientific evidence." This evidence must include data from well-designed studies conducted with recognized scientific procedures and principles.

OTC Drugs with Food Health Claims

Over-the-counter drugs that are also

Low-fat diets rich in fiber-containing grain products, fruits, and vegetables may reduce the risk of some types of cancer, a disease associated with many factors.

foods present complicating concerns for FDA. One such case is calcium antacids, which have been used as dietary supplements as well.

As drugs, such products are labeled for short-term problems, which, if persistent, may indicate a more serious condition, such as an underlying ulcer. Conse-

quently, the drug labeling directs users to see a doctor if symptoms persist. As food supplements, however, these products are labeled for long-term use at lower levels consistent with daily dietary guidelines. The labeling usually provides no directions to seek medical help and places no time limits on use.

---

fat and less than 300 mg cholesterol daily. The average American adult diet has 13 percent saturated fat and 300 to 400 mg cholesterol a day.

Typical foods. Fruits, vegetables, skim and low-fat milks, cereals, whole-grain products, and pastas (not egg pastas).

Requirements. Foods must meet criteria for "low saturated fat" (1 g or less of saturated fat per reference amount and 15 percent or less of calories from saturated fat); "low cholesterol" (20 mg or less of cholesterol per reference amount and, when a food has a small reference amount, per 50 g of the food); and "low fat." Fish and game meats must meet criteria for "extra lean." Claims must use "saturated fat and cholesterol" and "coronary heart disease" or "heart disease" in discussing the nutrient-disease link.

Fiber-containing grain products, fruits, and vegetables and cancer. Diets low in fat and rich in fiber-containing grain products, fruits, and vegetables may reduce the risk of some types of cancer. The exact role of total dietary fiber, fiber components, and other nutrients and substances in these foods is not fully understood.

Typical foods. Whole-grain breads and cereals, fruits, and vegetables.

Requirements. Foods must meet criteria for "low fat" and, without fortification, be a "good source" of dietary fiber. Claims must not specify types of fiber and must use "fiber," "dietary fiber," or "total dietary fiber" and "some types of cancer" or "some cancers" in discussing the nutrient-disease link.

Fruits, vegetables, and grain products that contain fiber, particularly soluble fiber, and risk of coronary heart disease. Diets low in saturated fat and cholesterol and rich in fruits, vegetables, and grain products that contain fiber, particularly soluble fiber, may reduce the risk of coronary heart disease. (It is impossible to adequately distinguish the effects of fiber, including soluble fiber, from those of other food components.)

Typical foods. Fruits, vegetables, and whole-grain breads and cereals.

Requirements. Foods must meet criteria for "low saturated fat," "low fat," and "low cholesterol." They must contain, without fortification, at least 0.6 g of soluble fiber per reference amount, and the soluble fiber content must be listed. Claims must use "fiber," "dietary fiber," "some types of dietary fiber," "some di-

etary fibers," or "some fibers" and "coronary heart disease" or "heart disease" in discussing the nutrient-disease link. The term "soluble fiber" may be added.

Fruits and vegetables and cancer. Diets low in fat and rich in fruits and vegetables may reduce the risk of some cancers. Fruits and vegetables are low-fat foods and may contain fiber or vitamin A (as beta-carotene) and vitamin C. (The effects of these vitamins cannot be adequately distinguished from those of other fruit or vegetable components.)

Typical foods. Fruits and vegetables.

Requirements. Foods must meet criteria for "low fat" and, without fortification, be a "good source" of fiber, vitamin A, or vitamin C. Claims must characterize fruits and vegetables as foods that are low in fat and may contain dietary fiber, vitamin A, or vitamin C; characterize the food itself as a "good source" of one or more of these nutrients, which must be listed; refrain from specifying types of fatty acids; and use "total fat" or "fat," "some types of cancer" or "some cancers," and "fiber," "dietary fiber," or "total dietary fiber" in discussing the nutrient-disease link.

—D.F.

Even though the label may separate such dual directions, FDA is concerned a person may incorrectly assume the medical dosage is safe for dietary usage.

"If firms want to market products with both food and drug instructions or with health claims," says FDA's Yetley, "they may need to provide data to show the agency that the labeling won't confuse consumers, that consumers can differentiate between drug instructions and food or health claim instructions, and that, therefore, the product won't be misused."

Guidelines for Using Health Claims

In labeling with approved health claims, all statements about the diet-disease relationship must be consistent with FDA conclusions. Claims must enable consumers to understand the relationship and the nutrient or food substance's importance in the relationship in terms of a total daily diet.

Required information must be of one type size and in one place, without intervening material. The main panel may refer to a claim located elsewhere, as in an attached pamphlet.

When a health-claim graphic, such as a heart symbol, is used, the claim or a reference to its location must be nearby.

The food label must list the content of the nutrient for which a health claim is made.

If a claim is about reduced levels of a nutrient, such as cholesterol, the content must be low enough to qualify for the approved claim or must meet the FDA definition for "low."

If a claim is made about a nutrient at increased levels, the content must be in an appropriate form and high enough to justify the claim. If a definition exists for the nutrient, the content must meet that definition's "high," unless the approved health claim specifies an alternative level.

Denied Claims

FDA denied a claim for omega-3 fatty acids in reducing the risk of coronary heart disease. Omega-3s are found in oily fish and sea mammals. John Wallingford, Ph.D., who led FDA's review of this claim, noted, "Results of studies relating fish intake and risk of coronary heart disease were conflicting and inconsistent. The most compelling evidence was a well-controlled study that showed fish consumption may reduce the chance of death from a second heart attack. However, these studies did not establish that the effects were due specifically to omega-3 fatty acids."

Data revealed that omega-3s may raise the blood LDL-cholesterol (the bad type) of people with high blood fats and may interfere with blood glucose control in diabetics.

FDA also denied a claim about zinc (an essential trace mineral) and immune function in the elderly. Some studies had suggested that older people consume less zinc than recommended and that intake declines as people age. FDA concluded the evidence did not support the theory that increased dietary zinc would improve the immune function in older Americans.

Some studies appeared to show zinc supplements improved immunity to disease in older people. But the number of study participants was limited, many studies were flawed, and reported improvements were small. In larger, well-designed studies in which older patients received either zinc or placebos (inert pills) in addition to multi-vitamin and mineral preparations, the greatest immune function improvements were among those taking placebos. Zinc supplementation not only did not improve immune system function in the elderly, at 100 mg or more a day, it actually suppressed immunity.

FDA denied a claim for folic acid and neural tube birth defects. The agency continues, however, to consider this issue. Neural tube defects occur within the first six weeks after conception, often before the pregnancy is known. Adequate daily folic acid intake (at least 0.4 mg, or 400 micrograms, but not more than 1 mg) has been recommended for women from puberty through menopause to reduce the risks of having a baby with these severe birth defects.

The agency convened an advisory committee of outside experts to resolve the remaining issues. "We are proceeding as quickly as possible to evaluate several potential safety issues," Yetley explains. "We don't want to have a health claim if it might cause harm."

FDA denied claims for fiber and cancer, fiber and cardiovascular disease, and antioxidant vitamins and cancer because the scientific evidence was inconclusive. It is impossible to adequately distinguish effects of fiber or antioxidants from those of other food components, the agency said.

Nevertheless, in approving the claim for fruits and vegetables and cancer, FDA incorporated information on vitamin A (as beta-carotene) and vitamin C. These nutrients are found in fruits and vegetables whose use as part of total dietary patterns is associated with reduced cancer risks.

As stated in the 1991 proposal, FDA considers a health claim on a food label "a promise to consumers that including the food in a diet . . . will be helpful in attaining the claimed benefit and will not introduce a risk of another disease or health-related condition."

ADA timely statement on proposed revision of US RDAs for use on food labels

One of the FDA's proposals under the authority granted by the Nutrition and Labeling Act of 1990 was to replace the U.S. Recommended Daily Allowances (U.S. RDAs), with U.S. Reference Daily Intakes (RDIs) that would enable consumers to compare the nutrient content of many foods. RDIs would be established for protein, 13 vitamins and 13 minerals, based mainly on the 1989 Recommended Dietary Allowances published by the National Academy of Sciences. Most RDI values are lower than their corresponding U.S. RDA values, which means that the percentages of vitamins and minerals on most food labels will generally be higher than they are now. The American Dietetic Association and other proponents favor this idea because the RDIs are closer than the U.S. RDAs to most people's actual requirements. The dietary supplement industry fears that the RDI system will decrease supplement sales by increasing people's perception that the foods they consume contain adequate amounts of nutrients. In December 1992 Congress enacted a moratorium preventing the FDA from implementing the RDI system for at least a year.

Editor

Since the Food and Drug Administration (FDA) published its proposed regulations implementing the National Labeling and Education Act of 1990, there has been some controversy regarding the establishment of the Reference Daily Intakes (RDIs) and the Daily Reference Values (DRVs) that would replace the US Recommended Daily Allowances (US RDAs). [1]

ADA supports FDA's proposed concept of using age-adjusted population mean values for the RDIs and DRVs in lieu of continued use of outdated US RDAs. The US RDAs were generally derived from the highest 1968 Recommended Dietary Allowances (RDA) value for each nutrient given. The proposed RDIs and DRVs use a population-adjusted average of all the age/sex groups of RDA values (excluding those for pregnant and lactating women). We do not believe the new, somewhat lower, values for the RDIs and DRVs are disadvantageous to the population.

Although use of the RDIs and DRVs result in a slight lowering of amounts, we believe these values are more realistic in view of the population's needs. Such values are also more congruent with today's scientific information, as they are based on the latest edition (1989) of the RDAs.

The ADA supports the proposed RDI levels for biotin, vitamin B-12, folate, and vitamin E even though the proposed levels, which are based on the 1989 RDAs, will be only half or less of the current US RDAs. However, we do recognize that the RDAs for older adults for some nutrients, such as vitamin B-12, may need to be revised and that levels for many other nutrients are 10% to 20% lower than their current US RDA. This modest shift is preferential to the continued use of the highest RDA value as the US RDA value, for several reasons:

■ nutrient content and health claims on food labels will be more consistent with today's dietary recommendations for healthful eating;

■ these lower values will encourage more prudent fortification and (re)formulation of foods per the FDA fortification policy and substitute foods standards; and

■ the highest value for nutrients is not always appropriate as the reference point.

Hence ADA believes the proposed new values for RDIs and DRVs are improvements over the present outdated US RDAs and these proposed values address America's actual nutrition-related health problems.

EFFECT ON FEDERAL FEEDING PROGRAMS

The effect that lower reference values would have on federal feeding programs has been a matter of concern. FDA's proposal addresses information that will be used exclusively on food labels. Therefore, the proposed lower values will not affect federal feeding programs such as the Special Supplemental Food Program for Women, Infants, and Children, Food Stamps, and school food programs. These programs depend upon the most current RDAs established by the Food and Nutrition Board of the National Research Council for the targeted age/sex groups they serve.

NEW TERMINOLOGY TO REPLACE THE US RDAS

We recognize that the proposed use of the acronyms "RDIs" and "DRVs" may contribute to the belief that there will be consumer confusion. However, these acronyms themselves would not appear on the label.

ADA recommends the term "Reference Value" instead of the proposed term "Daily Value." [2] US RDAs have long been confused with RDAs and a new term is needed. "Reference Value" is less likely to be misinterpreted as a daily goal. FDA supports the term "reference" describing it as "more harmonious with the terminology used in developed nations around the world." [3]

Regardless of whether the terminology changes or the term "US RDA" continues to be used, ADA believes the most important issue is updating the numerical values.

1. TRENDS TODAY AND TOMORROW

ADDITIONAL REMARKS

ADA provides these additional comments, which we believe would decrease consumer confusion:

1. The rounded figure of 2,000 kcal, instead of 2,350 kcal, is recommended as the basis for the calculation of some of the DRVs. Based on the incidence of obesity in Americans as reported in Healthy People 2000, we believe the 2,350-kcal value is too high for most Americans, particularly women and older adults, and that the 2,000-kcal figure more accurately reflects the recommended caloric intake levels for Americans.

The 2,000-kcal value facilitates calculation of a gender inclusive adult range of plus or minus 20% (1,600 for women and 2,400 for men). Use of this value would lower the likelihood of the 2,000-kcal level being misconstrued as a population goal since a round number has less implied specificity. The 2,000-kcal level would not affect the levels of the RDIs; however, it would lower the DRVs for fat, saturated fat, and cholesterol to more appropriate levels for much of the population.

2. There needs to be differentiation among reference values for nutrients to be minimized vs those to be maximized. ADA suggests that reference values be preceded by an indicator such as "no more than" for nutrients to be minimized in American diets (fat, saturated fat, cholesterol, and sodium) and "no less than" for nutrients to be maximized.

ADA has had long-standing concerns regarding food labels and nutrient values. We are aware that some of the criticism of the revision of the US RDAs has been led by interest groups concerned more with sales of vitamin/mineral supplements than with the nutrition status of Americans. Updated reference values presented in an understandable format are essential if food labels are to help Americans make more healthful food choices.

---

[1]The RDIs are based on a population-adjusted average of all the age/sex groups of RDA values, excluding those for pregnant and lactating women. Vitamins, minerals, and protein would be expressed on the label as a percentage of the RDI. The DRVs are based on either a 2,350-kcal basis or on discussions, recommendations, and guidelines presented in "Diet and Health, the Surgeon General's Report on Nutrition and Health" and the National Cholesterol Education Program's "Report of the Expert Panel on Population Strategies for Blood Cholesterol Reduction" (NCEP Report). Total fat, saturated fat, unsaturated fat, cholesterol, total carbohydrate, dietary fiber, sodium, and potassium would have DRV values.

[2]FDA proposed to use the two sets of reference values—RDIs and DRVs—as a single list of reference values known as the "Daily Values" for use in presenting nutrition information on the food label.

[3]The Food and Drug Administration's "Talk Paper: Revision of the US RDAs," page 4, paragraph 4.

Getting Information From FDA

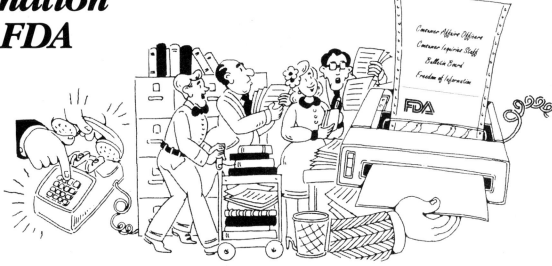

Dori Stehlin

Dori Stehlin is a staff writer for FDA Consumer. *Monica Arcarese, a student at Towson State University, also contributed to the article while a summer intern at FDA.*

A woman called the Food and Drug Administration's office in Orlando, Fla., to thank consumer affairs officer Lynne Isaacs for the nutrition and diet information Isaacs had sent a few weeks before.

"She told me that she was ready for a serious well-balanced diet," Isaacs said. "She had tried all the fad diets and knew they didn't work. Then she admitted there was one fad she had never tried—a product that claims to burn the fat off while you sleep. She said that because she was an insomniac she figured the product would never get a chance to work. Of course that product doesn't work anyway, but I think her reason for not trying it may have been unique."

Thousands of people call or write FDA each year wanting information on a gamut of FDA-regulated items, from aspirin, tongue depressors, and canned green beans to cancer drugs, heart pacemakers, and infant formula.

Exactly what information does FDA have for consumers, and how can they get it?

Consumer Affairs Officers

FDA has consumer affairs officers (also known as public affairs specialists) throughout the country who can respond to questions about the agency and what it regulates.

"Every time there's something in the news about infant formula or baby food, mothers start calling," says Marie Ekvall, FDA's consumer affairs officer in Chicago. "I can hear the baby crying; sometimes the mother's crying, too."

Ekvall can usually give enough information over the phone to help the mother determine if there is any risk for her baby. As a follow-up, Ekvall then sends a reprint from *FDA Consumer* that will give the mother detailed information on infant nutrition.

In addition to reprints of articles from *FDA Consumer*, CAOs also have brochures, posters, teacher kits, press releases, and background papers on all kinds of FDA-related topics.

Consumers interested in audiovisuals can borrow or buy agency-produced slide shows, videotapes and films. CAOs have information on the titles available, prices, and how to order audiovisuals.

CAOs are also available to speak to consumer and other groups on specific topics such as food labeling, health fraud, or AIDS.

To get in touch with your area's CAO, look for the Food and Drug Administration entry under the Department of Health and Human Services in the U.S. Government section of your local phone book.

Consumer Inquiries Staff

FDA's Consumer Inquiries Staff, located at agency headquarters in metropolitan Washington, D.C., is devoted solely to answering consumers' questions. The staff often consults various other FDA offices to find answers to detailed or complicated questions. Last year, Consumer Inquiries received an average of 2,400 requests per month for information.

Send requests for information to FDA, Consumer Inquiries Staff, HFE-88, Room 16-63, 5600 Fishers Lane, Rockville, Md. 20857; telephone (301) 443-3170.

Electronic Bulletin Board

Most people would describe a bulletin board as a piece of cork, some thumbtacks, and lots of papers with important information and announcements. But tacks and cork have been replaced by computers and modems on FDA's electronic bulletin board, which contains:
• press releases
• the *FDA Enforcement Report's* listing of recalls and litigations
• drug and device approvals
• congressional testimony
• speeches by FDA's commissioner
• FDA *Federal Register* summaries
• current information on AIDS, including published information on experimental drugs
• articles from *FDA Consumer*
• articles from the *FDA Drug Bulletin.*

"SORRY, I'LL HAVE TO REFER YOU TO . . ."

FDA doesn't have all the answers. Several other government agencies have responsibilities closely related to FDA's, so it isn't unusual for consumers to be confused about who watches over what. Here's a confusion-controlling list of subjects consumers often call FDA about, but which are under the purview of another agency. (All addresses listed below are for headquarters offices in Washington, D.C. Local offices are listed in the phone book under U.S. Government.)

Alcohol

The labeling and quality of alcoholic beverages are regulated by the Treasury Department's Bureau of Alcohol, Tobacco, and Firearms. ATF's address is Room 4402, Ariel Rios Federal Building, 1200 Pennsylvania Ave., N.W., Washington, D.C. 20226; telephone (202) 566-7135.

Information on drug and alcohol abuse, including counseling information, is available from the Alcohol, Drug Abuse, and Mental Health Administration's National Clearinghouse for Alcohol and Drug Abuse, P.O. Box 2345, Rockville, Md. 20852; (301) 468-2600.

Consumer Products

While FDA keeps watch over the quality of bread, the toaster used to brown it is the responsibility of the Consumer Product Safety Commission. Household appliances (except those that emit radiation), baby furniture, and toys are some of the more common products CPSC covers. Letters can be sent to CPSC, Washington, D.C. 20207, or the commission can be called toll free on 800-638-2772.

Drugs

Drugs of Abuse: Illegal drugs with no approved medical uses, such as heroin, are the sole responsibility of the Drug Enforcement Administration. Because some medically accepted drugs have a potential for abuse (for example, amphetamines, barbiturates and morphine), FDA assists DEA in deciding how stringent DEA controls on such drugs should

be. DEA also limits the amount of these drugs that can be manufactured each year. Everyone who markets controlled drugs, from manufacturers and distributors to pharmacists, must register with DEA. Questions about these responsibilities should be sent to the Drug Enforcement Administration, U.S. Department of Justice, Washington, D.C. 20537; telephone (202) 307-1000.

Nonprescription Drug Advertising: The Federal Trade Commission is the primary agency for regulating ads for nonprescription drugs. The commission's address is 6th St. and Pennsylvania Ave., N.W., Washington, D.C. 20580; telephone (202) 326-2180.

Child-Resistant Packages: The Consumer Product Safety Commission is responsible for child-resistant packages. See address above.

Food Stamps

The federal food stamp program is administered by local governments, usually as part of their social service departments.

Meat and Poultry

The U.S. Department of Agriculture's Food Safety and Inspection Service is responsible for the safety, labeling, and all other issues concerning meat and poultry. Consumers with questions on these issues, as well as how to safely handle, prepare and store chicken, beef and pork, should write or call the Food Safety and Inspection Service's Meat and Poultry Hotline, Room 1163S, Washington, D.C. 20250; telephone 800-535-4555.

Pesticides

FDA, USDA, and the Environmental Protection Agency share the responsibility for regulating pesticides. EPA determines the safety and effectiveness of the chemicals and establishes tolerance levels for residues on feed crops and raw and processed foods. These tolerance levels (the amount of pesticide allowed to remain on a crop after harvesting) are normally set 100 times below the level that might cause harm to people or the environment. To ensure that pesticide

residues do not exceed the allowable levels, FDA tests all foods except meat and poultry, which fall under USDA's jurisdiction. Questions for EPA can be sent to Room W311, Mail Code A-107, 401 M St., S.W., Washington, D.C. 20460; telephone (202) 382-4361.

Radiation

Environmental: EPA monitors radiation in the environment.

Nuclear Industry: Licensing and regulation of the nuclear industry is the Nuclear Regulatory Commission's responsibility. NRC also ensures that the public is protected from hazards arising from nuclear materials in power reactors, hospitals, research laboratories, or other commercial facilities. Questions for NRC should be sent to the NRC Office of Public Affairs, Washington, D.C. 20555; telephone (202)-492-7715.

Restaurants and Grocery Stores

Inspections and licensing of restaurants and grocery stores are usually handled by local health departments.

Tobacco

Collecting taxes on cigarettes and other tobacco products is ATF's responsibility. Information on the health effects of smoking is available from the Office of Smoking and Health, Centers for Disease Control, 5600 Fishers Lane, Rockville, Md. 20857; telephone (301) 443-5287.

Veterinary Products

EPA regulates products used directly on animals to control pests. USDA's Animal and Plant Health Inspection Service handles animal vaccines. The inspection service's address is APHIS, Veterinary Services, U.S. Department of Agriculture, Washington, D.C. 20090-6464; telephone (202) 447-5193.

Water

Depending on how it gets to consumers, water is regulated by either FDA or EPA. If the water comes through the tap, it must meet EPA's national standards for drinking water. Bottled water, however, is FDA's responsibility.

Consumers who have computers with modems can subscribe to FDA's bulletin board by contacting BT Tymnet, 6120 Executive Blvd., Rockville, Md. 20852; telephone 800-872-7654.

For more details on the types of information "posted" on the bulletin board, contact Karen Malone, FDA Press Office, HFI-20, Rockville, Md. 20857; telephone (301) 443-3285.

Freedom of Information Staff

The Freedom of Information Act makes most unpublished documents concerning FDA's regulatory activities available to the public. These include:

• enforcement records, including product recall notifications

• summaries of safety and effectiveness data from approved new drug applications

• regulatory letters telling companies to correct violations found during FDA inspections.

An FOI request for agency records can be denied only under set guidelines. Documents that may be exempt from public disclosure under the Freedom of Information Act include:

• trade secrets and confidential commercial or financial information

• certain interagency or intra-agency memos or letters

• personnel, medical and similar files that, if released, would constitute an invasion of privacy

• certain records compiled for law enforcement purposes

All FOI requests should be in writing. For consumers, there is a copying fee of 10 cents per page and a search fee of $10 per hour. No fee is charged if the total is less than $10.

For more information or to make an FOI request, contact the Freedom of Information Staff, HFI-35, FDA, Room 12A-16, 5600 Fishers Lane, Rockville, Md. 20857.

What Does FDA Regulate?

FDA's responsibilities include foods, drugs, cosmetics, biological products, medical devices, radiological devices, and veterinary products sold in interstate commerce. (For information about what FDA does *not* regulate, see box.)

Some of the agency's specific responsibilities include:

Drugs:
• new drug approval
• good manufacturing practices for all prescription and nonprescription drug manufacturers
• prescription drug advertising
• tamper-resistant packaging

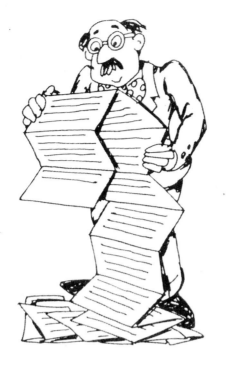

Biologics:
• human vaccine licensing
• blood banks
• allergenic product licensing
• licensing of test kits to screen blood for the AIDS virus

Foods:
• labeling
• safety of all food products except meat and poultry (see accompanying article)
• good manufacturing practices
• bottled water

Medical Devices:
• pre-market approval of new devices
• manufacturing controls
• medical device reporting of malfunctions or serious adverse reactions
• registration and device listing

Electronic Products:
• radiation safety performance standards for microwave ovens, television receivers, diagnostic x-ray equipment, cabinet

x-ray systems (e.g., baggage x-rays at airports), laser products, ultrasonic therapy equipment, mercury vapor lamps, and sunlamps

• guidance to health professionals and consumers about recommended practices to reduce unnecessary exposure to radiation

Veterinary Products:
• livestock feeds
• pet foods
• veterinary drugs and devices

Our Lips Are Sealed

Some of the hardest questions FDA has to deal with are ones about a specific drug, says Marie Ekvall, FDA's consumer affairs officer in Chicago. "I encourage [callers] to talk to [their] doctor or pharmacist, and I let them know about resource books like the *Physicians' Desk Reference,* but I have to be careful not to play doctor," she says.

"We get a lot of calls that, by law, we simply aren't allowed to answer," says Janet McDonald, San Francisco's CAO. For example, FDA employees cannot release any confidential information on unapproved drugs, including clinical trials, unless the manufacturer gives the agency permission or has already released the information to the public.

"This is information people usually have to get from their physicians or from private, nonprofit organizations such as those that deal with Alzheimer's disease or arthritis," says McDonald.

But there are some calls that just can't be answered by FDA or anyone else. For example, there's the boy who wrote Orlando's Isaacs to find out where he could buy a "hoverboard," one of those flying skateboards in the movie "Back to the Future II."

"Those things haven't been invented yet—I'd know because my 8-year-old would be begging for one," says Isaacs. "But if they were real, I guess they'd belong to the Consumer Product Safety Commission."

Nutrients

I've information on vegetable, animal, and mineral. . . .
—W. S. Gilbert in *The Pirates of Penzance*

Some aspects of nutrition have remained relatively unchanged in recent years. One of these is the list of nutrients. Even the specific vitamins and minerals have undergone little revision. Carbohydrates, lipids, and proteins are still identified as the nutrients that provide energy; vitamins, minerals, and water do not. Fiber is not a nutrient because it is not essential to life (note the traditional Eskimo diet), but it is included in this unit because it plays a significant role in maintaining normal physiological functioning.

Although the list of nutrients has remained the same, knowledge about each nutrient has not. Turnover in data on nutrition can be so rapid that information is obsolete before it is printed. Nor does the existence of voluminous data mean that theories are proved. Studies and experiments must be replicated, subjected to peer review, refined, and tried again. Conflicts in data must be considered and resolved. Furthermore, much of the evidence is epidemiological, which indicates a relationship but does not prove cause and effect. It is often years before sufficient evidence will support firm recommendations for either normal or therapeutic diets.

Compounding the problem of formulating recommendations is the fact that differences among human beings are truly remarkable; an average human being does not exist. Physiological variations in individuals preclude accurate predictions of nutrient amounts that cause the negative effects of either deficiency or excess. Moderation and variety are key words in advice about food or nutrient intake. The National Academy of Sciences tries very hard to establish recommendations that more than cover a person's actual requirement but that are not high enough to cause harm. The result is the periodically revised Recommended Dietary Allowances (RDAs).

Many Americans might agree that foods with high protein content are always better for them than foods with little or no protein. It is commonly believed that more protein means more muscle. In fact, it is just an expensive way to get calories for most people in the United States,

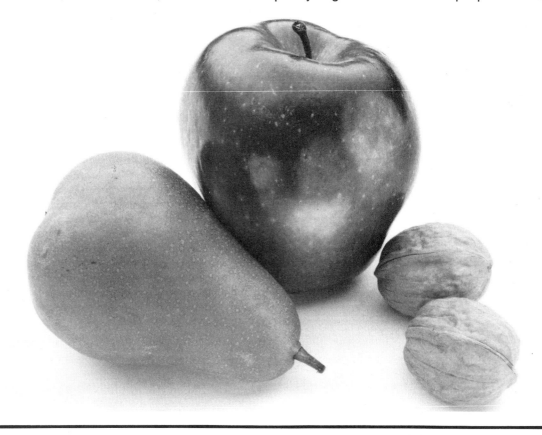

who frequently eat far more protein than they need. Protein recommendations and the benefits and risks of too much are identified in the article "Things Nobody Ever Told Rocky Balboa About Protein."

Fat-free, lower-fat, light, slim, and other similar terms are used to designate foods that are supposed to be healthier. Virtually everybody understands that fat and cholesterol have some connection to heart disease, and many people are eager to reduce the amounts of fat they consume. Published health guidelines for Americans recommend less than 30 percent of calories from fat and a maximum of 10 percent from saturated fat. Because of high interest and concern, two articles on this topic discuss lipid terminology, ways to reduce fat in one's diet, and the relationship of dietary fat to health. Current evidence indicates that it is saturated fat that negatively affects health and that unsaturated fat, especially mono-unsaturated fat, may even have positive effects. To further complicate the picture, interest has renewed in trans-fatty acids, those formed into a different chemical configuration when hydrogenation makes liquids into solids. Still, as the article "Fat for the Fit" points out, margarine remains a better health choice than butter.

Much mythology continues to revolve around the inherent values and dangers of sugar (see "The Sugar Bugaboo"). The repeated victim of near-vitriolic attacks, sugar is suggested as the cause of virtually every ill in society—juvenile delinquency and crime included. To date, sugar has been convicted only of causing dental caries.

Vitamins (articles 18–21) are nutrients that have been both wisely used and greatly abused. Once discovered, they were responsible for "miraculous cures" of terrible diseases known for centuries—pellagra, scurvy, and beri-beri. Although ample evidence supports a concern that excesses are sometimes as risky as too little, people often assume that more vitamins inevitably mean better health and use them inappropriately to "cure what ails you." As scientists continue to push the limits of knowledge, additional information is emerging about the role of vitamins in achieving and maintaining health. Of great current interest is the antioxidant potentials of vitamins C and E and beta-carotene. This is research to watch, as scientists wonder if these vitamins can positively influence the likelihood of strokes, heart attacks, cancer, or even cataracts. It is not known whether new knowledge will affect the next RDA revisions, or if there will simply be more support for the current recommended levels of intake. For now at least, most responsible scientists advise getting these vitamins from food, not pills.

Minerals are the topic in article 23. The function of iron in preventing anemia has long been known, and many women and children suffer from the fatigue of this deficiency. Since 6 milligrams of iron accompany each 1,000 kilocalories of the typical diet, it is difficult for many adult females to get even the lowered RDA. Thus, understanding how to increase the absorption of iron becomes important. But, in an interesting new twist, some researchers have become intrigued by an apparent relationship between high iron levels and risk of heart attacks. The full significance of this relationships is not known at this time.

A comparatively recent "miracle" has occurred with the discovery that fluoride can greatly reduce dental caries (see "Fluoride: Cavity-Fighter on Tap"). Fluoridated water supplies, necessary if the tooth structure is to be strengthened against decay, have not always been easily attained. Years ago, as a PTA president, I helped to promote action by a city council for fluoridation. As that became known, literature descended upon me that argued that fluoride caused cancer and was a Russian plot to poison our water supplies. The first argument is still made by those using scare tactics. The latter argument seems laughable now; it was not so in the 1950s.

While oat bran is a fad that has passed, the benefits of fiber remain. Few people consume the recommended amount of 20–35 grams daily. In "The Importance of Fiber," a summary of fiber facts will assist the convert in locating fiber sources and including them in meals.

Much as we would like them, there are few absolutes in the science of nutrition. Perhaps there never will be, but the present decade will be a period of great discovery. For those who marvel at the continued unfolding of the mysteries of human physiology, this is a tremendously exciting era in which to live.

Looking Ahead: Challenge Questions

Are some nutrients more important than others in maintaining health? Support your answer.

What claims are made for vitamins that you know to be false?

How should one decide whether or not to take supplements? Are the issues involving single supplements of a vitamin or mineral any different than for multivitamins?

How would you persuade someone opposed to fluoridated water that it is a good public health measure?

Should fiber be designated a nutrient?

Determine the percentage of your average daily calories that are contributed by fat.

Things nobody ever told Rocky Balboa about protein

Five raw eggs cracked into a blender. That was Rocky Balboa's idea of a power breakfast in the movie that catapulted Sylvester Stallone to star status. Presumably, he believed all the protein in that gloppy mixture would give him the extra strength he needed to win the championship fight. What Rocky was unaware of, however, is that eating huge amounts of protein doesn't have anything to do with building strong muscles. True, muscles are made of protein, and foods like eggs and milk supply substantial amounts of that nutrient, but there is no direct link between big muscles and "big" amounts of protein that go beyond the levels the average American takes in.

Rocky isn't the only "person" with misconceptions about how protein works in the body. Confusion about its role in maintaining good health abounds, not just among muscle builders but also among dieters as well as those who believe meat meals are a must for meeting protein needs. That's why it is particularly important to set straight what protein's functions are—and how much everyone needs on a day-to-day basis.

Yo, Rocky lost in the 15th round

If extra amounts of protein do not go to the muscles, as Rocky thought, where do they end up? Assuming they are not burned as fuel by the body (a fair assumption in the case of most Americans, who get plenty of "fuel" from carbohydrate and fat), in fat stores. It has to do with the fact that when protein is eaten it does not travel directly from the mouth to the parts of the body an ambitious muscle builder is trying to develop. Instead, it is digested into the 20 or so amino acids that serve as protein's building blocks. Then the body "decides" where and how protein is needed.

Consider that protein has a great many functions other than increasing brawn. One of them is to help maintain fluid balance. Different types of protein are also what make up antibodies, the anti-disease agents that help the body fight any organisms perceived as foreign, such as viruses that cause flu, smallpox, and measles. Then, too, special "pumps" made of protein move nutrients into and out of cells when necessary. The fact that the protein "pumps" keep more potassium inside the cells than out and more sodium outside the cells than in is what allows nerve impulses to travel—so that we can think, move, and breathe.

Even though protein performs in so many ways in the body, only 10 to 15 percent of calories need come from that nutrient. The lion's share—at least 55 to 60 percent of calories—should come from carbohydrates, and the rest should be contributed by fat.

Other ways in which protein supports life: It helps blood to clot when a cut or other wound is sustained; it makes scar tissue; it allows for the making of visual pigment that lets us see; and it creates new cells when old ones die.

When the body determines how the incoming protein must be utilized and where it must be supplied, it arranges the amino acids made available from digestion of the protein taken in with food to form the specific proteins called for. (It's the sequence of amino acids that distinguishes, for example, the blood-clotting protein known as thrombin from the visual pigment protein called opsin and from the proteins that make up muscle, insulin, hair, and nails.) The next step is to "send" them on their way. Once all the tissues' protein (as well as energy) needs are met, any amino acids left over are simply converted into fat and deposited in the abdomen, hips, thighs, or buttocks, according to the propensity of the particular body.

If "megadoses" of protein are used simply to meet the body's many protein needs and any extra is stored as fat, a bodybuilder may well ask: How, then, can I increase the size of my muscles? The only way is to put stress on them through exercises such as weight lifting.

Ironically, although bodybuilders looking specifically for bulging biceps will not benefit by eating more protein than anyone else, people who engage regularly in aerobic exercises that require moving around vigorously, such as running, biking, or swimming (as opposed to standing in one spot and lifting weights), do require higher levels according to the results of research conducted by Tufts scientist William Evans, PhD. For a 150-pound man, the difference amounts to about five extra

From *Tufts University Diet & Nutrition Letter,* Vol. 8, No. 12, February 1991, pp. 3-6. *Tufts University Diet & Nutrition Letter,* 53 Park Place, New York, NY 10001.

ounces a day of meat, milk, cheese, fish, or some combination of those foods. But since Americans in general eat much more protein than they need (about twice the recommended dietary allowance), that higher requirement is usually nothing for athletic people to be concerned about. The only ones who tend to be at risk for protein deficiency are people who are trying to lose weight or maintain a rigidly low weight as they exercise and cut back too far on their protein/calorie intake.

Is it possible to eat too much protein?

Can the body become overburdened with much more protein than it could possibly make use of? Emerging scientific evidence would suggest yes, at least for people with kidney disease. A high-protein diet is not known to *cause* kidney problems, but it may worsen an already existing one. The kidneys are the organs that filter waste products from the blood, including nitrogen, which is contained in protein but not in carbohydrate or fat. Excess amounts of nitrogen are excreted in the urine as part of a substance called urea. The hypothesis is that since much of the waste the kidneys end up filtering are products that result from the breakdown of protein, the more protein eaten, the greater the stress on the already faltering kidneys and the faster their deterioration.

Researchers in Melbourne, Australia, have tested the hypothesis on about 60 patients in the initial stages of kidney disease by feeding some of them diets containing protein in amounts about equal to the RDA and giving others diets containing only half the RDA. A year and a half later, fully one in four of the patients eating the more "typical" amounts of protein ended up with end-stage renal (kidney) disease, the most severe form of the illness, for which the only alternatives are a kidney transplant or several days a week of being hooked up to a dialysis machine that does the filtering the kidneys are no longer capable of. But only 6 percent of those on the relatively low-protein diet had become that sick. . . .

It should be pointed out that a low-protein diet cannot reverse or perhaps even halt the process of kidney disease, but it may slow it enough to give kidney patients many more fruitful years before having to undergo surgery or becoming forever dependent on a machine. That's especially promising news in light of the fact that 34,000 Americans fall victim to end-stage renal disease annually. It's also promising for the millions of Americans who do not suffer from kidney failure but who pay health insurance premiums. The yearly cost of taking care of people with severe kidney disease is $4 to $5 billion.

Metabolic disorders

A small number of people are at risk of problems with protein because of an inborn error of metabolism in which one or another amino acid does not work in the body the way it is supposed to. One of these "errors," called phenylketonuria, or PKU, is actually an enzyme defect that allows too much of the amino acid phenylalanine to build up in the tissues of the central nervous system.

No symptoms are apparent at first. A newborn infant with PKU who is not treated will behave like any other baby. Within a few months, however, he will become irritable and perhaps hyperactive as well. As time passes, he may also suffer convulsions and develop an abnormal gait and posture. But the most devastating effect is irreversible brain damage so severe he will never even learn to talk.

Today nearly all hospitals screen newborns for PKU—about one in every 12,000 to 15,000 people is estimated to have it. The treatment for those who are afflicted is straightforward. It involves eating special nutritional supplements and foods that contain enough phenylalanine to help build the proteins in which it is needed but not enough to damage body tissues. . . .

How much protein are *you* getting?

Individuals with particular amino acid disorders obviously must know exactly how much protein is in the food they eat. But how can anyone else figure out the amount of protein he or she takes in and whether it's more than required?

First, it's necessary to determine your individual needs. If you are an adult and not pregnant, compute the number of grams in your recommended dietary allowance for protein by multiplying your body weight (in pounds) by 0.36. Children and pregnant and lactating women need more protein than others because they are laying down new tissue as well as maintaining what they already have. That's why, for example, the protein RDA for infants up to six months of age is their body weight (in pounds) multiplied by 1 (almost three times the 0.36 figure) and for boys and girls 11 through 14, body weight multiplied by 0.45.

Pregnant women are supposed to take in about 10 grams more protein a day than usual by the time they reach their third trimester. And women who are breast-feeding should consume an extra 10 to 15 grams, especially during the first six months after they give birth.

Once you compute your protein RDA, it's necessary to learn how much protein is in the foods you eat. The chart above should help, but an even easier device is to remember that an ounce of most animal foods contains about seven grams, while plant foods contain considerably less.

What that means in practical terms is that a 120-pound woman who eats a cup of yogurt in the morning, three ounces of canned tuna at lunch, and four ounces of beef or chicken at dinner (as much as in a quarter-pound hamburger and less than many people are accustomed to) is taking in 57 grams a day, more than 130 percent of her 43 gram RDA (120 x .36 = 43). And that's without

---

The protein in the foods you eat

	Protein (grams)
1 oz meat, poultry, or fish	7
1 oz cheese	7
1 egg	7
1 cup milk/yogurt	8
½ cup vanilla ice cream	2
½ cup beans	6
2 tablespoons peanut butter	9
1 cup rice	9
1 cup spaghetti	5
1 cup cooked vegetables	4
1 potato, baked with skin	5
1 slice bread	3

---

counting the protein in any bread, cereal, or vegetables she might eat or in the milk with which she lightens her coffee, all of which could easily add at least 15 to 20 grams more! Clearly, it's easy to take in plenty. Even American vegetarians who have been surveyed have been shown to consume 100 grams of protein a day.

And they do not have to be concerned that the proteins in the plant foods they eat are not "complete," meaning that unlike most proteins in flesh foods and dairy products, they do not contain the nine essential amino acids that the body is unable to make and therefore must be in the diet in adequate quantities in order to synthesize whatever amino acid chains—proteins—are necessary.

Plant proteins are better than some assume, and unless the vegetarian diet is extreme (leaving out whole groups of foods, for instance, or concentrating too much on one type of food), the amino acids they provide are likely to complement each other and thereby provide protein that is as high in quality as the protein found in the usual diet.

Which foods specifically complement which? Beans go with grains or cereals, cereals match with leafy vegetables, peanut protein is coupled with wheat, oats, corn, or rice, and soy protein (which in itself is of high quality) is combined with corn, wheat, rye, or sesame. In other words, many vegetarian dishes you probably eat anyway—rice and beans, a peanut butter and jelly sandwich, split pea soup with a piece of bread— all contain complete proteins. Even a vegetarian who pays no attention to the complementarity of his proteins is likely to meet his quota. And lacto-ovo vegetarians, who eat dairy products and eggs but no other animal proteins, will certainly have no trouble.

There are a couple of advantages to taking in more protein from plant foods and a little less from certain kinds of animal foods. One is that less fat will be consumed, since with many cuts of meat and poultry and some dairy products, high quality amino acid makeup is accompanied by more fat than is found in grains and vegetables. Consider that earlier in this century, when Americans obtained half their protein from animal foods and half from plant foods, they were eating less fat than they are today, a time when at least two thirds of the protein in the average diet comes from animal foods and only one third from plants. A second bonus of taking in more protein from plants: plant protein is often less expensive than animal protein, as any comparison between prices at the butcher counter and the produce aisle will show. Of course, animal foods are often richer in many vitamins and minerals than plant foods, so you need to be careful about taking in enough of certain nutrients, such as iron, calcium, and zinc, when constructing a high-plant, low-animal product diet.

Getting less fat along with animal proteins

Although animal foods are generally fattier than plant foods, it is definitely possible to choose at least some high-protein foods of animal origin— which also supply plenty of other nutrients—and limit fat at the same time. Low-fat, high-protein choices are in bold type.

	Protein(g)*	Fat(g)⁺	Total calories
1 cup whole milk	8	8	150
1 cup skim milk	**8**	**0**	**86**
3½ oz roasted chicken with skin	27	14	239
3½ oz roasted chicken without skin	**29**	**7**	**190**
3 oz broiled T-bone steak (choice cut)	24	9	182
3 oz broiled top round steak (select cut)	**27**	**5**	**156**

* A gram of protein contains 4 calories. ⁺ A gram of fat contains 9 calories.

Special K for those on weight-loss diets?

Many dieters were reared on weight-loss regimens that were high in protein (and often fat) and low in carbohydrates. The Stillman Diet, popular in the early 70s, was one of them. It allowed as much high-protein beef and poultry as the dieter wanted, but severely limited carbohydrates such as bread, pasta, fruits, and vegetables.

A good number of today's weight-conscious eaters know better. They are aware that the recommended way to lose weight is to fill up on starchy foods like bread and pasta as well as on high-fiber fruits and vegetables and eat potentially high-fat flesh foods in limited amounts. But some people still mistakenly believe that when it comes to dieting, protein is the nutrient to focus on. Advertisements for Kellogg's Special K cereal have played on that misconception with their "keep the muscle, lose the fat" slogan. The ads are intended to make dieters think that if they eat the product, they will shed pounds of fat rather than muscle. The reasoning: the protein in Special K will "spare" the protein in the tissues and not let it break down to supply the body with energy while calorie intake is restricted, leaving fat alone to break apart. Hopeful weight-losers buy into it, believing that if the cereal keeps the body's protein from disintegrating, their decreased calorie consumption will affect their fat stores only and thereby make the loss of fat all the more rapid.

But unless a dieter restricts calories so severely that he ends up on a crash diet or a modified fast, not enough protein in the body will be lost to worry about. Furthermore, if someone *were* on a modified fast and needed to insure that the protein in his or her vital organs would remain intact, Special K would not be the food to reach for. Granted, it contains more protein than most breakfast cereals, but a serving still supplies only 10 percent of the U.S. Recommended Daily Allowance for that nutrient. It is for those reasons that the Iowa Attorney General recently filed suit against Kellogg, calling the Special K ads "deceptive" and "misleading."

The bottom line for people who watch their weight: You don't need more protein than anyone else. Protein intake has to be sufficient to cover the body's losses of that nutrient, to replace dead cells with new ones, and to keep them working properly, but as with Americans who are not restricting calories, dieters' protein needs are generally met without any special precautions.

When protein is in short supply

Hair, nails, antibodies, hemoglobin, insulin, bones, teeth, connective tissue, skin. All of these, along with other body parts, are made with protein. Indeed, proteins are essential for the growth and upkeep of every single body tissue. In many third-world countries, that lesson has often been learned tragically.

On the west coast of Africa in Ghana, for instance, when a mother has a second baby, her first child frequently becomes very sick. His growth is stunted, his hair loses its color, his skin turns patchy and scaly, and his body becomes swollen with edema or water retention. He also falls ill easily and becomes very weak and listless. In many cases he eventually dies.

Ghanaians once attributed the illness to "the evil spirit that infects the first child when the second child is born." They called that spirit kwashiorkor. Today's scientists know that kwashiorkor—a problem in third-world countries across the globe—is the result of a protein deficiency that can occur when a mother weans her first born from the breast to make way for her newborn but is not able to serve her older child foods that contain the same high quality protein found in her breast milk. Ghanaian children are often given a porridge made mostly of starch and very little protein.

People who are starving are also at great risk for protein deficiency, but not necessarily because they are not taking in enough protein. A lack of calories could cause a protein deficit in itself. The reason is that if the body does not receive a sufficient supply of calories or energy from the three energy-giving nutrients—carbohydrate, fat, and protein—it will digest its own protein-containing tissues and use the calories "released" in the process to make up for the lack. The casual observer may observe only a change in hair and skin at first, but protein from other more vital tissues, which include the muscle of the heart, lungs, and brain, will be broken down even earlier.

By and large, Americans are fortunate enough not to be at risk for protein deficiency. It's true there are some groups of people in the United States who may fall near or into the danger zone: children in very poor families, pregnant women who do not get enough to eat, senior citizens with low incomes or disabilities that prohibit them from shopping for themselves, and alcoholics who squeeze out protein calories from their diet with calories from alcohol. But even they are generally not in severe enough trouble to suffer from full-blown kwashiorkor. And as for the overwhelming majority of Americans, they take in much more protein than they need.

Consider that the adult recommended dietary allowance for protein is in the neighborhood of 50 grams (.36 grams for every pound of body weight). Consider too that the RDA is set above the needs of most people. Add to that the fact that many adults in the U.S. take in an average of about 100 grams of protein a day—two to three times the RDA—and it's clear that few people need worry about taking in too little protein.

A Basic Primer On Fats In The Diet

(Excerpted from material provided by the Human Nutrition Information Service of the U.S. Department of Agriculture)

On average, people in the U.S. eat about 37% of their total calories as fat. Many nutrition authorities have suggested it is best to restrict fat intake to no more than 30% of total calories, limiting saturated fatty acids to about a third of this amount. Limiting cholesterol is also important to your health. Here's a basic overview of what those terms mean – and some good advice to follow...

What is fat?

Fat is the most concentrated source of food energy (calories). Each gram of fat supplies about 9 calories, compared with about 4 calories in a gram of protein or carbohydrates. In addition to providing energy, fat aids in the absorption of certain vitamins. Some fats provide linoleic acid, an essential fatty acid which is needed by everyone in small amounts.

Butter, margarine, shortening and oil are obvious sources of fat. Well-marbled meats, poultry skin, whole milk, cheese, ice cream, nuts, seeds, salad dressings and some baked products also provide a good deal of fat.

Cholesterol

Cholesterol is not a fat, but a fat-like substance, found in the body cells of humans and animals. It is needed to form hormones, cell membranes and other body substances. The body is able to make the cholesterol it needs for these functions. Cholesterol is not needed in the diet.

Cholesterol is present in all meat, poultry and fish, in milk and milk products and in egg yolks. It is not found in foods of plant origin such as fruits, vegetables, nuts, grains and seeds.

Fatty acids

Fatty acids are the basic chemical units in fat. They may be either "saturated," "monounsaturated" or "polyunsaturated." All dietary fats are made up of mixtures of these fatty acid types.

Saturated fatty acids are found largely in fats of animal origin, including whole milk, cream, cheese, butter, meat and poultry. They are also found in large amounts in some vegetable oils, including coconut and palm.

Monounsaturated fatty acids are found in fats of both plant and animal origin. Olive and peanut oil are the most common examples, along with most margarines and hydrogenated vegetable shortening.

Polyunsaturated fatty acids are found largely in fats of plant origin including sunflower, corn, soybean, cottonseed and safflower oils. Some fish are also good sources.

From *Nestlé Worldview*, Vol. 2, No. 4, Winter 1990/1991. *Nestlé Worldview*, prepared by the Nestlé Information Service, 1133 Connecticut Avenue, NW, #310, Washington, DC 20036.

To your health...

Eating a diet high in fat – especially saturated fatty acids – and cholesterol causes elevated blood cholesterol levels in many people. High blood cholesterol levels increase the risk of heart disease. Reducing fat is an especially good idea for those people who are limiting calories. Not only do fats provide more than twice the calories of proteins and carbohydrates, but they also contain few vitamins and minerals.

Moderation is the key

Eliminating *all* fats is not good for you either. For example, milk, meat, poultry, fish and eggs all contribute fat, saturated fat and cholesterol to your diet – but they also provide essential nutrients such as calcium, iron and zinc. So the key is moderation. Focus on a *balanced* overall diet and avoid too much fat where possible by using lower fat dairy products and lean meats and reducing the amount of fats added at the table.

How Does Your Diet Score?

Do the foods you eat provide more fat than is good for you? Answer the questions below, then see how your diet stacks up.

How often do you eat:

	seldom or never	1-2x per week	3-5x per week	almost daily
Fried, deep-fat fried or breaded foods?	☐	☐	☐	☐
Fatty meats such as bacon, sausage, luncheon meats and heavily marbled steaks and roasts?	☐	☐	☐	☐
Whole milk, high-fat cheeses and ice cream?	☐	☐	☐	☐
High-fat desserts such as pies, pastries and rich cakes?	☐	☐	☐	☐
Rich sauces and gravies?	☐	☐	☐	☐
Oily salad dressings or mayonnaise?	☐	☐	☐	☐
Whipped cream, table cream, sour cream and cream cheese?	☐	☐	☐	☐
Butter or margarine on vegetables, dinner rolls and toast?	☐	☐	☐	☐

Take a look at your answers. Several responses in the last two columns mean you may have a high fat intake. Perhaps it's time to cut back.

Cutting Back On Fat

Here are 15 tips to help you avoid too much fat, saturated fat and cholesterol in your diet:

1. Steam, boil or bake vegetables; or for a change, stirfry in a small amount of vegetable oil.

2. Season vegetables with herbs and spices rather than with sauces, butter or margarine.

3. Try lemon juice on salads or use limited amounts of oil-based salad dressing.

4. To reduce saturated fat, use margarine instead of butter in baked products and, when possible, use oil instead of shortening.

5. Try whole-grain flours to enhance flavors of baked goods made with less fat and cholesterol-containing ingredients.

6. Replace whole milk with skim or lowfat milk in puddings, soups and baked products.

7. Substitute plain lowfat yogurt, blender-whipped lowfat cottage cheese or buttermilk in recipes that call for sour cream or mayonnaise.

8. Choose lean cuts of meat.

9. Trim fat from meat before and/or after cooking.

10. Roast, bake, broil or simmer meat, poultry or fish.

11. Remove skin from poultry before cooking.

12. Cook meat or poultry on a rack so the fat will drain off. Use a non-stick pan for cooking so added fat will be unnecessary.

13. Chill meat or poultry broth until the fat becomes solid. Spoon off the fat before using the broth.

14. Limit egg yolks to one per serving when making scrambled eggs. Use additional egg whites for larger servings.

15. Try substituting egg whites in recipes calling for whole eggs. For example, use two egg whites in place of each whole egg in muffins, cookies and puddings.

Fats and Cholesterol – True or False?

And finally, here's a chance to test your general knowledge on the subject:

	True	False
1. Fruits, vegetables and most breads and cereals have little fat.	☐	☐
2. Fruits contain cholesterol.	☐	☐
3. Chicken without skin contains less fats than chicken with skin.	☐	☐
4. Cholesterol is found in both the lean and fat of meat.	☐	☐
5. Skim milk has almost no fat.	☐	☐
6. Cholesterol is found in both egg yolk and egg white.	☐	☐
7. Mozzarella cheese (part skim milk) has less fat than natural Cheddar cheese.	☐	☐
8. Chicken is a better choice than lean beef or pork to moderate dietary cholesterol.	☐	☐

Answers:
1-True. 2-False: Fruits, vegetables and grains contain no cholesterol. Cholesterol is found only in foods of animal origin. 3-True: Chicken without skin contains only half as much total fat as chicken with skin. 4.-True. 5-True. 6-False: Cholesterol is found only in egg yolk. 7-True. 8-False: In the same size serving, the cholesterol contents of lean beef or pork and chicken are about the same.

FAT FOR THE FIT

Not all fats clog the arteries. Here's how to recognize the right types for hearty appetites.

For years, health experts have urged Americans to eat less fat. So it came as a shock a few months ago when The New England Journal of Medicine published an editorial suggesting that Americans need not cut down on fat if only we'd get the fat from a different source.

Two Harvard researchers, Walter Willett, M.D., and Frank Sacks, M.D., recommended that we emulate the "Mediterranean diet." Greeks and Southern Italians, like Americans, derive 35 to 40 percent of their calories from fat. Unlike Americans, they have had very low rates of coronary heart disease.

The difference? Americans get much of their fat from meat and dairy products; Mediterranean people get most of theirs from olive oil.

This epidemiological information is not likely to change the standard recommendation that we should get no more than 30 percent of our total calories from fat; that recommendation is based not only on the known connection between dietary fat and coronary disease but on the connection between fat and obesity, diabetes, and possibly cancer. However, the researchers' proposal does dramatize an essential point: Not all fats are necessarily bad for the heart. We need to pay attention not only to how much fat we eat but to which fat.

The science of fat

The difference between fats that are hazardous to the heart and those that are relatively safe stems from a simple chemical distinction between them. Fats that have a hydrogen atom at every available site, like those in meat, dairy products, and tropical oils, are saturated fats—so called because they are "saturated" with hydrogen. Fats with one pair of hydrogen atoms missing, like the main fats in olive oil, are *mono*unsaturated. Fats with two or more pairs of hydrogen atoms missing are *poly*unsaturated fats, found in corn, soybean, and other vegetable oils.

Because changing even a single atom in a molecule can profoundly affect its chemical

properties, these fats may have strikingly different effects on health.

The clearest difference is that saturated fats, unlike unsaturated fats, increase the risk of coronary disease. Eating saturated fats raises blood levels of cholesterol, which accumulates in deposits in the arteries that can eventually restrict blood flow to the heart. Saturated fat in the diet has a far greater effect on blood levels of cholesterol than dietary cholesterol does.

Olive vs. corn

Unsaturated fats do not raise blood-cholesterol levels. In fact, several studies have indicated that both polyunsaturated and monounsaturated fats can actually re-

duce those cholesterol levels. Some evidence also suggests that monounsaturated fats have an advantage in that regard: Polyunsaturated fat tends to lower HDL cholesterol (the "good" cholesterol) along with LDL (the "bad" kind), while monounsaturated fat appears to cut LDL only. That difference, much ballyhooed by the olive-oil industry, is the main reason for recent advice that people should replace highly polyunsaturated oils with monounsaturated ones whenever possible.

Consumers Union's medical consultants believe that the evidence on HDL is too weak on its own to justify choosing one oil over another. But there may be a different

---

CHOOSING AND USING OILS

No vegetable oil is made purely from one kind of fat; all contain a mix of monounsaturated, polyunsaturated, and saturated fats. The label should tell you the number of grams of each kind of fat in a one tablespoon serving. All oils have the same number of calories: 9 per gram, or 120 per tablespoon.

If you want to start using a highly monounsaturated oil, olive oil is not your only choice. Canola oil is high in monounsaturates, too, and has a milder flavor than olive oil, so it's often a better choice for baking. Peanut oil, also mainly monounsaturated, can be heated to a somewhat higher temperature before it smokes, making it a good choice for stir-frying.

Here are some ways to cut down on your total fat intake by using less oil when you cook:

■ Steam, boil, poach, bake, microwave, or broil foods instead of sautéing them.

■ If you do sauté, grease a non-stick pan lightly with oil. Or try a vegetable-oil spray, which allows you to use less oil. You could also sauté foods in broth or wine instead of using oil.

■ Make your own salad dressings, using more vinegar than oil. Balsamic or red-wine

vinegar may be mild enough that you can skip the oil entirely. Or you could replace some of the oil with chicken broth.

Better than butter

While the hydrogenated oils in margarine make it worse for your arteries than unsaturated oils, it's still a healthier choice than butter. That's because only 10 to 30 percent of the fats in margarine are hydrogenated; 60 percent or more of the fats in butter are saturated. (Margarine and butter each get virtually all their calories—100 per tablespoon—from fat. That's fewer calories than oil provides, simply because they contain a bit of water.)

If you want to eat as little hydrogenated oil as possible, try a tub or squeeze margarine. Those types generally have more liquid oil—usually corn, safflower, or soybean oil—and less hydrogenated oil than stick margarine does. Check the label to be sure; liquid oil should be listed as the first ingredient. You might also consider one of the newer "light" margarines, which cut calories and total fat by replacing some of the oil with additional water. However, that makes them less suited for certain types of cooking, particularly pan frying.

---

reason—safety—for leaning toward mono-unsaturates.

Some animal studies have raised the possibility that a high intake of polyunsaturated fats may increase the risk of certain kinds of cancer. While most experts believe that polyunsaturates probably do not pose such a threat in humans. there's no way to test that belief directly, since no group of people in the world has a diet that's high in poly-unsaturated fats.

There is ample evidence, however, that *monounsaturated* fats are safe: Millions of Mediterranean people have long soaked their food in olive oil, which is mainly monounsaturated, without developing high levels of cancer. If you want to add some oil as you cut back on saturated fats—for example, to substitute for butter in cooking—your most prudent course might be to use a highly monounsaturated oil, such as olive oil, peanut oil, or canola oil.

Some people cook with margarine that contains hardened or partially hardened

BREAKING DOWN THE FATS

This chart gives you the key facts about the fat content of many common foods—the total amount as well as the breakdown into saturates, polyunsaturates, and monounsaturates. The most important information for your heart is the saturated-fat content. A quarter-cup of cashew nuts, for example, has more fat than a cup of ice cream. The ice cream has far more saturated fat, however, and is thus worse for your arteries. In fact, its 9 grams of saturated fat are about a third of the average daily limit—30 grams for men, 26 for women—that most experts recommend. Total fat is significant largely as a contributor to obesity. (A gram of fat contains 9 calories.)

Note that the figures for meat may understate how much fat meat-centered meals actually add to the diet. We used the modest 3-ounce serving size recommended by the National Academy of Sciences. Many Americans consume twice that much—two pieces of chicken, for example—in a meal.

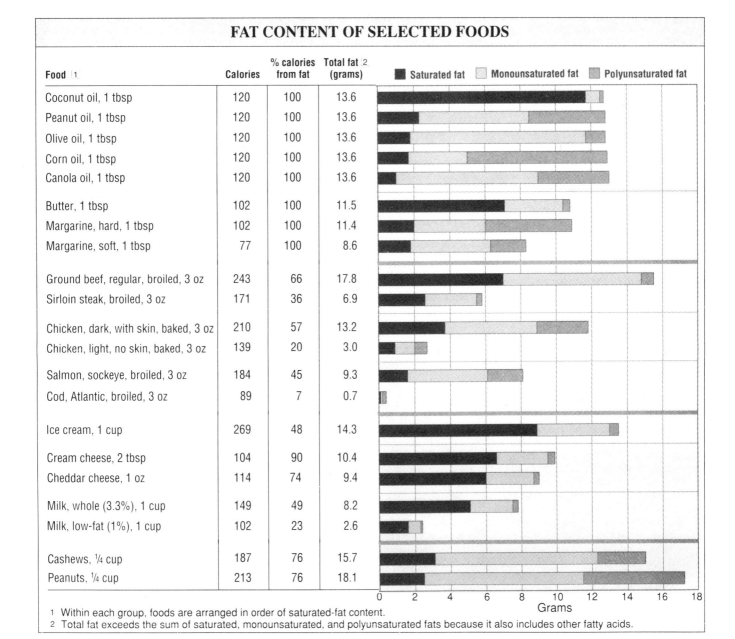

FAT CONTENT OF SELECTED FOODS

Food [1]	Calories	% calories from fat	Total fat [2] (grams)	■ Saturated fat □ Monounsaturated fat ▨ Polyunsaturated fat
Coconut oil, 1 tbsp	120	100	13.6	
Peanut oil, 1 tbsp	120	100	13.6	
Olive oil, 1 tbsp	120	100	13.6	
Corn oil, 1 tbsp	120	100	13.6	
Canola oil, 1 tbsp	120	100	13.6	
Butter, 1 tbsp	102	100	11.5	
Margarine, hard, 1 tbsp	102	100	11.4	
Margarine, soft, 1 tbsp	77	100	8.6	
Ground beef, regular, broiled, 3 oz	243	66	17.8	
Sirloin steak, broiled, 3 oz	171	36	6.9	
Chicken, dark, with skin, baked, 3 oz	210	57	13.2	
Chicken, light, no skin, baked, 3 oz	139	20	3.0	
Salmon, sockeye, broiled, 3 oz	184	45	9.3	
Cod, Atlantic, broiled, 3 oz	89	7	0.7	
Ice cream, 1 cup	269	48	14.3	
Cream cheese, 2 tbsp	104	90	10.4	
Cheddar cheese, 1 oz	114	74	9.4	
Milk, whole (3.3%), 1 cup	149	49	8.2	
Milk, low-fat (1%), 1 cup	102	23	2.6	
Cashews, ¼ cup	187	76	15.7	
Peanuts, ¼ cup	213	76	18.1	

0   2   4   6   8   10   12   14   16   18
Grams

1 Within each group, foods are arranged in order of saturated-fat content.
2 Total fat exceeds the sum of saturated, monounsaturated, and polyunsaturated fats because it also includes other fatty acids.

vegetable oils instead of cooking with butter or lard. But oils are hardened by hydrogenation, or adding hydrogen atoms, which makes unsaturated fats chemically closer to saturated fats.

A major international study known as the Seven Country Study—one of the first to draw the connection between saturated-fat intake and coronary disease—recently found that heavy consumption of hydrogenated oils is associated with higher blood-cholesterol levels and more deaths from coronary disease. A Dutch study also showed that feeding volunteers a diet very high in hydrogenated oils raised their levels of LDL cholesterol and lowered HDL—just as a diet high in saturated fats did. Always check labels for the words "hydrogenated" or "partially hydrogenated" oil.

Heart-healthy eating

Over the years, some researchers have suggested that just consuming more unsaturated oils, regardless of the rest of the diet, would help lower blood-cholesterol levels. But any such effect would be small at best—and would add needless calories. Boosting your intake of vegetable oils makes sense only if you're substituting those oils for saturated fats.

The average American now gets about 14 percent of calories from saturated fat, more than a third over the maximum of 10 percent recommended by most health experts, and double the 7 percent maximum recommended by some authorities.

Cutting down on saturated fat is the most important dietary step you can take to protect your heart. In a study published in March, Columbia University researchers put men on one of two diets that reduced their total intake of fat from the usual 37 percent of calories to 30 percent. One diet kept saturated-fat intake the same, while the other reduced it sharply. Blood-cholesterol levels fell only in the men on the diet that cut saturated fat.

To reduce your intake of saturates, you'll need to eat less meat and dairy foods (except for reduced-fat products, such as milk, cheese, and yogurt), and replace those foods with grains, fruits and vegetables, fish, and poultry. If you use butter often, substitute oil or margarine instead (see box, page 59).

Beware of so-called tropical oils—palm oil, palm kernel oil, and coconut oil—as substitutes. Although they're of vegetable origin, they're highly saturated. Some coffee creamers, in particular, contain nearly a gram and a half of saturated fat from coconut oil per tablespoon—an amount that could add up for someone who drinks several cups of coffee a day.

In addition to trimming the saturated fat from your diet, it's still important to watch your total fat intake. Several prominent nutrition experts have recently proposed that a limit of 25 percent of calories from fat would be an even better goal than the current 30-percent standard.

The sugar bugaboo

Marketers are cashing in on fears about sugar. But there's little to fear.

In May, *NutraSweet* ran TV commercials and took out ads in USA Today and The Wall Street Journal to announce a milestone: America's most popular artificial sweetener—now found in more than 4000 food products—had just reached its 10th anniversary. According to the manufacturer, *NutraSweet* owes its success not just to dieters' fear of calories but to the public's fear of sugar. The sweetener, the ads proclaim, is used by "active, health-conscious people who really care about what they eat."

Whether or not *NutraSweet* has really "made the world a better place to eat," as the company claims, it's certainly demonstrated America's appetite for sugar substitutes. Chemical companies, poised for the expiration of *NutraSweet's* patent, are preparing a flock of new noncaloric sweeteners. And health-food manufacturers are exploiting sugar fears to grab a toehold on mainstream grocery shelves with their fruit-juice-sweetened products—cereals, fruit bars, yogurts, and cookies. . . .

Fueling this national flight from sugar is the popular belief that it not only makes you fat but causes hyperactivity, hypoglycemia, diabetes, and a host of other health problems. Nearly all those beliefs—including even the notion that it's fattening—are wrong.

Sugar and fat

Actually, sugar's main drawback is that its calories are "empty"—that is, sugar contributes nothing but calories to the diet. A can of sugar-sweetened soda contains about 160 calories. If you drank three cans of soda a day and otherwise maintained your usual diet and exercise habits, you could gain about a pound a week.

But sugar is not the main caloric culprit in such sweets as candy bars, cookies, and ice cream. The fat in such items contributes far more calories than sugar does. A plain donut, for example, gets

---

A natural tranquilizer?

Researchers Judith J. Wurtman, Ph.D., and Richard J. Wurtman, M.D., at the Massachusetts Institute of Technology believe that many people crave sugar more for its soothing effect than its sweet taste. Their research suggests that sugar and other carbohydrates cause the brain to absorb more of the amino acid tryptophan, which is then converted into serotonin. That chemical seems to promote calmness, sleepiness, and a sense of well-being.

"When certain people feel hostile or anxious," Richard Wurtman told CRHL, "they'll use carbohydrates like a drug." Sugar is the carbohydrate of choice, he says, because users associate its distinctive taste with the change in mood. Sweets are also less likely to be eaten with protein, which blocks the effect of carbohydrates on brain chemicals.

The University of Michigan's Adam Drewnowski, Ph.D., agrees that some sweet foods may promote those mood changes. But he contends that the combination of sugar and fat in those foods is just as likely to be responsible. Drewnowski suggests that the combination could produce a calming effect by promoting the release of opium-like endorphins in the brain.

Other preliminary research supports the pacifying effects of both sugar and fat. In rat studies conducted by Cornell University's Elliott M. Blass, Ph.D., both substances reduced signs of pain. That effect disappeared when an endorphin blocker was used, suggesting that sugar and fat may both work through the endorphin system.

---

52 of its 105 total calories from fat but only 17 from sugar. Even a chocolate bar gets more calories from fat (126) than from sugar (90).

University of Michigan nutrition researcher Adam Drewnowski, Ph.D., believes that many overweight people actually suffer not so much from a "sweet tooth" as from a "fat tooth" (see box). In studies using special confections containing varying proportions of fat and sugar, Drewnowski has found that heavier people tend to favor foods with the highest fat content. Similarly, epidemiological studies suggest that overweight people eat more fat than thin people—and that they actually eat less sugar as well.

Does it make kids hyperactive?

To test the hyperactivity theory, several researchers have studied children whose parents are convinced it's true. In these studies, the children are observed after downing a high-sugar drink and, on another occasion, an artificially sweetened drink. Neither the children, their parents, nor the observers know which drink is which until after the experiments. In one such study of 50 hyperactive children, Chicago Medical School researcher Mortimer D. Gross, M.D., found no difference in activity after serving lemonade sweetened with sugar and lemonade sweetened with saccharin. Other studies similarly have found no evidence of "sugar hyperactivity."

Some accused criminals have invoked the so-called *Twinkie* defense, claiming that sugary junk food caused their violent behavior. And some prison administrators have gone so far as to cut sugar in prison diets. But the idea that sugar causes violence is based on anecdotal evidence and a few poorly designed studies. Other studies dispute that link.

Does it spark hypoglycemia?

Because blood-sugar levels can fluctuate after you eat sugar, some people believe that sugar can trigger symptoms of hypoglycemia, or low blood sugar. The fluctuations can occur when the pancreas secretes the hormone insulin in response to a hefty dose of sugar. Ordinarily, insulin prevents blood sugar from rising too high. In a few people, that insulin release can cause blood sugar to fall below normal levels.

But such drops in blood sugar almost never cause symptoms. The rare exceptions are people with a condition called reactive hypoglycemia, who can experience such symptoms as sweating, trembling, rapid heartbeat, and hunger. Many other people mistakenly blame hypoglycemia when they experience such symptoms, but there's almost always some other cause. If you think you have hypoglycemia, your physician can help you determine if your symptoms coincide with a drop in blood-sugar level.

Hypoglycemia is more common among people with diabetes. But in those people, hypoglycemia has nothing to do with eating too much sugar. Instead, it happens only when they eat too little food, inject too much insulin, or exercise too much.

Does it cause diabetes?

Diabetes is characterized by high blood-sugar levels, so people with the disease should monitor their sugar intake as well as the rest of their diet. That may explain the popular belief that sugar causes diabetes. But sugar is not to blame.

> ## The only real risk from sugar for most people is tooth decay.

Suspicions have focused on type II diabetes, the most common form of the disease, which is usually discovered after age 40. Actually, type II diabetes is caused by genetic factors, too little insulin, or resistance to insulin. Obesity is also a risk factor.

The other form of diabetes, type I, which usually strikes before age 20, is caused by an immune-system disorder. Like type II, it has nothing to do with consuming sugar.

One charge that has teeth

The only real risk from sugar for most people is tooth decay. But fluoride, plastic sealants for children's teeth, and improved oral hygiene have dramatically reduced the incidence of cavities. So avoiding sugar is not as important as it once was. Still, some precautions are in order.

The acid that causes tooth decay comes from the breakdown of sugars and other carbohydrates by bacteria in your mouth. You can minimize the risk by limiting sweets to mealtime. That way, the bacteria churn out their acid only a few times a day. And eating a meal increases production of saliva, which may wash sugars away from your teeth and help neutralize the acids. Certain foods such as aged hard cheese and peanuts may also counter the effects of the acids.

Sweets that cling to the tooth surface—including baked goods, caramels, syrups, and even dried fruits—are the most damaging. Soft drinks can be harmful, too, since they bathe the teeth in sugar, unless you use a straw. Safe snacks include seeds, nuts, peanut butter (without sugar), cheese, plain yogurt, raw vegetables, and popcorn.

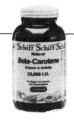

THE SUPPLEMENT STORY
CAN VITAMINS HELP?

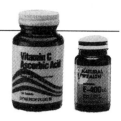

For a long time, the only voices endorsing nutritional supplements belonged to the people who sold them. In the opposite camp stood the guardians of the nation's well-being, including the Surgeon General, the National Research Council, and the U.S. Department of Health and Human Services (HHS). Their position remains that a balanced diet provides all the nutrients needed for good health.

In recent years, however, some scientists have jumped ship. They point to mounting evidence that certain vitamins and other nutrients may offer protection against cancer, cataracts, Parkinson's disease, and other disorders. They speculate that extra doses of those nutrients may slow the aging process. And, while few go so far as to make public recommendations, they freely admit that popping pills has become part of their own daily routine.

The pills they take are antioxi-dants—for the most part, vitamin C, vitamin E, and beta-carotene, a substance partially converted to vitamin A in the body. (Vitamin A itself does not have antioxidant activity.) Antioxidants are thought to be protective largely because they can inactivate free radicals, destructive molecules that can damage cells.

Those who take antioxidants to slow the aging process admit they're on somewhat shaky ground. "It's banking on an aging mechanism that hasn't been proven," says biologist David Harrison of The Jackson Laboratory in Bar Harbor, Maine. Nonetheless, like several scientists we contacted, he takes a supplement regimen that includes vitamins C and E, beta-carotene, and a multiple-vitamin tablet. "I'm not sure it does any good, but I'm certainly not sure that it doesn't."

The case for antioxidants as an anti-aging remedy is still speculative. Attempts to use them to extend lifespan in animals have been largely unsuccessful. But several converging lines of evidence suggest antioxidants may help stave off diseases of aging.

Free-radical damage has been implicated by some studies in diseases such as cancer, rheumatoid arthritis, cataracts, and cardiovascular disease. High levels of antioxidants—measured both in the diet and in the blood—have been associated with lower rates of these illnesses. "Whether we look at animal or cell culture studies, at population comparisons or intervention trials, we see the same relationship between antioxidants and protection from disease," says Dr. Jeffrey Blumberg, associate director of the U.S. Department of Agriculture Human Nutrition Research Center on Aging at Tufts University.

Moreover, he notes, it appears that the higher the antioxidant level, the lower the risk of disease, and vice-versa. In some studies of diet and cancer, for instance, people with the lowest intake of beta-carotene had up to seven times the lung-cancer risk of those with the highest intake. In other reports, people with the diets richest in vitamin C were at the lowest risk for cancer of the stomach, oral cavity, and esophagus. And in a large study of 16 European populations, there was a strong correlation between high blood levels of vitamin E and a lower risk of death from coronary disease.

The next step is to give volunteers antioxidants in experimental programs and see whether their rates of disease are lower than average. Many such trials, including a dozen sponsored by the National Cancer Institute, are now attempting to provide that link.

The Physicians Health Study, a major ongoing project administered by Harvard Medical School,

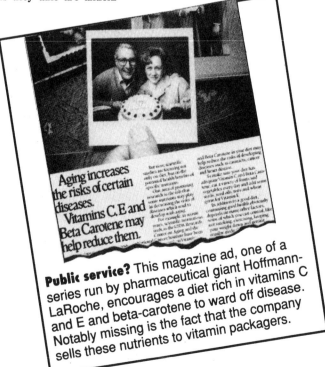

Public service? This magazine ad, one of a series run by pharmaceutical giant Hoffmann-LaRoche, encourages a diet rich in vitamins C and E and beta-carotene to ward off disease. Notably missing is the fact that the company sells these nutrients to vitamin packagers.

recently turned up an unexpected, hopeful finding about beta-carotene and heart disease—a finding the researchers stumbled on while testing beta-carotene as a cancer preventive. The investigators gave beta-carotene to half of the 22,000 physicians in the study. After six years, the researchers found that in a subgroup of 333 men who had signs of coronary disease before entering the study, those receiving beta-carotene experienced half as many cardiovascular "events" such as heart attack and stroke. It's premature to conclude that beta-carotene protects the heart, but the study offers a tantalizing lead for further testing.

In another promising intervention study, at Tufts University, healthy elderly individuals given vitamin E supplements showed significant improvements in immune function, which typically declines with age.

How much is enough?

Even at this early stage, the evidence raises important questions about how much of those nutrients we need and the best way to get them. Traditionally, vitamins have been recommended in amounts sufficient to prevent deficiency diseases such as scurvy and rickets. Those levels, determined by a National Academy of Sciences committee, are the Recommended Dietary Allowances (RDAs).

While the RDAs vary by age and sex, the U.S. RDA—the number used on most food and supplement labels—gives the level that should be enough to prevent deficiency in most healthy people. The U.S. RDA for vitamin C is 60 milligrams; for vitamin E, 30 I.U. (international units). While there is no U.S. RDA for beta-carotene, the U.S. RDA for vitamin A is 5000 I.U.—which can also be provided by about six milligrams of beta-carotene.

Current work on antioxidants suggests to some researchers that doses higher than the RDAs may be best for disease prevention. Most clinicians advise that we get those extra nutrients from our diets, because most studies have examined antioxidants in foods rather

than supplements. "We know that vegetables high in beta-carotene are protective, but we don't know if the benefit is from the beta-carotene or some other component," explains Dr. Judith Hallfrish, research leader of the carbohydrate nutrition lab at the U.S. Department of Agriculture.

Loading up on fruits and vegetables is certainly good advice. Yellow and green leafy vegetables, such as carrots, sweet potatoes, squash, cantaloupe, spinach, and broccoli, are rich in beta-carotene; green leafy ones are also high in vitamin E. Good sources of vitamin C include citrus fruits and juices, strawberries, broccoli, brussels sprouts, and sweet red peppers.

The Dietary Guidelines for Americans, a joint effort of the Department of Agriculture and Health and Human Services, recommends at least three daily servings of vegetables and two of fruit. By one estimate, those intakes can provide as much as two to four times the U.S. RDAs for vitamins E and C, plus five or six milligrams of beta-carotene. However, some researchers believe even those levels are too low to afford optimal protection from disease.

Moreover, for most Americans, obtaining those nutrients from food alone would entail a profound dietary change. In one large national food-consumption survey, only 9 percent of participants met the fruit and vegetable guidelines cited above. Other surveys indicate a substantial gap between the typical daily intake of antioxidants and the levels Dr. Blumberg estimates may be optimal for disease prevention, based on the scientific literature. The average intake of beta-carotene is approximately two milligrams, well below the 25-mg level that he believes may be protective and that other researchers are using in clinical trials. The average intake of vitamin C, about 100 mg, is also well below the 500 mg Blumberg says may be optimal.

It's virtually impossible to get what appears to be an optimal dose of vitamin E—between 100 I.U. and 400 I.U. daily—by diet alone. In some population studies, notes Dr.

Blumberg, individuals with the lowest risk of disease had blood levels of vitamin E high enough to suggest they were taking supplements.

"It may be true you can get the RDAs if you improve your diet," says Dr. William Pryor, a biochemist at Louisiana State University, Baton Rouge, and a prominent free-radical researcher. "But if you believe pharmacologic levels of vitamins can protect against disease, you're talking about supplements."

What to do?

A growing number of researchers now believe that, in addition to loading your diet with fruits and vegetables, taking antioxidant pills may be a reasonable move. Even the relatively high doses used by these scientists appear to be safe; the levels of vitamin C, vitamin E, and beta-carotene they consider optimal have not been associated with adverse effects. (In contrast, higher doses of vitamin C—more than 1000 milligrams a day—may cause diarrhea and other problems. And high doses of some other vitamins, notably vitamin A and vitamin D, have been shown to cause harm.)

As for price, an RDA-level multivitamin and mineral supplement, plus additional doses of vitamins E and C and beta-carotene, totals about a quarter a day.

Nevertheless, CU's medical consultants are not yet ready to recommend supplements for the general population. No one has yet proven the theory that antioxidants slow aging and fight disease by protecting the body from free radicals, although evidence is accumulating. Very few studies so far have examined the effects of supplement intake directly, and prospective clinical trials are still essential.

In addition, there's the nagging fact that the vitamin industry remains completely unregulated: No Government safeguard guarantees that the doses in pills match what's promised on the label. Researchers have found many vitamin supplements contain lower doses than the label claims.

WHAT CAN E DO FOR YOU?

Over the past year, several studies looking at a variety of different ailments have all reached the same conclusion: Vitamin E appears to offer protection against disease. Most notably, two studies involving more than 130,000 people reported that vitamin E helps prevent coronary heart disease. A third new study found that the vitamin cuts the risk of certain cancers. Meanwhile, other recent research has hinted at a beneficial effect on everything from cataracts to immune function.

Many researchers believe that it takes lots of vitamin E to provide that protection. Unfortunately, you can't get a lot of the vitamin from food alone. That's why some of those researchers are already taking vitamin-E supplements. Should you do the same?

Beyond deficiency

Your body needs vitamin E to maintain the integrity of its cell membranes. But that doesn't take much: Only some premature infants and a few people whose bodies have difficulty absorbing vitamin E run low enough to develop cellular defects. For that reason, the National Academy of Sciences has set its Recommended Dietary Allowance (RDA) at just 8 mg for women and 10 mg for men. That's about what the typical American consumes.

But preventing outright deficiency may not be enough. The recent flurry of studies on vitamin E suggests that higher doses—at least several times higher than the RDA—might provide much more than basic cell maintenance.

That's because vitamin E is a powerful antioxidant, a compound that protects cells against molecules called free radicals. Lacking part of their molecular structure, free radicals try to snatch that part from other molecules, a process known as oxidation. That damages the cells and is believed to be a first step in the development of coronary disease and cancer, as well as many other diseases.

Protecting the heart

Researchers believe that vitamin E could help prevent coronary disease by exerting a positive influence on low-density lipoprotein, or LDL, cholesterol, the ordinarily "bad" kind. Apparently, LDL promotes clogged arteries only when it's oxidized by free radicals. And since vitamin E travels through the bloodstream attached to LDL molecules, it has ample opportunity to shield them from oxidation.

In one recent study, volunteers who took supplements to load their bloodstream with high levels of vitamin E did indeed have fewer oxidized LDL molecules circulating through their arteries than people with lower blood levels of the vitamin. So, in theory at least, higher vitamin-E blood levels should reduce the risk of developing coronary disease.

Just last month, Finnish researchers supported that theory with the results from a year-long study of some 200 men with elevated LDL levels. Using special sound-wave tests to measure fatty deposits in major arteries, they documented slower progression of coronary disease among those with the most vitamin E in their blood.

Further evidence that vitamin E can protect the heart came last November at an American Heart Association conference, where Harvard researchers presented the latest findings from their ongoing studies of 87,000 female nurses and 46,000 male health professionals. When the studies began, the researchers collected information on the subjects' typical intake of vitamin E from both diet and supplements. The researchers then compared that initial

E FOR EVERYTHING?

As a powerful antioxidant, vitamin E has the potential to help prevent or treat not only coronary heart disease and cancer, but also many other health problems caused by the cellular reaction called oxidation. Here's a look at some possibilities:

■ **Arthritis.** A few small studies have tested daily doses of up to 1200 mg of vitamin E among patients with osteoarthritis or rheumatoid arthritis. In general, the vitamin relieved pain, swelling, and morning stiffness nearly as effectively as a commonly prescribed anti-inflammatory drug. Those findings now need to be tested in larger, longer trials.

■ **Cataracts.** Several recent population studies have suggested that people who consume the most vitamin E have the lowest risk of cataracts, which cloud the lens of the eye and can cause blindness. In December, for example, a large Finnish study found that people with the most vitamin E in their blood had only half as much risk of cataracts requiring surgery as those with the lowest blood levels. Researchers are currently testing that observation in trials of vitamin-E supplements.

■ **Immune function.** Population studies suggest that people with the highest blood levels of vitamin E are less likely to acquire several common infectious diseases. And one experiment found that giving large doses of vitamin E to healthy older people can strengthen certain measures of immunity. However, no trial has yet directly tested whether such improved immunity actually confers better health. (For more on antioxidants and immunity, see CRH, 11/92.)

■ **Muscle protection.** Tufts University researchers have found that vitamin-E supplements may protect overworked muscles during exercise. In a pair of studies, sedentary men took either a placebo or 530 mg of vitamin E every day for seven weeks. They then performed a vigorous 45-minute treadmill workout. After the workout, blood samples from the men who took vitamin E contained lower amounts of chemicals that promote inflammation. That effect, the researchers speculate, should limit both soreness and injury after strenuous exercise.

■ **Parkinson's disease.** A few laboratory and population studies have suggested that large doses of vitamin E could delay or even halt the loss of brain cells in patients with Parkinson's disease. However, a recent randomized trial involving 800 patients found that daily doses as high as 1300 mg taken for nearly five years failed to slow the progression of the disease. Still, some researchers speculate that the vitamin might slow the disease in its earlier stages.

■ **Skin protection.** Preliminary research has hinted that certain forms of vitamin E applied to the skin might help protect against skin cancer caused by sun exposure. However, it's unclear whether the types or amounts of the vitamin sometimes included in lotions and sunscreens would be at all effective.

vitamin-E intake with the chance of subsequently developing coronary disease.

Over eight years, the nurses who took daily supplements containing at least 65 mg of vitamin E (the lowest dose available in a single-nutrient supplement) had about one-third less risk of heart attack or death from coronary disease than those who didn't take supplements. And over four years, the male health professionals who took daily vitamin-E supplements

had about one-quarter less risk of heart attack or advanced coronary disease. Both studies also found some evidence that getting 25 mg or more of vitamin E from foods each day might have a protective effect as well.

While those recent studies are all promising, the results from earlier research have been mixed: Two investigations found a correlation between blood levels of vitamin E and low risk of coronary disease, but at least half a dozen others failed to find a similar trend.

In a recent review of the evidence to date, Harvard researchers concluded that the notion that vitamin E protects against coronary disease is "promising but clearly unproven." A more definitive answer should form over the next few years as results become available from several ongoing or planned prevention trials including vitamin-E supplements.

Preventing cancer

In addition to possibly helping prevent cancer by keeping cells from becoming oxidized and turning cancerous, vitamin E might fight the disease indirectly by boosting the immune system. Whatever the explanation, animal trials have found that vitamin E can sometimes halt the development of tumors.

The possibility that vitamin E might help fight cancer has been studied more extensively in humans than the link with coronary disease. And a few studies have yielded strong positive findings.

Last year, for example, National Cancer Institute researchers reported that people who had taken vitamin-E supplements for at least six months were half as likely to develop cancers of the mouth and throat. (The researchers didn't ask about key dietary sources of vitamin E, so they were unable to determine whether or not diet alone might also have had a protective effect.)

In 1991, a Finnish study of some 36,000 people also found an apparent anti-cancer effect. Over an eight-year period, the subjects with the lowest blood levels of vitamin E were 50 percent more likely to develop any sort of cancer than were those with the highest levels.

Other human studies have also found that vitamin E may help prevent cancer, but the protective effect has generally been weaker. According to one comprehensive review, the evidence to date suggests that people who consume the most vitamin E may have a slightly lower risk of cancers of the colon, rectum, esophagus, and lung. The vitamin's cancer-fighting potential should become clearer over the next few years as results become available from several ongoing trials.

Supplemental insurance?

Coronary disease and cancer are the two leading killers in the U.S. So anything that might help prevent them deserves serious consideration. The possibility that vitamin E may have several other health

2. NUTRIENTS

benefits as well only adds to its appeal (see box, previous page).

It certainly makes sense to include as much vitamin E in your diet as you can. That's trickier than with other antioxidants, such as vitamin C or beta-carotene, since the foods that contain the most vitamin E are concentrated plant fats like vegetable and seed oils, as well as vegetable-oil products such as margarine and salad dressing. But with wise choices from among the foods in our table, most people can get much more vitamin E and still keep their fat intake low.

Indeed, one recent analysis found that a typical low-fat, high-produce diet provides a daily intake of about 25 mg of vitamin E—roughly three times the RDA. Some of the studies that found a beneficial effect from the vitamin suggest that such a relatively modest intake alone could be enough to deliver the benefit. By adding a daily bowl of fortified cereal, you could more than double that level.

However, some of the most encouraging studies performed to date have looked at higher levels of vitamin E than can be had through diet alone. That's why some researchers and physicians are already hedging their bets by taking supplements.

"I wouldn't argue with anyone who wants to wait for firm evidence before taking vitamin-E supplements," Harvard researcher Walter Willett, M.D., told CRH. "But I also think it's perfectly rational to take supplements now because there's a good chance they will help and there seems to be no danger."

Indeed, taking vitamin-E supplements does appear to be safe. The largest and longest experimental trial to date, lasting nearly five years and involving some 800 subjects, found no adverse effects from a daily dose of more than 1300 mg of vitamin E—well over 100 times the RDA. While it's still theoretically possible that problems could eventually crop up over many decades of daily supplements, most researchers think that's unlikely.

If you do decide to take a vitamin-E supplement, stay within a modest range. A typical low-level multivitamin provides 30 mg of vitamin E, along with moderate amounts of various other vitamins and minerals. (On some product labels, that 30-mg dosage may also be listed as 45 IU, or International Units.) If you choose a single-nutrient vitamin-E supplement, stick with a relatively low dosage of 65 to 260 mg (100 to 400 IU).

But don't use vitamin-E supplements as an excuse to neglect a healthy diet. Other nutrients in such a diet—particularly vitamin C and beta-carotene—appear to have a protective effect of their own. Those nutrients may also enhance the effect of vitamin E. And there are likely to be other, still unidentified substances in foods that could be equally important. In fact, more than any single nutrient, whole foods—especially fruits and vegetables—have consistently shown the most potential for reducing the risk of coronary disease and cancer.

VITAMIN-E CONTENT OF SELECTED FOODS

Food	Serving size	Vitamin E (mg)	Vitamin E (IU) [1]
FORTIFIED CEREALS			
Just Right	1 oz	30	45
Total Corn Flakes	1 oz	30	45
Most	1 oz	30	45
Product 19	1 oz	30	45
Total Wheat	1 oz	30	45
Crispy Wheat 'N Raisins	1 oz	8	11
Nutri Grain Corn	1 oz	7	11
Nutri Grain Wheat	1 oz	7	11
NUTS AND SEEDS			
Sunflower seeds	¼ cup	16	24
Filberts	¼ cup	8	12
Wheat germ, toasted	¼ cup	7	11
Peanuts	¼ cup	3	4
Peanut butter	2 tbsp	3	4
Almonds	¼ cup	2	3
OILS, SPREADS, AND DRESSINGS			
Wheat germ oil	1 tbsp	26	39
Sunflower oil	1 tbsp	7	10
Safflower oil	1 tbsp	5	7
Mayonnaise, regular	1 tbsp	4	6
Margarine spread, light	1 tbsp	3	5
Corn oil	1 tbsp	3	4
Cod liver oil	1 tbsp	3	4
Vegetable shortening	1 tbsp	2	3
Canola oil	1 tbsp	2	3
Margarine spread, regular	1 tbsp	2	3
Olive oil	1 tbsp	2	2
French salad dressing	1 tbsp	1	2
Italian salad dressing	1 tbsp	1	2
Mayonnaise, low-fat	1 tbsp	1	1
PRODUCE [2]			
Sweet potato, baked	1 medium	5	8
Avocado	1 medium	3	4
Dandelion greens	1 cup	1	2
Dandelion greens, boiled	½ cup	1	2
Cabbage, boiled	½ cup	1	2
Turnip greens	1 cup	1	2
Turnip greens, boiled	½ cup	1	2
Cabbage	1 cup	1	2
Tomato paste	¼ cup	1	2
Spinach	1 cup	1	2
Olives, black or green	10 large	1	2
POULTRY AND SEAFOOD			
Abalone, steamed/poached	3 oz	7	10
Escargot	6	3	4
Turkey liver, braised	3 oz	2	4
Atlantic salmon, baked/broiled	3 oz	2	2
Chicken liver, braised	3 oz	1	2

[1] Vitamin-E content is sometimes listed in International Units. (1 milligram of vitamin E equals approximately 1.5 IU.)
[2] Raw unless otherwise specified.

Source: ESHA Research, Salem, Ore.

CAN MEGADOSES OF VITAMIN C HELP AGAINST COLDS?

Charles W. Marshall, Ph.D.

Dr. Marshall, a retired biochemist, is author of Vitamins and Minerals: Help or Harm?, *which won the American Medical Writers Association award for the best book of 1983 for the general public. The book can be obtained for $14 postpaid from LVACHF, Inc., P.O. Box 1747, Allentown, PA 18105.*

Few things have stirred the imagination and hopes of the public in matters of nutrition or vexed nutrition scientists as much as Linus Pauling's 1970 book, *Vitamin C and the Common Cold.* The book's main claim is that taking 1 gram (1,000 mg) of vitamin C daily will reduce the incidence of colds by 45% for most people, but that some persons might need much larger amounts. It recommends that if symptoms of a cold do start, you should take 500 or 1,000 mg every hour for several hours—or 4 to 10 grams daily if symptoms don't disappear with smaller amounts. Without question, publication of this book, combined with Pauling's reputation as a Nobel Prize–winning scientist, has made vitamin C a best seller. When his theory was announced, millions of Americans rushed to try it for themselves. The second edition of the book, issued in 1976 as *Vitamin C, the Common Cold and the Flu,* suggests even higher dosages.

Pauling has also suggested that most people need a daily vitamin C intake of 2,300 mg or more for "optimum" health and to meet stresses, including infections. In *How to Live Longer and Feel Better* (1986) he states that individual biochemical variability is so great that optimum intake may be as high as 250 mg to 20 grams or more per day.

Many concerned persons have wondered whether Pauling's advice is prudent, and millions have experimented upon themselves to see if they can tell. Pauling himself reportedly takes 12,000 mg daily and raises it to 40,000 mg when symptoms of a cold appear! Pauling presumably has adapted to such dosage, but most people would suffer chronic diarrhea and the risk of kidney stones.

HOW SCIENTIFIC FACTS ARE DETERMINED

The "scientific community" consists of thousands of scientists throughout the world, most of whom operate under a strict set of rules known as the scientific method. Simply stated, this is a system of logical steps designed to separate cause-and-effect from coincidence. This method is used to answer such questions as: "If you do a particular thing, will something else take place?" and "If two things follow one another, are they related?"

A scientific "fact" is determined by analyzing the results of all the experiments that bear on that particular fact. In the case of vitamin C, there are two key questions. First, does vitamin C prevent colds? And second, does it reduce their severity? Before discussing experiments on these questions, however, we should note that not all experiments are created equal. *To be valid, an experiment must be well designed, and its data must be honestly collected and interpreted with good techniques of statistical analysis.* One hallmark of a good experiment is that others can repeat it and get the same results.

Experimental studies of the possible value of vitamin C in the prevention of infections have been conducted by medical investigators ever since preparations of the pure crystalline vitamin became commercially available during the 1930s. By 1982, about thirty of these were reported and the majority of medical scientists had concluded that supplementation with vitamin C does not prevent colds and, at best, may slightly reduce the symptoms of a cold. Two subsequent reports have not altered these conclusions.

Linus Pauling remains steadfast in his belief that the scientific community is wrong—basing his ideas on the same experiments but interpreting their results differently. Moreover, he suggests the following way to determine one's correct vitamin C dosage: "If you are taking 1 gram per day, and find that you have developed two or three colds during the winter season, it would be wise to try taking a larger daily quantity." Presumably, if you have fewer colds than expected, you should believe that vitamin C has been responsible for the decrease.

Unfortunately, in the real world, scientific facts cannot be determined that simply. Consider the following questions:

1. Is it possible that you actually had a different number of colds than you recall? This would be faulty data collection.

From *Nutrition Forum,* September/October 1992, pp. 33-36. Reprinted with permission of Stephen Barrett, M.D., Publishers, P.O. Box 1747, Allentown, PA 18105.

2. Is it possible that you would have had only one cold this year anyway? If so, what happened to you would be a mere coincidence.

3. Is it possible that you had a very mild cold but wish so strongly for a favorable result that you didn't count it? If so, this would be an effect of bias.

Scientific experiments must be designed to overcome these possible sources of error. The problem of faulty memory can be overcome by keeping close track of the individuals involved in an experiment. The problem of coincidence can be overcome by using large numbers of people and following them for significant lengths of time. The problem of bias, however, is far more complicated. Use of the double-blind method is critical, but as you will see, experiments with vitamin C have encountered some very curious results when subjects were able to figure out whether they were getting the vitamin or the placebo during experiments intended to be double-blind.

So far, at least 30 experiments have tested the ability of vitamin C to protect against colds in large groups of people. Five review articles by biomedical scientists have found Pauling's claims unsupported, except for slight reduction in severity, in most of those trials that were scientifically properly designed and executed. Now let's examine the evidence.

INOCULATION TRIALS

One way to test whether high-dosage vitamin C prevents colds is to inoculate the throats of volunteers with cold viruses. Two studies of this type found that everyone got colds whether they took vitamin C or not. Dr. Walker and co-workers in 1967 and Drs. Schwartz, Hornick and associates in 1972–73 gave half of their volunteers a placebo and the rest 3,000 mg of vitamin C daily for several days before inserting live cold viruses directly into their noses; and then continued 3,000 mg of vitamin C (or placebo) for seven more days. All of the volunteers got colds, which were of equal severity.

PRETREATMENT WITH VITAMIN C TRIALS

Another way to test vitamin C is to see what happens to matched groups over a period of time. Two teams of investigators have done this more than once, one team led by Dr. John L. Coulehan and the other by Dr. Terence Anderson.

Dr. Coulehan's first study was done on 641 Navajo Indian children, half of whom received a placebo while the rest received 1,000 mg of vitamin C daily. A complicated system of judging the severity of head, throat and chest symptoms was used. The Coulehan team reported in 1974 that the vitamin C group had less severe colds, but other scientists who reviewed the study criticized the method of judging the severity of symptoms.

So in 1976 the Coulehan team repeated their study with 868 Navajo children but used a better system of scoring severity. The children receiving vitamin C averaged 0.38 colds per person while the placebo group averaged 0.37. The average duration of the colds was 5.5 days in the vitamin group and 5.8 in the placebo group. Thus, in this test, vitamin C neither prevented colds nor shortened their duration. In 1979, Dr. Coulehan published his analysis of vitamin C versus the common cold and concluded that extra vitamin C is not worth taking.

THE ANDERSON TRIALS

In 1972, Dr. Terence Anderson and colleagues at the University of Toronto published the results of a 3-month double-blind study of 818 volunteers aged 10 to 65. Half received 1,000 mg of vitamin C daily before colds and 4,000 mg per day during the first 3 days of a cold, while the other half received "equivalent" placebos. This study was designed to test Pauling's claims that ingestion of 1,000 mg of vitamin C daily would reduce the frequency of colds by 45% and the total days of illness by 60%. These claims were certainly not supported by the study's outcome. In the vitamin group, 74% had one or more colds during the study period, while 82% of the placebo group had one or more colds. The difference, which amounted to "one-tenth of a cold per person," was judged by Dr. Anderson to be "of no practical importance." The severity, as measured by days confined indoors, averaged 1.36 days for the vitamin group and 1.87 days for the placebo group—a 30% difference that Anderson decided to explore further. At the end of this trial, before the double-blind code was opened, all volunteers were asked whether they had experienced any unusual feelings of well-being [euphoria] during the trial. Nineteen percent of both groups said yes—an interesting example of the placebo effect.

In 1974, the Anderson team reported on a larger trial to see what results would be obtained with different amounts of vitamin C. Some 3,500 volunteers were divided into eight groups, six of which received various daily dosages of vitamin C while the others received placebos for three months. No difference in the incidence of colds was found among the groups taking no vitamin C, 250 mg, 1,000 mg or 2,000 mg daily. A possible slight reduction in severity of symptoms was found in the vitamin C groups, but volunteers taking dosages of 4,000 or 8,000 per day when a cold began did no better than those taking only 250 mg per day.

The third Anderson trial, reported in 1975, covered 16 weeks and used 488 volunteers (ages 14 to 67), with one-third receiving a pill of vitamin C as its sodium and calcium salts, and one-third given vitamin C in slow-release capsules, and one-third getting a placebo. The vitamin C dosage was 500 mg once a week (equivalent to about 70 mg daily) before colds, but 1,500 mg the first day of a cold followed by 1,000 mg on the second and third days. No reduction in the incidence of colds was observed, but those taking vitamin C averaged less time at home (1.62 vs. 1.12 days indoors). Do you think that a half-day's less confinement is of practical significance?

Taken together, the Anderson studies suggest that extra vitamin C may slightly reduce the severity of colds, but that it is not necessary to take the high dosages suggested by Pauling to achieve this result. Nor is there anything to be gained by taking vitamin supplements year-round in the hope of preventing colds.

OTHER STUDIES

In 1975, Carson and co-workers told of treating company employees with 1,000 mg of vitamin C or a placebo daily during colds. The number of colds per person, the duration of colds and their severity were the same in both vitamin and placebo groups.

In 1975, Karlowski and associates at the National Institutes of Health reported treating volunteers as follows: 25% received placebos; 25% took 3,000 mg of vitamin C daily before colds but placebos during colds; 25% were given placebos daily before colds and 3,000 mg of vitamin C daily during colds; and 25% got 3,000 mg daily before colds and 6,000 mg daily during colds.

The experiment was supposed to be double-blind, but the doctors had failed to make the placebo taste the same as the vitamin C pills as is done in most trials. As a result, half of the volunteers correctly guessed which pill they were getting and therefore became unblinded. When the results were tabulated with all volunteers lumped together, the average number of colds per person was 1.27 colds for the vitamin group and 1.41 for the placebo group. But among those who remained blinded, no differences in the incidence or severity were found. This fascinating result shows how many people who think they are taking a positive step (such as taking a vitamin) may report a favorable result even when none really exists!

TWO TRIALS WITH IDENTICAL TWINS

In 1977, Miller and colleagues treated 44 pairs of identical twins for 5 months as follows. One twin in each pair received a vitamin C capsule while the other got a placebo. The daily vitamin C dosages before and during colds ranged from 500 for younger children to 1,500 mg for older ones. The investigators noted "no significant overall benefit on cold symptoms" as reported by the children's mothers, but the responses varied among the subgroups when the children were divided according to

sex and age. After the data were analyzed, four mothers admitted tasting the capsules in an attempt to figure out which twin was getting the vitamin C! Thus it is possible that the ratings of these mothers and possibly others were influenced by guessing which twin was getting the vitamin C.

A double-blind Australian trial with 95 pairs of identical twins was reported in 1981. One of each pair took 1,000 mg of vitamin C for 100 days while the other received a placebo. The vitamin C group had slightly more colds but a shorter duration of colds (5 days instead of 6).

In 1977, Tyrell and co-workers reported treating 743 men and 758 women for 5 months as follows. Half received placebo pills daily. The others took vitamin C but only during colds at dosages of 4,000 mg on the first and second days of a cold and 200 mg on the third day. There was no benefit from taking vitamin C. The incidence and duration of colds were the same for both men and women in the vitamin and placebo groups. Men in both groups missed an average of half a day's work while women missed a day.

An 8-week trial with 764 U.S. Marine recruits carried out by Pitt and Costrini was reported in 1979. Half of the recruits received 2,000 mg of vitamin C daily, while the others took placebo pills on the same schedule. No benefit from vitamin C was found. Ninety percent of both groups got colds, and no difference in severity or duration of colds was found.

In a 1984 study Dr. M. H. Briggs gave half of 528 volunteers 1,000 mg vitamin C daily and the other half a daily placebo for three months. In the vitamin C group 47% got colds, and 46% of the placebo group. Severity of symptoms lasted an average of 3.1 days for the vitamin C group and 3.3 days for those getting placebos. Briggs concluded: No prevention and no benefit.

In 1990 Dr. Elliot Dick and co-workers summarized the methods and results of their three double-blind controlled trials to test methods of transmission of viruses, by contaminated fingers or inhaling viruses in the air, and to test the protective effect of vitamin C. They used 24 volunteers (8 donors and 16 recipients). The recipients were non-smoking men who tested negative for antibodies to the RV16 type cold virus. Half of these were pretreated for 3.5 weeks with 2,000 mg of vitamin C daily (4 × 500 mg), and the other eight were given four placebos daily. The eight donors were infected with RV16 cold virus by direct inoculation into the nose and then were housed with the recipients 24 hours a day for a 7-day interaction period. All donors developed colds first and then all 16 of the recipients. The vitamin C or placebo pills were continued during the week of interaction and for the following two weeks. During the 7-day interaction period the men were supervised and slept, ate and played cards in the same room. All got colds, but the authors claim that the vitamin C group suffered significantly less "symptoms and signs" such as coughs and mucus production.

2. NUTRIENTS

DO ADDED BIOFLAVONOIDS HELP?

In 1979, Dr. I. M. Baird and co-workers reported a 10-week experiment with 350 volunteers (ages 17 to 25) who were divided into three groups. One-third of them, as the placebo group, received a daily "supplement" of a synthetic orange drink containing no vitamin C. A second group got a synthetic drink containing 80 mg of synthetic vitamin C. The third group was given enough pure orange juice daily to provide 80 mg of natural vitamin C plus bioflavonoids. The incidence of colds was the same for all three groups. Both vitamin C groups had slightly less severe colds than the placebo group. Thus the synthetic vitamin C was as effective as the natural vitamin C and the presence of bioflavonoids had no apparent effect.

ANTIHISTAMINE EFFECT OF VITAMIN C

Histamine in varying amounts is almost always released in the tissues of the respiratory tract by an allergic-like response to the stress of common cold infections. Perhaps the first clue that animals and humans might use vitamin C to combat stress that involves histamine release came in 1940 from the research team led by the co-discoverer of vitamin C, Dr. Charles Glen King of Columbia University.

Dr. King's group showed that stressing rats with certain drugs stimulated their bodies to synthesize extra vitamin C. Later, evidence was presented to support the belief that animals, such as the rat, who can make their own supply of vitamin C, react to histamine by producing extra vitamin C.

In 1974, two other research teams found that rats given vitamin C along with histamine-releasing drugs had a reduction in stress symptoms and reduced histamine in the urine. They concluded that vitamin C can act like an anti-histamine drug. However many physicians believe that reducing infection-caused inflammation (nature's defense reaction) slows recovery.

TWO RECENT REVIEWS

Two comprehensive reviews covering just about all of the published reports about testing vitamin C against colds in humans are those of Dr. A. Stewart Truswell of the University of Sydney, Australia, and Dr. Harri Hemila, Institute of Biotechnology, University of Helsinki. In 1986 Dr. Truswell concisely summarized the results of 27 trials conducted since 1970. Of these, five were treatment trials with vitamin C or a placebo given only at the onset of a cold and for only several days—all of which found no benefit. The other 22 were doubled-blind controlled trials giving daily vitamin C or placebo before and during colds. Of these twelve trials showed no prevention and no reduction in duration or severity, five trials showed no prevention and only slight, statistically non-significant lessening of severity, and the other five trials reported no prevention and a small but significant reduction of duration of the colds. Dr. Truswell concluded: "It is now fairly clear that for preventing colds, vitamin C has no worthwhile effect," but there is "a little more evidence for a small therapeutic effect." However, as Dr. T. W. Anderson's second trial in 1974 revealed, 250 mg of vitamin per day reduced severity as much as did 1,000 mg or 4,000 mg.

In his 1992 review entitled, "Vitamin C and the Common Cold," Dr. Harri Hemila concluded: "Vitamin C has consistently decreased the duration of cold episodes and severity of symptoms." Yet Dr. Truswell found no reduction in severity in 17 of 27 trial reports he analyzed.

And finally, let us note that Dr. Richard Cutler at the National Institute on Aging and Dr. R. S. Sohal claim there is evidence that an excess supply of antioxidants like vitamins C and E from outside the body (exogenous) suppresses the body's own unique endogenous (from within) antioxidants such as catalase and superoxide dismutase.

OVERVIEW

Does it make sense to supplement with vitamin C? If so, should it be done daily or only at the first sign of a cold or other infection? And what dosage should be used?

The many studies done in the last thirty years clearly prove that daily vitamin C supplements, whether 100 mg or 5,000 mg, do not prevent colds and provide, but only for some people, only a slight reduction in duration and severity of colds. Dr. Thomas Chalmers, a prominent medical educator and researcher, concluded in 1975: "I, who have colds as often and as severe as those of any man, do not consider the very minor potential benefit that might result from taking vitamin C three times a day for life worth either the effort or the risk, no matter how slight the latter might be."

If you choose to supplement when a cold strikes, there is no reason to take more than 250 mg per day, as shown in the 1974 Anderson study. This amount is easily obtained from the age-old "remedy," fruit juices. Supplementation with larger amounts of vitamin C has not been shown to be more effective, and it may cause diarrhea or have other adverse effects.

What about other infections? It is known that the body's pool of vitamin C in the blood plasma and white cells declines rapidly the first day or two in the presence of stresses such as severe infections, burns or surgery. Some doctors believe that under these circumstances, a supplement of 250 mg, but never more than 500 mg, per day for a few days may aid in recovery.

Folic Acid: New Findings Renew Old Debate

If all women of childbearing age consumed adequate amounts of the B vitamin folic acid, the incidence of life-threatening neural tube defects (NTDs) could be reduced 50 percent in this country, according to a report released last fall by the Centers for Disease Control and Prevention (CDC).

Currently the average American woman consumes one-half the recommended amount of folic acid, reviving a familiar debate among nutritionists on the best way to obtain recommended vitamin levels.

Should women be encouraged to more carefully select folic-acid rich foods, or take a vitamin supplement with the recommended amount? Should the Food and Drug Administration (FDA) allow more foods to be fortified with folic acid? Should health claims for folic acid-rich foods be permitted?

NTDs, which include anencephaly and spina bifida, account for about five percent of all U.S. birth defects annually. Infants born with anencephaly are missing most or all of their brain and die shortly after birth. Most babies born with spina bifida, in which the spinal cord is exposed, grow to adulthood but do so with severe paralysis or other disabilities.

Getting Enough Folic Acid

According to CDC, a daily intake of 0.4 milligrams (mg) of folic acid potentially can eliminate one-half of all NTDs. To achieve this reduction, however, all women of childbearing age are advised to consume recommended amounts of the vitamin, because the defects occur during the first month after conception—before many women realize they're pregnant. And over one-half of U.S. pregnancies are unplanned.

Each day, the average American woman consumes about 0.2 mg of folate, the generic term for food compounds with the biologic activity of folic acid.

To obtain recommended intakes of folic acid through diet requires careful selection of foods consistent with the U.S. Dietary Guidelines and the Food Guide Pyramid. Good sources of folate include leafy dark-green vegetables, legumes, citrus fruits and juices, whole grains and peanuts. Some grain products such as breakfast cereals also are fortified with folacin.

But because many American women do not eat enough of these foods, CDC identified additional fortification of the food supply as one way in which to ensure an adequate intake of folic acid.

"We don't have rickets in this country anymore because we fortified milk with vitamin D," said Godfrey Oakley, M.D., director of CDC's Division of Birth Defects and Developmental Disabilities. "With fortification, people who need folic acid would get it without even thinking about it. Plus it's an extremely inexpensive way to obtain the nutrient," Oakley said.

Dietary supplements with folic acid are another potential means to achieve recommended intakes. Some 20 percent of American women currently take vitamins containing folic acid daily. But this approach may not be realistic for women of lower socioeconomic status, who are among those with the lowest folic acid intakes.

As with many other nutrients, there are also risks associated with consuming too much folic acid. Although the scientific evidence is limited, excessive folic acid can complicate the diagnosis of vitamin B-12 deficiency, causing anemia and permanent nerve damage.

"The dose at which we see positive effects in reducing the risk of neural tube defects is uncomfortably close to the doses at which we begin to have safety concerns," said FDA Commissioner David Kessler, M.D. "FDA's mandate is to ensure that women of childbearing age get enough folic acid. But the agency must also do everything in its power to see that no one is exposed to excessive amounts of the nutrient," Kessler said.

Balancing Risks and Benefits

To examine CDC's recommendations and FDA's current regulatory policy on folic acid, the agency convened an advisory committee last November. After hearings and public debate, the panel recommended a public education program and modest fortification of the food supply with folic acid. An upper level of one mg of folate from dietary sources and supplements was advised.

However, the panel recommended against allowing any health claims about the vitamin on food or supplement labels. The experts generally agreed that stronger scientific evidence on folic acid and NTDs is still needed.

In December, FDA followed the panel's advice and denied a health claim for folic acid and NTDs. In publishing its final regulations on food labeling, the agency said it will permit health claims for seven nutrient-disease relationships, but not for folic acid and birth defects. FDA is still reviewing the recommendations on food fortification and other areas and is expected to announce a decision in the near future.

Fluoride
Cavity-Fighter on Tap

Dodi Schultz

Dodi Schultz is a freelance writer in New York City and a contributing editor of Parents *magazine.*

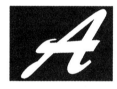

A decade ago, the National Institutes of Health called it "the leading chronic disease of childhood." An editorial published in the *Journal of the American Medical Association* just a few years before that, in 1975, went further, terming it "the most common disease of mankind."

The scourge referred to, dental caries (non-dentists call it tooth decay), is a malady that may well be on its way out, thanks mostly to fluoride, a remedy supplied by nature in some parts of our nation and applied by human ingenuity in others. It's now a major ingredient in 95 percent of the toothpaste we purchase. It's also an ingredient in the community water supplies serving most of our citizens.

Interest in the role of fluoride arose when it was observed that people in some parts of the country had a surprisingly low incidence of tooth decay. The areas, it turned out, were those in which fluorides occur naturally in the drinking water.

By the mid-1950s, the results of decade-long controlled studies of water-supply fluoridation had established beyond a doubt both the effectiveness and the safety of fluoridation in reducing tooth decay. The practice was—and continues to be—endorsed by the American Medical Association, the American Dental Association, the U.S. Public Health Service, and the National Research Council.

Exceeding Expectations

Every 10 years, PHS (of which FDA is a part) determines national health objectives for the decade ahead. In setting dental health goals in 1980, PHS declared that by 1990, the proportion of 9-year-olds who had never had cavities in their permanent teeth should rise to 40 percent.

At the time, 40 percent seemed a sensible expectation (the most recent data then available showed that in the mid-70s, the figure was under 30 percent). Yet, even then a new survey was under way, and it soon became clear that at the time the goal was set, it had already been not only achieved, but surpassed.

In 1982, the National Institute of Dental Research released the results of its 1979-80 survey, based on a sampling of 40,000 children nationwide, showing that more than half of the 9-year-olds (51 percent) were decay-free. In fall of 1988, PHS announced that, according to preliminary results from a 1986-87 survey, over *65 percent* of American 9-year-olds had never had decay in their permanent teeth. And the trend continues.

How Fluoride Helps . . .

There are three requirements for the creation of cavities: teeth, which are extremely susceptible to attack by certain acids; bacteria—notably *Streptococcus mutans*—that produce those acids; and food on which the bacteria can feed. Carbohydrates, especially sucrose (ordinary sugar), make fine fare for *S. mutans* and kin.

No vaccine against caries-causing bacteria is in sight. Nor has anyone found a way to enforce immediate after-meals tooth-brushing to remove the bacteria-nourishing nutrients. Enter fluoride, which structurally bolsters the teeth's resistance to acid invasion. If babies receive fluoride from the start (even when still in the womb), while their teeth are still developing, and continue to do so all through formation of both their baby teeth and the permanent set, stronger teeth will erupt, teeth that are more resistant to attack by decay-causing bacteria.

To achieve resistance, children growing up in an area where the water is neither naturally nor artificially fluoridated may need to receive supplements (see "Fluoride Supplements for Young Teeth").

Only fluoride taken internally, whether in drinking water or dietary supplements, can strengthen babies' and children's developing teeth to resist decay. Once the teeth have erupted, they're beyond help from ingested fluoride.

For both children and adults, fluoride applied to the surface of the teeth can nonetheless add protection, at least to the outer layer of enamel, and it has unquestionably also played a role in reducing decay. The most familiar form, of course, is fluoride-containing toothpaste, introduced in the early 1960s. Fluoride rinses are also available, as are applications by dental professionals. All these

Reprinted from *FDA Consumer,* January/February 1992, pp. 34-38.

products are regulated by FDA. They are considered effective adjuncts to ingested fluoride—and they are the only useful sources of tooth-strengthening fluoride for teenagers and adults.

... And (Sometimes) Hurts

There is one proven adverse effect of fluoride on the teeth: Too much fluoride can cause a condition called dental fluorosis. In its mildest form, this condition causes small, white, virtually invisible opaque areas on teeth. In its most severe form, it causes a distinct brownish mottling. However, dental fluorosis doesn't result from artificial fluoridation alone, because the levels are kept low enough to avoid this effect.

Over the years, many studies of dental fluorosis patterns have established optimal levels for fluoride in drinking water—levels that will provide protection against decay but will cause no, or negli-

Dental caries is a malady that may well be on its way out, thanks mostly to fluoride.

gible, fluorosis. Fluoride levels are stated in parts per million (ppm) concentrations. About 1 ppm is ideal. Less than 0.7 ppm isn't adequate to protect developing teeth; more than about 1.5 to 2.0 ppm can lead to mild fluorosis. Artificial fluoridation of water uses an optimum standard set by the Environmental Protection Agency of 0.7 to 1.2 ppm, depending on locality (a lower amount is needed in warmer parts of the country, where people drink more water).

Dental fluorosis affects only the teeth. In its mildest form, it isn't at all apparent

to the untrained eye and can be detected only by an experienced dentist or specially trained technician. Somewhat greater discoloration does become a cosmetic problem, a condition that an individual may feel mars his or her appearance even though it's not truly harmful. Severe fluorosis poses a threat to health, since the discoloration may be accompanied by actual pitting of dental enamel—rendering affected teeth possibly more, rather than less, susceptible to decay. As with the benefits of fluoride, once permanent teeth have erupted, there is no longer any threat of dental fluorosis.

A study reported in the *Journal of the American Dental Association* in 1983 by

a team from the National Institute of Dental Research clearly described the impact of excess fluoride. Seven Illinois communities where water consumption was likely to be similar were compared; their natural fluoride concentrations ranged from an optimal 1.06 ppm up to an excessive 4.07 ppm. Experienced clinicians examined the teeth of youngsters aged 8 to 16. Where the fluoride level was optimal, the examiners could find no fluorosis in 86 percent and detected only mild signs in another 12 percent; severe fluorosis was found in 0.6 percent. At two to three times optimal levels, severe cases were found in 5 to 8 percent. At the highest level, the figure jumped to a

---

When to Give Fluoride Supplements

To be sure that teeth incorporate decay-fighting fluoride during structural development, infants and children need to receive fluoride on a regular basis. Whether or not supplements are needed, and how much, depends on both the local water supply and sources in a child's diet.

Fluoride supplements, which are regulated by FDA as drugs, may take the form of drops or, for older youngsters, chewable tablets. They are available both alone and in combination with vitamins.

The daily requirement rule of thumb suggested by the American Dental Association and the American Academy of Pediatrics is 0.25 milligrams per day up to age 2, 0.5 mg for ages 2 and 3, and 1 mg after age 3 and until the teen years. Children who consume tap water with a fluoride concentration of less than 0.3 parts per million (ppm) need full supplementation. At water supply levels between 0.3 and 0.7 ppm, only half the need is met; if the water supply provides 0.5 ppm, for example, an average 5-year-old should receive 0.5 milligrams of supplemental fluoride per day. Breast-fed infants are exceptions to the rule, since breast milk contains almost no fluoride (nor do ready-to-drink formulas).

Further, doctors need to consider both the local water supply and the baby's diet as a whole in calculating needs and prescribing supplements, points out Katherine Karlsrud, M.D., a clinical instructor in pediatrics at Cornell University Medical College.

The process can be complicated for physicians in some "mixed" geographical areas. Karlsrud practices in New York City, which offers what she pronounces a "perfect" fluoride level—but she also cares for children from surrounding counties where the level is zero.

"Each baby's need," she says, "has to be individually figured out. If a baby in Manhattan, for example, is being partly breast-fed, but half that baby's diet consists of formula reconstituted with tap water, half the child's need for fluoride is being met." That would not be true, though, for an infant in nearby Suffolk County, on Long Island, where the citizenry at this writing continues to reject health officials' recommendation that the water supply be fluoridated.

In areas where the drinking water provides protective fluorides, over 0.7 ppm, breast-fed babies who have been weaned need no further supplementation.

—*D.S.*

O nly fluoride taken internally can strengthen babies' and children's developing teeth to resist decay.

disturbing 23 percent—almost a quarter of the youngsters examined.

EPA is the federal authority responsible for ensuring that naturally occurring fluoride levels meet safety standards. Above the concentration that protects against tooth decay, fluoride is considered a contaminant, and the states must report local levels to EPA.

As Edward V. Ohanian, Ph.D., of the human and environmental criteria division in EPA's Office of Water explains, the agency has established two "maximum contaminant levels (MCLs)" for fluoride, 2 ppm and 4 ppm. The first MCL is considered the point above which *cosmetic* effects—in the form of a degree of dental fluorosis—can occur and is intended to ensure public awareness of that possibility. Although EPA cannot compel the states to hold fluorides to this level, the 4-ppm MCL is legally enforceable, since it is based on the possibility of adverse *health* effects above that level. Local authorities may be ordered to defluoridate the water if levels exceed that figure.

In accordance with the Safe Drinking Water Act, EPA periodically reexamines its standards and is currently reviewing information that has become available since 1985. A report is expected by late 1992 or 1993.

A Community Decision

Along with caries reduction, PHS set another dental health objective a decade ago—that by 1990, at least 95 percent of the population using community water systems would be drawing optimally

Tips for Parents

While parents should be sure that their children are getting fluoride's protection for their teeth, they should also be aware of what FDA's Ronald Coene calls the "total body burden of fluoride" and be sure their children aren't ingesting unneeded amounts. (Only ingested fluoride, not topical application, has been associated with dental fluorosis or any other systemic effect.)

Some guidelines on various fluoride sources:

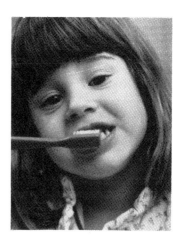

• Drinking Water: Find out from local health officials the fluoride concentration in your community's water supply. If it's below protective levels, see that your children receive supplements until their teen years. If the level's just right and a physician or dentist prescribes supplements, question him or her about it (exceptions would be breast-feeding babies who drink very little or no water). If the level is naturally too high, contact your local EPA office.

Some promoters of bottled water, which some families choose for drinking instead of tap water, claim their products come from springs of remarkable purity. According to Neil Sass, Ph.D., a science policy advisor in FDA's Center for Food Safety and Applied Nutrition, "Perhaps 50 percent of bottled waters are taken from municipal water supplies, which may or may not be fluoridated. Some are put right into the bottles; others are filtered. In many cases, any fluoride content may be removed before bottling."

One researcher who checked out a number of popular bottled water brands reported in the *New England Journal of Medicine* in 1989 that, except for three imported carbonated brands, none had fluoride levels above 0.25 parts per million; of those three, two fell short of the cavity-fighting range and one exceeded it (the fluoride level of the sample tested was 1.9 ppm).

• *Fluoride Supplements:* If they're needed, be sure the doses are appropriate, taking into consideration, for example, such factors as an infant's varied diet.

• *Toothpaste:* The fluoride concentration in toothpaste is high, and toothpaste is meant to be applied to the surface of the teeth, not swallowed. According to Assistant Secretary for Health James O. Mason, M.D., if the average 2-year-old brushing twice a day swallows the toothpaste, it could add 0.5 milligrams per day to the child's fluoride intake—full supplement dosage for a child of this age. He suggests that children be carefully taught never to swallow toothpaste and to use only a pea-sized amount on the brush.

• *Rinses:* FDA has concluded that these nonprescription products can indeed boost the anti-cavity effect of fluoride toothpaste. They are best used after brushing but should not be used by children under 6 unless recommended by a dentist. (Nor should they be used by anyone who may be apt to swallow some of the product.)

• *Dental-Office Application:* This is the most concentrated topical form of fluoride, and can be quite helpful in preventing cavities in children and adults alike. The likelihood of harm from proper application is virtually nil, says Jack Klatell, D.D.S., chairman of the department of dentistry at Mount Sinai School of Medicine: "The application is usually in the form of a paste or gel inside a mouth guard, which is placed in the mouth and left in contact with the teeth for a period of time and then removed."

—D.S.

fluoridated water from their taps. But by 1985, that figure was only 62 percent, and growth in community water fluoridation had slowed to 1 to 2 percent a year. Why are so many fluoride-deficient water supplies still unfluoridated?

There is no national law requiring fluoridation, and the question must be decided locally. Although most Americans are aware that many substances are routinely added to our water to ensure that it's safe and drinkable, there are still some apprehensions about the addition of chemicals that don't occur naturally. And some misunderstandings have arisen.

Four Ill-Fated Rats

The most recent misunderstanding occurred in the spring of 1990, with the news of an experimental animal study. Some abbreviated reports of the study were interpreted as confirming a "weak link" between fluoride and cancer. However, a more detailed look at the study results shows this was not the case. In the study by PHS's National Toxicology Program, four male rats given very high doses of fluoride developed osteosarcoma, a rare form of bone cancer.

They were among 50 rats and mice of both sexes given the highest doses of fluoride they could tolerate in their drinking water for two years. One rat that developed cancer received fluoride at a level of 45 ppm; the other three received it at a level of 79 ppm. There were no cancers found in female rats, or in mice of either sex, at these fluoride levels; nor were cancers found in any animals at lower levels.

Despite the weakness of the association, the Department of Health and Human Services assembled a panel to review all current and past research relating to fluoride safety. The group, the Ad Hoc Subcommittee on Fluoride of the Committee to Coordinate Environmental Health and Related Programs, included scientists from more than a dozen federal agencies and was chaired by former FDA Commissioner Frank E. Young, M.D., Ph.D.

The subcommittee's report, released in February 1991 after months of examining the evidence, concluded there was no cause for alarm and no reason to link fluoridation of water with any human disorder or disease, including osteosarcoma or other malignancies. And a study published in the April 1991 issue of the *American Journal of Public Health,* comparing the incidence of osteosarcomas in fluoridated and unfluoridated areas of

New York state, found no difference in the rates.

The PHS report did observe that there are multiple sources of fluoride and commented that, "In accordance with prudent health practice of using no more than the amount necessary to achieve a desired effect, health professionals and the public should avoid excessive and inappropriate fluoride exposure."

Clearly, the levels of fluoride added to water supplies do not represent a public health hazard. But the risk of adverse effects, specifically of fluorosis in young teeth, is real if infants and children ingest appreciably more fluoride than they need for decay prevention.

Ronald F. Coene, an engineer and water supply specialist at FDA's National Center for Toxicological Research, who served as executive secretary of the special subcommittee, points out that, "It is possible for a child to get too much fluoride. That can happen when more than maximum allowable levels occur naturally in drinking water, or from swallowing toothpaste. It can also result from unneeded dietary supplements. Sometimes, dentists have been known to recommend fluoride tablets when the local water supply is fluoridated. Too much fluoride can cause fluorosis. That was the concern of the committee when it comes to overexposure—fluorosis, not cancer."

Might Americans be taking in too much iron?

When Art Linkletter warned television viewers 30 years ago that "that worn-out feeling may be due to iron-poor blood," few people watching him make his pitch for Geritol supplements containing "twice the iron in a pound of calves' liver" would have taken issue. After all, iron deficiency was often referred to as one of the country's most prevalent nutritional problems. It's still considered a major nutritional concern today. In the last few months, however, widespread media attention devoted to research results suggesting that high levels of iron stored in the body may be a significant risk factor for the development of heart disease has some consumers wondering.

"High Level of Iron Tied to Heart Risk" is the way one major newspaper put it. "Bad News for the Geritol Set" proclaimed a well-respected magazine, which then went on to say that it may be prudent to avoid meat and fortified cereals, both important contributors of iron to the diet.

The headline-making research that led to the advice was conducted on almost 2,000 middle-aged men in eastern Finland. Scientists there found that every 1 percent increase in the men's levels of a substance which indicates how much iron the body has stored was associated with an increase of over 4 percent in heart attack risk. That risk was more than doubled for those with the highest measurements, helping to make iron stores a greater predictor of heart attack in the study than several well-accepted factors such as high blood cholesterol and high blood pressure.

The name of the substance the scientists measured is serum ferritin. Ferritin is a protein that stores iron in the tissues, and the amount in blood serum provides an indirect measure of the total amount of iron stores the body has on hand.

Some researchers, intrigued by the findings, believe they shed new light on many aspects of the heart disease story, including why women are much less prone to heart attacks early in life. The prevailing theory has been that women are protected by the hormone estrogen and that their risk of having a heart attack goes up when their estrogen levels decrease at menopause. But, the scientists say, it may be that younger women are protected because of iron losses that occur during menstruation. They point to research showing that after menopause, when women's heart attack rates begin to catch up with men's, their levels of stored iron catch up as well. With that research in mind, a few scientists have gone so far as to suggest that people consider donating blood, the iron-rich body fluid, two to three times a year to lower their iron stores.

Other proponents of the iron/heart disease theory point out that iron promotes formation of very damaging forms of oxygen that can work to make the "bad" LDL-cholesterol in the blood even more prone to accumulate as part of plaque on artery walls. In other words, iron could be contributing to atherosclerosis and clogged blood vessels.

Before you start practicing blood-letting

Provocative as the results from Finland may be, most scientists believe it is far too soon to draw any definitive conclusions about iron's effects on the risk of heart disease and certainly too soon for Americans to make any changes in their iron-related behavior, either through changes in diet or frequency of blood donation for the purpose of depleting iron stores. Says Jeffrey Blumberg, PhD, Associate Director of the USDA Human Nutrition Research Center on Aging at Tufts as

From *Tufts University Diet & Nutrition Letter,* Vol. 10, No. 11, January 1993, pp. 3-6. *Tufts University Diet & Nutrition Letter,* 53 Park Place, New York, NY 10001.

Muscling more iron into your diet

The Recommended Dietary Allowance for iron for men and for women beyond their childbearing years is 10 milligrams. For younger women, the RDA is set at 15 milligrams to make up for their iron losses during menstruation each month. (In both cases, the RDA takes into account the fact that the body absorbs relatively little of the iron we eat; most of it passes out of us rather than makes its way to the tissues.)

The foods listed below give an idea of how iron needs can be met. Animal sources of the mineral—beef, poultry, and fish—contain a form of iron known as heme iron that the body absorbs better than it does other forms. Fruits, vegetables, and legumes contain non-heme iron, of which much less is assimilated. However, eating those foods with others that contain vitamin C will enhance absorption, so that, for instance, adding some vitamin C-containing tomato slices to a salad that has beans will allow the body to hold onto a greater amount of the beans' iron. The presence of heme iron can increase the absorption of non-heme iron as well. For instance, the non-heme iron in potatoes used in making a stew will

be absorbed better if the stew contains some heme iron-containing beef.

Also worth keeping in mind: coffee and tea taken with food can decrease iron absorption significantly. Thus, iron seekers should consider forgoing those beverages at mealtime.

	Iron (milligrams)
oysters, cooked, moist heat, 3 oz	11.4
beef, top round, choice, broiled, 3 oz	2.3
beef liver, braised, 3 oz	5.8
chicken, breast meat, roasted, 3 oz	0.9
turkey, breast meat, roasted, 3 oz	1.3
pork tenderloin, roasted, 3 oz	1.3
flounder, cooked in dry heat, 3 oz	0.9
tuna, light, canned in water, 3 oz	1.3
lima beans, boiled, ½ cup	2.1
broccoli, boiled, 1 spear	1.5
potato, baked	2.8
enriched spaghetti, cooked, 1 cup	2.0
enriched white bread, 1 slice	0.7
whole wheat bread, 1 slice	0.9
raisins, ⅓ cup (packed)	1.1
peas, boiled, ½ cup	1.2
peanut butter, 2 tablespoons	0.5

well as a prominent scientist in the field of antioxidant research, "the press has made far too

Menstruating women in the U.S. generally have only one fourth to one half of the stored iron men have. Thus, men are in a better position than women to donate "the gift of life." That's not to say it's unsafe for women to donate blood. They simply will have less stored iron afterward.

much of this single study. Much remains to be addressed. For instance," he says, "it needs to be kept in mind that the subjects constituted an unusual population. Eastern Finnish men may be very different from most Americans."

That's certainly true in terms of iron status. Consider that the average iron intake among the Finns was 19 milligrams per day, considerably more than the 10 to 15 milligrams American men are estimated to consume. Furthermore, the Finns' measurements of serum ferritin—the substance that indicates how much iron is stored throughout the body—averaged up to 50 percent higher than serum ferritin in American males. More than one in four had levels that were up to 100 percent higher than those found in American men. In comparison with American women, the Finnish men's serum ferritin was 300 to 600 percent higher. In other words, even if iron *were* found to have something to do with the develop-

ment of heart disease, Americans may not have levels high enough to trigger any kind of significant problem.

The differences between Finnish and American subjects constitute just one reason to hesitate before trying to cut down on iron. Although a drop in that mineral may not be significant enough to cause iron-deficiency anemia, it could conceivably compromise the proper functioning of the immune system as well as take away from optimal work performance and the ability to concentrate when learning. That is, if people made a concerted effort to cut down on their iron stores to stave off heart disease, they might hurt themselves in other ways.

Clearly, the research community has a lot to do before any new recommendation concerning iron can be made with assurance. As the Harvard heart disease expert Charles Hennekens, MD, puts it, "if other investigators using different techniques and different populations—some men, some women—all show the same thing, we've got a message for the general public." Until then, he says, the public should concentrate on making the proven lifestyle changes that we *know* will decrease heart disease risk, such as eating less fat and quitting smoking. Adds Tufts University mineral researcher James Fleet, PhD, "whatever is eventually learned about iron, adding or subtracting a single nutrient from the diet will never make or break heart disease risk by itself. It's a set of lifestyle factors—total diet and exercise patterns—that counts, along with whether the illness runs in the family."

Does all this mean that for now, at least, no Americans should be concerned about taking in too much iron? If only it were that simple.

A known risk for iron overload

The body guards its iron stores very jealously, as well it should. Without an adequate supply of iron, our red blood cells do not have enough of an iron-containing protein called hemoglobin, which functions by picking up oxygen in the lungs each time we take a breath and carrying that life-sustaining substance to all the tissues of the body. Of the one-ninth to one-sixth of an ounce of iron present in each adult (about a teaspoonful), 70 percent can be found in hemoglobin.

One way our bodies help insure that enough iron is on hand is to absorb more from the food we eat when stores become deficient; iron absorption can increase dramatically if necessary. Unfortunately, some people have a condition that causes them to absorb a relatively large amount of iron even if they don't need it. And since there is no way to get rid of it other than by bleeding—via menstruation, childbirth, injury, or blood donations (the inability to lose significant amounts of iron any other way is a second mechanism our systems have for making sure we don't run low)—their internal organs become iron overloaded and thereby cause problems like liver disease, congestive heart failure, diabetes, arthritis, and without early enough intervention, death.

The condition, a hereditary disease called hemochromatosis, is estimated to afflict more than a million Americans. That comes to about one in every 200 to 250 people, far fewer than suffer from iron *deficiency* but still more than all those afflicted with cystic fibrosis, Huntington's disease, and muscular dystrophy combined.

Fortunately, many people with hemochromatosis never develop any problematic symptoms that endanger their health. Tragically, however, those who do are often not diagnosed correctly until somewhere in mid-life, when iron stores are five to 50 times the norm and the illness has ravaged their bodies. A 1988 survey of a group of people with iron overload revealed, in fact, that one in three had met with more than 11 doctors before receiving a proper diagnosis.

The delay is largely due to the fact that many of the initial symptoms—weakness, fatigue, achy joints, decreased sexual desire—are so variable and nonspecific that it is all too easy to attribute them to other conditions, including iron-deficiency anemia! Some patients suffering from the disease are actually instructed to take iron supplements, which only make their condition worse.

That hemochromatosis frequently escapes early detection is very troubling, particularly in light of the simplicity of its treatment: periodic phlebotomy or blood-letting to get rid of excess iron stores (the more iron lost in blood, the more the body's storage tissues must give up to make new red blood cells) and avoidance of iron supplements and foods highly fortified with the mineral.

How can you tell that you may have too much stored iron? Only certain blood tests, two of which are the serum ferritin test and the transferrin saturation test, provide the answer. The full series of blood tests that check for iron overload costs about $75 to $100 and is worth considering for anyone who has a family history of hemochromatosis or suffers from what might be the early symptoms of the disease, but has not been treated successfully for his or her complaints and has not yet been told that iron overload might be the culprit.

The more common iron-based affliction

While hemochromatosis is no small matter, iron deficiency is much more prevalent. In fact, a lack of iron is the most common nutrient deficiency worldwide, affecting more than a billion people. The groups at particular risk: children six months to four years old, whose iron reserves may not be sufficient to meet the needs of their rapid growth; pre- and early adolescents, who are also growing and often have poor diets; women of childbearing years, who lose iron in the blood during menstruation; and pregnant women, who in order to deliver healthy babies must have sufficient iron to cover the requirements of the fetus, the placenta, their own expanded blood volume, and the blood losses that occur during childbirth.

If an iron "deficit" is dramatic enough, the result is full-blown iron-deficiency anemia, a condition in which iron stores are so low and, consequently, the number of hemoglobin molecules so diminished that not enough of them are available to pick up an adequate amount of oxygen from the lungs and distribute it to the rest of the body. Such cases are akin to a lack of air, which is why many people with anemia may feel like people often do at very high altitudes where the air is "thin": weak and woozy and easily fatigued.

Fortunately, the incidence of iron-deficiency anemia is relatively rare. But some researchers estimate that one out of every 10 to 15 people in the at-risk groups have at least some degree of impaired iron status. The practical upshot of "low-grade" iron deficiency: Basic functioning may not be up to par. That could mean anything from too little energy to perform everyday tasks in an efficient manner to difficulties staying alert, say, in school or on the job.

Does that signify that the tens of millions of people in the at-risk segments of the population should automatically take iron supplements? Absolutely not. It would not be prudent for anyone to swallow iron pills unless a demonstrated need for them has been shown with a true iron deficiency as diagnosed by a physician. Even when iron pills are prescribed, there should be adequate follow-up so that what might only be a need for short-term supplementation doesn't turn into unnecessary "chronic" iron therapy without end.

Those who are drawn to the idea of swallowing iron supplements without proof of need should consider that they can cause unpleasant side effects, including constipation, diarrhea, and gastric upset. They can also contribute to nutrient imbalances. Specifically, too much iron can interfere with the availability of the essential nutrients copper, manganese, and zinc. Furthermore, if supplemental iron is not truly needed but taken overzealously anyway, iron toxicity can occur in the form of liver damage as well as damage to other organs.

None of this is to say people shouldn't make every effort to eat adequate amounts of iron-containing *foods*: an average of up to six ounces a day of meat, poultry, and/or fish, the richest sources of iron in the diet, along with beans, enriched breads and the like, and for smaller iron contributions, vegetables and fruits. In the absence of blood tests for iron status ordered by a physician, following such a balanced diet will safely help minimize the risk of an iron shortfall in people predisposed to deficiencies of that mineral as well as cause the least potential damage to those Americans at risk of iron overload.

What your doctor may not have told you

A woman walks into her physician's office complaining of persistent fatigue and a general lack of stamina. Her doctor takes a sample of her blood, sends it off to a lab for tests and, based upon the results, diagnoses her as having iron-deficiency anemia. His cure: iron supplements.

Simple, right? Not if the doctor didn't order all the right tests. And that's a possibility. According to at least a couple of accounts, iron-deficiency anemia has been overdiagnosed in the U.S. precisely because some physicians have used too few blood tests to detect it. The reason goes back to the definition of anemia. Simply put, anemia is a reduction in the number of hemoglobin molecules and/or in the number or size of the red blood cells. But too little hemoglobin or too few red blood cells may result from many things that have nothing to do with whether the body is taking in or storing enough iron. For instance, anemia can be caused by too little of a number of other nutrients: folic acid; vitamin B_6; copper; and, usually due to malabsorption, B_{12} (anemia brought on by a B_{12} defi-

ciency is known as pernicious anemia)—all are necessary for proper red blood cell formation. Trauma and illnesses that cause internal bleeding can lead to anemia as well.

What it comes down to is that anemia is better off regarded as a symptom, a clue to a problem, rather than *the* problem in and of itself. And the way to find out whether that problem has anything to do with iron status is to go beyond simply confirming the presence of anemia, which doctors do by ordering blood tests that measure hemoglobin levels and what is known as the hematocrit (the percentage of blood made up of red blood cells) and test specifically for iron deficiency. For that purpose, specialists recommend a serum ferritin test, which indirectly measures the amount of the mineral stored away in the body tissues. If stores are low enough or nonexistent, a lack of iron can be considered the anemia-causing culprit and iron supplements generally prescribed. (Of course, iron-deficiency anemia can be a symptom in itself, as in the case of internal bleeding in the gastrointestinal tract due to an ulcer or to a more serious problem such as cancer; the more bleeding, the more iron that leaves the body. Because iron-deficiency anemia can result from many conditions other than a lack of iron, it is important for physicians to make sure iron-deficient patients, particularly from middle age on, are not suffering from an underlying illness.)

Many doctors order blood tests in addition to the one that measures serum ferritin in order to make sure their diagnosis of iron-deficiency anemia is correct. One of those is the transferrin saturation test. Transferrin is a protein that takes iron absorbed from foods as well as from broken down red blood cells and carries it to whatever body tissues need it. If very little of it is saturated with the mineral, it could indicate that iron stores are low and/or that not enough iron is currently being taken in.

These same tests can also determine the presence of hemochromatosis, the disease of iron overload. If the readings are too high, a diagnosis of hemochromatosis can be made and patients can periodically have blood withdrawn to reduce their bodies' iron content.

The figures below show what is "normal" and what indicates the presence of iron-deficiency anemia and hemochromatosis. Bear in mind that the cut-off points are not "hard and fast" for a variety of reasons. One is that someone could be "outside" the normal range yet not have any problems with iron status. Conversely, someone could be "inside" normal yet be at some kind of risk. Consider that a 65-year-old man with a serum ferritin reading of 20, while technically within the desired parameters for that measurement, would be considered "low" by a physician because the patient presumably had been adding to his iron stores throughout his life. And a 19-year-old menstruating woman with a serum ferritin of 250 would be considered "high." Her age combined with her monthly blood loss would not normally allow her to build up such significant iron stores.

Various disease states can affect blood measurements as well. Even altitude influences readings. The "normal" hemoglobin range included here is for people living at sea level. In Denver, a city with a high altitude, "normal" is one half to one gram higher. (And in the very high Andes, hemoglobin levels can reach as high as 20 or 21.)

Tests for iron deficiency

Serum ferritin
normal: 20-250 (micrograms per liter of blood)
    low: 12-19
iron-deficiency: fewer than 12
iron-deficiency anemia: fewer than 12 *and* hemoglobin levels below normal (see below)

hemochromatosis: greater than 400; victims are often in the 1,000 to 2,000 range

Transferrin saturation
normal: 16-55 (as a percentage of total iron binding capacity of serum)
iron-deficiency: less than 16
iron-deficiency anemia: less than 16 *and* hemoglobin levels below normal
hemochromatosis: around 62 and above

Tests for anemia (but not specifically iron-deficiency anemia)

Hemoglobin
normal: men, 13.5-18 (grams per 100 milliliters of blood); women, 12.5-17
anemia: levels below normal

Hematocrit
normal: men, 40-54 (as the percentage of red blood cells in the total blood volume); women, 37-47
anemia: levels below normal

The importance of fiber

A healthy diet is usually described negatively—eat less fat, cholesterol, and salt, for instance, or less red meat, eggs, and chips. Yet the same diet can be given a positive slant: eat more fiber in the form of whole grains, fruits, and vegetables. Though interest in high-fiber foods goes back to Hippocrates, our understanding of fiber's health benefits has been greatly enhanced by research done during the last 25 years. Formerly called roughage or bulk, fiber was once thought of primarily as filler—in other words, if you eat high-fiber foods, you'll have less room for high-fat, high-calorie items. That is still seen as one of fiber's potential benefits, as is the fact that it is generally found in foods rich in vitamins and minerals. But scientists now recognize that fiber itself may play a role in reducing the risk of the leading chronic diseases—heart disease, cancer, and diabetes.

To many people, fiber is synonymous with oat bran, thanks to all the ads for oat cereals in recent years. But if you depend on oat bran alone to create a high-fiber diet, you are short-changing yourself. Fiber is hard to pin down because it isn't a single substance, but rather a large group of widely different compounds with varied effects in the body. What all types of fiber have in common is that they are the parts of plants that can't be digested by enzymes in the human intestinal tract. For simplicity, fiber can be divided into two broad categories: those that are insoluble in water and those that are soluble (see chart below). Most foods contain both types in varying amounts, but certain foods are particularly rich in one or the other.

Its benefits

In the late 1960s the British epidemiologist Dr. Denis Burkitt began to link a high-fiber intake among rural Africans with a low incidence of diseases all too common in industrialized Western countries. It has been difficult, however, to prove the protective effects of fiber because fiber isn't consumed in isolation. High-fiber foods may be beneficial because they tend to be low in fat and calories and usually replace meats and other fatty foods that may increase the risk, for instance, of colon cancer or coronary artery disease. Foods rich in fiber also tend to be high in antioxidants (such as beta carotene and vitamin C) and other substances that may protect against a variety of cancers, and it is hard to separate the effect of fiber from the effects of these other components. People who eat high-fiber diets may also make other healthy choices in their lives, such as exercising regularly and not smoking, that may lower their risk for some chronic diseases. In many studies, scientists use statistical techniques to adjust their data for some or most of these complicating factors, but even the best studies can't control for all known variables. Though extremely promising, the evidence concerning fiber's protective effects remains inconclusive, and research is continuing.

Here are some of fiber's proposed benefits:

Colon and rectal cancer. This is one of the leading causes of cancer deaths in the U.S., but is rarer in countries with a diet low in meat and rich in high-fiber foods. Dozens of studies have supported the hypothesis that a fiber-rich diet protects against colon cancer (a few studies have not). One of the strongest pieces of evidence came from New York Hospital in 1989 in a four-year study that found that a diet high in insoluble fiber significantly inhibited the development of precancerous colon and rectal polyps (which tend to gradually enlarge and become malignant) in subjects with an inherited predisposition to them. In January 1992 the *Journal of the National Cancer Institute* published a large study also showing that a high-fiber, low-fat diet helps prevent the growth of precancerous polyps.

No one knows exactly how insoluble fiber may protect against colon cancer, but several theories have been proposed. By moving foods faster through the system, fiber may lessen the exposure of colon walls to potential carcinogens. Or fiber may dilute the carcinogens or inactivate them in some way. Studies have also confirmed that insoluble fiber reduces bile acids in the intestines as well as bacterial enzymes, both of which are possible cancer promoters.

Breast cancer. Research into the effects of fiber on the risk of breast cancer is still in its early stages. A recent study at the American Health Foundation in New York City found that wheat bran (rich in insoluble fiber) reduces blood estrogen levels, which, the researchers theorize, may affect the risk of breast cancer. However, there has been no conclusive evidence from population studies to support this hypothesis. Another theory: when people eat more fiber they tend to eat less fat, and it has been proposed (though never proven) that a high-fat diet increases the risk of breast cancer.

Constipation. Insoluble fiber, consumed with adequate fluids, is the safest, most effective way to prevent or treat

2. NUTRIENTS

TYPE	MAJOR FORMS	EFFECTS	SIGNIFICANT SOURCES
Insoluble fiber	Cellulose, lignin, some hemicellulose	Increases stool bulk, alleviates some digestive disorders, may help prevent colon cancer.	Bran (outer layer) of wheat and corn; skins of fruits and root vegetables; leafy greens.
Soluble fiber	Pectin, gums, some hemicellulose	Lowers blood cholesterol, may help control blood sugar.	Oats, beans, barley, psyllium; many fruits and vegetables, such as apples and citrus fruit.

constipation—by increasing the frequency, bulk, and ease of bowel movements. This fiber is like a sponge: it absorbs many times its weight in water, swelling within the intestines and producing a larger, softer stool that the digestive system can pass quickly and easily. Also, when fiber enters the large intestine, some of it is broken down by bacteria, yielding compounds that in turn produce intestinal gas and initiate bowel movements.

Diverticulosis. About one American in 10 over age 40 and at least one in three over 50 suffers from diverticulosis, a condition in which tiny pouches form within the wall of the colon. When the pouches trap food, they may become painfully inflamed (diverticulitis). Insoluble fiber may help prevent or relieve this painful condition by reducing constipation and strained bowel movements, thus reducing pressure in the colon.

Heart disease. Numerous studies have indicated that soluble fiber (as in oat bran, barley, and fruit pectin) helps reduce total blood cholesterol, primarily by lowering LDL ("bad") cholesterol. The debate continues, however, about how much soluble fiber you have to consume to get a significant reduction—and, again, the typical high-fiber diet is low in fat and that alone may reduce blood cholesterol. Most attention has focused on oatmeal or oat bran, thanks to research funding (and ad campaigns) from cereal companies, but there have also been studies about other sources of soluble fiber, such as grapefruit pectin and apples. Most have shown modest positive effects. But rather than looking at any single food as a magic bullet against cholesterol, you should get your fiber from a variety of sources. Reducing your intake of saturated fat (from fatty meats, whole milk, cheese) and maintaining a healthy weight are even better ways to control blood cholesterol.

Diabetes. Some studies have suggested that soluble fiber improves control of blood sugar and can thus reduce the need for insulin or medication in people with diabetes. Exactly why isn't clear, but soluble fiber (specifically gums and pectin) seems to delay the emptying of the stomach and slow the absorption of glucose in the intestine.

Obesity. Most high-fiber foods are also high in complex carbohydrates (starch) and low in fat—a good combination for weight control. Many take longer to chew, which slows you down at the table. Fiber also fills you up temporarily without adding calories.

Is it safe?
Yes, although eating a large amount of fiber in a short time can result in intestinal gas, bloating, and cramps caused by fermentation of fiber and indigestible sugars in the colon. Usually this isn't serious and subsides once the bacteria in your system adjust to the fiber increase. You can reduce the chances of gas or diarrhea by adding fiber-rich foods *gradually* to your diet.

One potential problem of an extremely high-fiber diet is fiber's ability to bind some trace minerals, such as zinc, iron, magnesium, and even calcium, thus lessening their absorption by the body. This effect is minimal, however, and high-fiber foods tend to be rich enough in minerals to more than compensate for any losses. In contrast, fiber pills, which contain no nutrients, are more likely to create mineral deficiencies in people whose diet is nutritionally poor.

Increasing your intake
Even though it's too early to say for sure whether fiber can cure or even prevent disease, it's clear that a high-fiber, low-fat diet is healthful. Most authorities agree that, on average, Americans should at least double their consumption of dietary fiber—to 20 to 30 grams a day. Some even recommend 40 to 50 grams a day, an amount many vegetarians safely consume. While it helps to be aware of the amount of fiber in various foods (see chart below), these general steps will help ensure an adequate fiber intake:

1. Eat a variety of foods. This will give you both kinds of fiber and all their benefits.

2. Each day eat at least five servings of fruits and vegetables and three to six servings of whole-grain breads, cereals, and legumes (beans). This is likely to give you at least 20 grams

GOOD SOURCE OF INSOLUBLE FIBER	GOOD SOURCE OF SOLUBLE FIBER
More than 5 grams total fiber	
High-fiber wheat-bran cereal (1 oz)	Pinto, kidney, navy beans (dried, cooked, 1/2 cup)
Lentils (dried, cooked, 1/2 cup)	
2 to 5 grams total fiber	
Whole-wheat crackers (6)	Oat bran, oatmeal (dry, 1 oz)
Banana (medium)	Barley (dry, 1 oz)
Potato (medium, with skin)	Berries (1/2 cup)
Buckwheat groats (dry, 1 oz)	Apple, pear (medium, with skin)
Shredded-wheat cereal (1 oz)	Orange, grapefruit (medium)
Brown rice (cooked, 1/2 cup)	Figs, prunes, dried (3)
Brussels sprouts, broccoli, spinach (cooked, 1/2 cup)	Okra, cabbage, peas, turnips, sweet potato (cooked, 1/2 cup)
Wheat germ (3 Tbsp)	Chickpeas, split peas, lima beans (cooked, 1/2 cup)
Whole-wheat flour (1 oz)	
1 to 2 grams total fiber	
Whole-wheat bread (1 slice)	Carrots (cooked, 1/2 cup)
Pasta (cooked, 1 cup)	Peach, nectarine (medium)
Rye bread (1 slice)	Apricots (2)
Corn (1/2 cup)	
Low-fiber wheat cereal (1 oz)	
Cauliflower (cooked, 1/2 cup)	

of fiber a day. **Note:** A serving is not large—just one slice of bread, for instance, or half a cup of beans.

3. The less processed the food, the better. Opt for whole-grain products, such as whole-wheat flour and brown rice. (Remember, "wheat bread" is not whole-wheat unless the label says "whole wheat.") An apple has about twice as much fiber as an equal serving of applesauce, while apple juice has almost none. However, chopping or cooking fruits or vegetables, such as broccoli, won't affect fiber content to any significant degree.

4. Eat the skin of fruits and vegetables, when possible. A potato with skin has twice as much fiber as one without. Fruits with edible seeds, such as raspberries and figs, tend to contain lots of fiber.

5. Get your fiber from food, rather than from pills or powders. Bulk laxatives (high in fiber) may be safe and effective against constipation, but lack the nutrients found in fiber-rich foods.

6. Spread out your fiber intake. Getting all your fiber at one meal may reduce the benefits and increase the chance of unpleasant side effects.

7. Drink plenty of liquids.

High-fiber foods

Until a few years ago, chemists could measure only insoluble fiber, and the result was called "crude fiber." Better laboratory techniques now provide a more complete measurement of fiber, called "dietary fiber," which includes the soluble as well as the insoluble kind. Still, there is as yet no single "correct" way to measure dietary fiber, so results from different labs can vary substantially. Currently, manufacturers are not required to list fiber on nutrition labels unless they make a claim concerning it. New labeling regulations proposed by the FDA would require dietary fiber content to be listed on more labels.

Virtually all fruits, vegetables, and whole-grain products contain some of both types of fiber. The foods [in chart] are particularly good sources.

Through the Life Span: Diet and Disease

Food improperly taken, not only produces diseases, but affords those that are already engendered both matter and sustenance; so that, let the father of disease be what it may, intemperance is its mother.

—Richard E. Burton

When someone says "You are what you eat," is it literally true? In *Let's Eat Right to Keep Fit* (New York: The New American Library, 1970), Adelle Davis claims that one will not age on the days one eats right. Present evidence disagrees. Still, scientists believe that, within limits, what we eat affects what we are in both direct and indirect ways. An illustration from World War II is provided by Harry Golden (*Only in America*, Cleveland, Ohio: The World Publishing Company, 1958, p. 308):

When the Nazis took Denmark they requisitioned everything the Danes produced. The Danes, as you know, are famous dairy farmers and the Nazis took all their butter, animal fats, cheese, and allied products for their own armies. During that period the Danes were forced to lead an austere life and lived mostly on black bread and fish. What they have found out since is that during that austere period the incidence of degenerative diseases went way down— the Danes lived longer—but when the Danes got their butter, cheese, and animal fats back, the health chart went back to "normal" with a tremendous increase in stomach, heart, blood, and vein diseases. It is all a matter of diet, and I should hang my head in shame, being as fat as I am, and with no fewer than eleven thousand stories yet to write.

Studies of populations in other countries, as in the quote above, often provide clues to diet/disease connections. Researchers must interpret them cautiously, however, as such studies cannot prove cause and effect relationships and sometimes appear contradictory.

It is commonly agreed that a good (balanced) diet is important throughout life. But what is it? Many popular admonitions about what to eat and what to avoid have led to a good food/bad food philosophy. Chocolate is bad for you and will make you fat, but carrots are good. A thoughtful person may realize that no food is inherently good or bad, that it is quantity eaten that is problematic or beneficial. Thus moderation is a key concept. Add variety in what is eaten, and one is well on the way to a good diet. For more information, review the new food guide pyramid in article 5, unit 1.

The articles in this unit were selected because they concern the health of specific groups of people. In all cases, knowledge and commitment can help one avoid the health and dietary pitfalls of either omission or commission. Eating disorders (see article 25), in their many variations and combinations of bulimia and anorexia, are a particular hazard for teenage females, but younger and younger children, as well, are showing strong compulsions to diet. While causation is still theoretical, such behavior clearly becomes obsessive and may lead to permanent body damage as well as starvation and suicide.

Today most of us can look forward to living longer than our parents. About 13 percent of the U.S. population is age 65 or older; by the year 2000 it will be 15 percent or more. People hope to reach their genetic potentials and avoid disease, premature aging, and untimely death. Article 26 discusses the higher risks of malnutrition in the elderly and the challenges to find solutions as aging people lose interest and resources.

From childhood we have been admonished to eat a good breakfast, and we have responded with various degrees of enthusiasm. There is scientific support for this practice. Among children, breakfast improves the total daily nutrient intake, enhances the ability to learn and do well on tests, and reduces tardiness and absenteeism. For the rest of us, breakfast improves our strength and endurance in the late morning and promotes a better work attitude as well (see article 27).

Increasing numbers of Americans in all age groups are turning to vegetarian diets in the hope of avoiding whatever excesses contribute to chronic diseases. Since 1985 the numbers of vegetarians have risen from 6.5 million to 12.4 million, or 5 percent of the population. Certain benefits appear to be quite conclusive, as indicated in "Benefits and Risks of Vegetarian Diets," but there are risks that must be considered and avoided.

Disease, as well as health, is part of life, and some diseases have a clear association with nutrition. Nutrition may be only one factor, but, where a connection to food and nutrition is proved or suspected, prevention is clearly the emphasis today. One obvious example is heart disease, which is still a major concern, although mortality rates have declined over 20 percent since 1980. Consumers know that there is a link to cholesterol, but they are still confused about the relationship of dietary and blood cholesterols and the greater effects of saturated fat. Add terms such as HDLs and LDLs, mono- and polyunsaturated fats, and tropical oils to the discussion, and total confusion is likely. Article 29 is very useful in clarifying these issues.

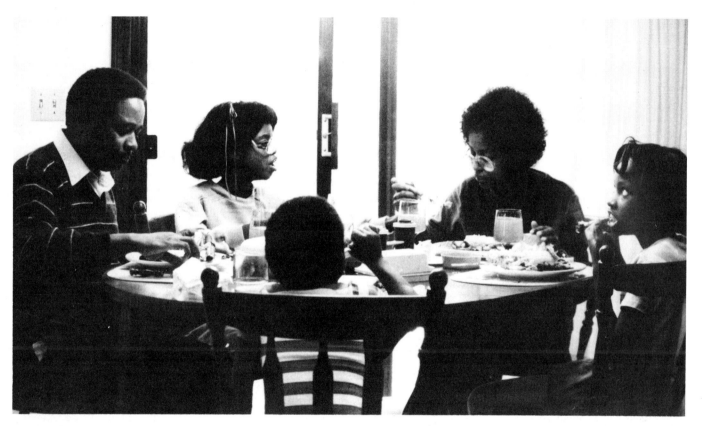

"A Lifelong Program to Build Strong Bones" addresses the connection between calcium and osteoporosis, the bone disease resulting in body stoop, porous bones, and hip fractures. Popular news sources and advertising constantly advise taking supplements. Calcium, especially dietary calcium, is important as a means of prevention, although its greatest contribution (when bone density can be increased) occurs well before menopause. After menopause, replacement estrogen appears to be the primary key to bone preservation in women, but calcium intake is still important and exercise must be emphasized.

Articles on two more significant health issues, hypertension and cancer, conclude this unit. Controversy remains over the practical significance of some of the current research, and critics often argue that avoiding excesses and eating a well-rounded diet is still the only sensible approach. One should remember that there is still much we do not know and that people are physiologically different. Connections between food/nutrition and health can be found in other units in this book.

Articles on vitamins and other nutrients are in unit 2, food-borne illness is dealt with in unit 5, and unit 6 discusses misinformation leading to harmful dietary practices. The reader should also review articles in previous *Annual Editions* and in reliable periodicals to fully appreciate the extent of the information and the confusion.

Looking Ahead: Challenge Questions

Pretend that you are planning research relative to nutrition and your age group. Rank order your top three priorities and defend them.

If you suspect that a friend has an eating disorder, what steps should you take?

Plan healthful breakfasts that you would eat and could eat "on the run."

What changes should you make in your daily diet to conform to the best current knowledge about heart disease, cancer, hypertension, and osteoporosis? Make a plan to do this.

EaTing DisOrdeRS
Require Medical Attention

Dixie Farley

Dixie Farley is a staff writer for FDA Consumer.

For reasons that are unclear, some people—mainly young women—develop potentially life-threatening eating disorders called bulimia nervosa and anorexia nervosa. People with bulimia, known as bulimics, indulge in bingeing (episodes of eating large amounts of food) and purging (getting rid of the food by vomiting or using laxatives). People with anorexia, whom doctors sometimes call anorectics, severely limit their food intake. About half of them also have bulimia symptoms.

The National Center for Health Statistics (NCHS) estimates that 10,000 bulimia cases and 11,000 anorexia cases were diagnosed in 1989, the latest year for which statistics are available. Studies indicate that by their first year of college, 4.5 to 18 percent of women and 0.4 percent of men have a history of bulimia and that as many as 1 in 100 females between the ages of 12 and 18 have anorexia.

Males account for only 5 to 10 percent of bulimia and anorexia cases. While people of all races develop the disorders, the vast majority of those diagnosed are white.

Most people find it difficult to stop their bulimic or anorectic behavior without professional help. If untreated, the disorders may become chronic and lead to severe health problems, even death. NCHS reports 67 deaths from anorexia in 1988, the latest year for which it has figures, but does not have similar information on bulimia.

As to the causes of bulimia and anorexia, there are many theories. One is that some young women feel abnormally pressured to be as thin as the "ideal" portrayed by magazines, movies and television. Another is that defects in key chemical messengers in the brain may contribute to the disorders' development or persistence.

The Bulimia Secret

Once people begin bingeing and purging, usually in conjunction with a diet, the cycle easily gets out of control. While cases tend to develop during the teens or early 20s, many bulimics successfully hide their symptoms, thereby delaying help until they reach their 30s or 40s. Several years ago, actress Jane Fonda revealed she had been a secret bulimic from age 12 until her recovery at 35. She told of bingeing and purging up to 20 times a day.

Many people with bulimia maintain a nearly normal weight. Though they appear healthy and successful—"perfectionists" at whatever they do—in reality, they have low self-esteem and are often depressed. They may exhibit other compulsive behaviors. For example, one physician reports that a third of his bulimia patients regularly engage in shoplifting and that a quarter of the patients have suffered from alcohol abuse or addiction at some point in their lives.

While normal food intake for a teenager is 2,000 to 3,000 calories in a day, bulimic binges average about 3,400 calories in 1 1/4 hours, according to one study. Some bulimics consume up to 20,000 calories in binges lasting as long as eight hours. Some spend $50 or more a day on food and may resort to stealing food or money to support their obsession.

To lose the weight gained during a binge, bulimics begin purging by vomiting (by self-induced gagging or with an emetic, a substance that causes vomiting) or by using laxatives (50 to 100 tablets at a time), diuretics (drugs that increase urination), or enemas. Between binges, they may fast or exercise excessively.

Extreme purging rapidly upsets the body's balance of sodium, potassium, and other chemicals. This can cause fatigue, seizures, irregular heartbeat, and thinner bones. Repeated vomiting can damage the stomach and esophagus (the tube that carries food to the stomach), make the gums recede, and erode tooth enamel. (Some patients need all their teeth pulled prematurely). Other effects include various skin rashes, broken blood vessels in the face, and irregular menstrual cycles.

Complexities of Anorexia

While anorexia most commonly begins in the teens, it can start at any age and has been reported from age 5 to 60. Incidence among 8- to 11-year-olds is said to be increasing.

Anorexia may be a single, limited episode with large weight loss within a few months followed by recovery. Or it may develop gradually and persist for years. The illness may go back and forth be-

Reprinted from *FDA Consumer,* March 1992, pp. 27-29.

Disorders' Definitions

According to the American Psychiatric Association, a person diagnosed as bulimic or anorectic must have all of that disorder's specific symptoms:

Bulimia Nervosa
• recurrent episodes of binge eating (minimum average of two binge-eating episodes a week for at least three months)
• a feeling of lack of control over eating during the binges
• regular use of one or more of the following to prevent weight gain: self-induced vomiting, use of laxatives or diuretics, strict dieting or fasting, or vigorous exercise
• persistent over-concern with body shape and weight.

Anorexia Nervosa
• refusal to maintain weight that's over the lowest weight considered normal for age and height
• intense fear of gaining weight or becoming fat, even though underweight
• distorted body image
• in women, three consecutive missed menstrual periods without pregnancy.

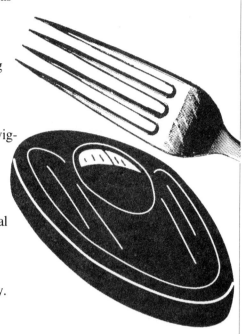

tween getting better and getting worse. Or it may steadily get more severe.

Anorectics may exercise excessively. Their preoccupation with food usually prompts habits such as moving food about on the plate and cutting it into tiny pieces to prolong eating, and not eating with the family.

Obsessed with weight loss and fear of becoming fat, anorectics see normal folds of flesh as "fat" that must be eliminated. When the normal fat padding is lost, sitting or lying down brings discomfort not rest, making sleep difficult. As the disorder continues, victims may become isolated and withdraw from friends and family.

The body responds to starvation by slowing or stopping certain bodily processes. Blood pressure falls, breathing rate slows, menstruation ceases (or, in girls in their early teens, never begins), and activity of the thyroid gland (which regulates growth) diminishes. Skin becomes dry, and hair and nails become brittle. Lightheadedness, cold intolerance, constipation, and joint swelling are other symptoms. Reduced fat causes the body temperature to fall. Soft hair called lanugo forms on the skin for warmth. Body chemicals may get so imbalanced that heart failure occurs.

Anorectics who additionally binge and purge impair their health even further. The late recording artist Karen Carpenter, an anorectic who used syrup of ipecac to induce vomiting, died after buildup of the drug irreversibly damaged her heart.

Getting Help

Early treatment is vital. As either disorder becomes more entrenched, its damage becomes less reversible.

Usually, the family is asked to help in the treatment, which may include psychotherapy, nutrition counseling, behavior modification, and self-help groups. Therapy often lasts a year or more—on an outpatient basis unless life-threatening physical symptoms or severe psychological problems require hospitalization. If there is deterioration or no response to therapy, the patient (or parent or other advocate) may want to talk to the health professional about the plan of treatment.

There are no drugs approved specifically for bulimia or anorexia, but several, including some antidepressants, are being investigated for this use.

If you think a friend or family member has bulimia or anorexia, point out in a caring, nonjudgmental way the behavior you have observed and encourage the person

to get medical help. If you think you have bulimia or anorexia, remember that you are not alone and that this is a health problem that requires professional help. As a first step, talk to your parents, family doctor, religious counselor, or school counselor or nurse.

For More Information

If you want more information about bulimia and anorexia, send your request and a stamped, self-addressed, business-size envelope to:

American Anorexia/Bulimia
 Association, Inc.
418 E. 76th St.
New York, NY 10021
(212)734-1114

Bulimia, Anorexia Self-Help
6125 Clayton Ave., Suite 215
St. Louis, Mo. 63139
(1-800)227-4785

National Association of Anorexia
 Nervosa and Associated Disorders,
 Inc.
P.O. Box 7
Highland Park, Ill. 60035
(708)831-3438

Nutrition and the Elderly

Alexandra Greeley

Alexandra Greeley is a freelance writer in Reston, Va., who has written on nutrition for Time-Life Books, The New York Times, Newsday, *and the* South China Post.

We all know a Norma Kramer—an older person whose life has slowly started to come apart—a widow living alone who in her depression eats sparsely. Her adult son drops by for dinner one night a week, but that may be her only substantial meal until his next visit. Finally, because she can no longer live well enough alone, Norma Kramer moves into a senior citizen's residence.

Outgoing now and healthy except for painful arthritis—72-year-old Kramer lives at the Har Sinai West senior highrise in Baltimore, Md. She looks forward each day to the Eating Together in Baltimore breakfast and lunch program at the residence—for there, not only can she gossip with friends, she also can eat wholesome, hot meals that fortify her.

Kramer's story is true, and altogether too common, repeated in varying versions everywhere by people who worry about aging relatives or friends. Without proper supervision, many millions of older Americans exist in a nutritional twilight zone, grappling with the daily challenge of eating—and often not eating well-balanced meals or any meals at all.

A recent survey completed for the new Nutrition Screening Initiative (sponsored by Ross Laboratories)—targeted at improving the nutritional health status of the aging—shows that while 85 percent of seniors surveyed believe nutrition is important for their health and well-being, few act on their beliefs. Further, 30 percent admit they skip at least one meal a day. These numbers may well soar, as America continues to gray at an escalating rate.

"Twelve percent of the population of the United States is now age 65 or older," says Jeffrey Blumberg, Ph.D., associate director of the USDA Human Nutrition Research Center of Aging at Tufts University. "But in 30 years, the figure will be closer to 20 percent."

Higher Risk of Malnutrition

Sound nutrition plays a major role in good health for people of any age. But, says Paul Kerschner, senior vice president of the National Council on the Aging in Washington, D.C., seniors tend to be at a disproportionate risk of poor nutrition that can adversely affect their health. He describes the unacceptably high levels of poor nutrition and malnutrition among the elderly, which range from 15 to 50 percent. He says the problem is particularly pronounced among those living in institutional settings.

To make matters worse, often the signs and symptoms of malnutrition can baffle and mislead even the professionals. For example, weight loss, lightheadedness, disorientation, lethargy, and loss of appetite are often diagnosed as illness, says Colleen Pierre, American Dietetic Association ambassador and director of the Eating Together in Baltimore program. "What the person really needs is to eat better," she says.

Responding to the widespread gap in nutrition knowledge, the American Academy of Family Physicians, the American Dietetic Association, and the National Council on the Aging have joined forces to promote the Washington, D.C.-based Nutrition Screening Initiative.

Kerschner says that the hoped-for goal of this five-year initiative is to "start good nutritional habits that will forestall inappropriate acute and institutional care and will help people age well and keep in better health." The campaign was initiated, he continues, because the nutritional status of older people was being ignored, not only by older people themselves, but also by the health-care community.

One other goal of the program, he continues, is to point out to institutions that eating is a major part of people's lives. "Even institutions that serve good meals don't present them as part of therapy," Kerschner says. Dietitians and nurses need to realize that meals at any age are an important part of daily life, whether people live at home or in an institution. So just presenting food, then taking it away when a person is finished, doesn't help the person learn good nutritional habits, he says.

A Complex Challenge

Unfortunately, encouraging older citizens to eat well and to pay serious attention to sound nutrition is a complex challenge with no single, simple solution. For one thing, the aging process itself becomes a real barrier, explains Blumberg. As many people age, he says, their biological clock winds down and they also start to lose lean body mass.

Consequently, their interest in food—and their appetites for it —tends to diminish so people cut back on calories. But that's not okay, says Blumberg. "Requirements for many nutrients don't diminish," he says, "and they may even increase with age. Eating less presents real problems leading to deficiency." For example, he says, requirements for vitamin B_6 actually increase for older people. "We find that when people are in a depleted but not a deficiency state, there are cognitive changes, changes in the immune systems, and deficits in sensitivity to insulin," he says. But an increase in B_6 intake corrects the problems.

Health declines have "a cascading effect," says pathologist Philip Garry, professor at University of New Mexico School of Medicine. But after studying 300 older adults from the ages of 65 to 93, Garry has concluded that even the process of aging itself may be retarded through behavioral changes.

"You really can slow aging down through eating well, exercising properly, keeping positive, and staying active," he says. "We don't see much change in them [the people in the study] due to aging," he continues, because very few of the people in his New Mexico Aging Process study are sedentary, have memory loss, or are on medications or overweight. "So they are going on in life like they did when they were much younger," he says, telling of a spry 80-year-old man in the study who works as a ski instructor. "The only time we see a dramatic change in someone is when something acute happens, such as a fall. That

Reprinted from *FDA Consumer*, Vol. 24, No. 8, October 1990, pp. 25-26, 28, by permission.

may precipitate a change in the dietary lifestyle," he says.

The reasons seniors shun balanced fare results from more than natural metabolic changes, of course: Some of these other factors are not so obvious. Loneliness, for example, can cripple the person who has always lived with a spouse or other family members, and it seems to hit older men particularly hard, reports Suzanne Murphy, nutritionist at University of California at Berkeley, and co-researcher of a study on the living arrangements and dietary quality of older adults in the United States, funded by the National Institute on Aging.

Without cooking or shopping skills, men may eat less or skip meals altogether. Women living alone may simply grow tired of kitchen duty and lose interest in eating. "Older Americans are at risk," she says, "but single older Americans are at greater risk." Depression—often linked to loneliness—may likewise curtail a person's interest in food.

Sensory Decline

Another roadblock to eating well is the decline in the sense of smell that directly affects a person's ability to taste—and enjoy—food. "We once believed that older people didn't eat well because of their decline in taste and taste buds," says James Weiffenbach, Ph.D., research psychologist, Clinical Investigation and Patient Care Branch, National Institute of Dental Research, National Institutes of Health in Bethesda, Md. "Taste and smell as a sensory system do affect eating. But the ability to taste remains fairly intact with age. It's the decline in the ability to smell that seems to be responsible for 'taste' complaints," he says.

Weiffenbach points out that older people have trouble identifying puréed foods. Though younger people do much better under usual circumstances, when holding their noses while eating, they are no better at identifying foods than older people. In essence, he says, you can't taste if you don't smell—smell is the real factor in the enjoyment of food.

Money worries play a large role, too. After people retire, their incomes often dwindle, forcing them to make some hard cutbacks in their budgets. The one area that usually cuts most easily is the food allowance.

In addition, certain medications can kill appetites or taste sensations. Or people may wear ill-fitting dentures that make chewing meats and fibrous vegetables difficult. Perhaps failing eyesight

causes meals to look less appealing and makes reading food labels difficult. Perhaps, too, disease or broken bones limit mobility so that shopping or cooking becomes an unwelcome chore.

Weakness is another factor. How, asks Gail Martin, assistant administrative director of the National Association of Meal Programs (which represents Meals on Wheels), Washington, D.C., can a frail elderly person carry home a heavy bag of groceries, particularly if that home is six blocks away and that person has no cab fare?

Unlike years ago, when all tradesmen came to the door, she continues, shopping today is more difficult. Shoppers generally must leave home, usually by car, to buy their provisions. "If you are 85 years old and have a car," she says, "you must be able to drive it and handle it well enough to maneuver shopping mall parking lots. And you'll probably have to park at a distance from the store. There are obstacles for those even in the best of health. Our society has not thought through how older people are going to live and make it."

Practical Suggestions

While most experts express dismay at the situation, they all offer practical suggestions that almost every aging American can follow. For one, Blumberg suggests, simply taking supplements can help. "By the time someone is old, the consequences of inappropriate nutrition are hard to void," he explains. "But it's not too late to start to reduce the risk. I know of only one ready alternative, and that's to take supplements. Others talk about fortifying foods. But if the vitamin D requirement for an older person really is two to three times higher than the current allowance, it may not be realistic to tell a 65-year-old woman to drink five glasses of milk a day." Of course, he cautions, supplements in large amounts can be toxic.

Another expert, however, does not advise the use of supplements. "I hate to make a recommendation for supplements," says Jean Pennington, associate director for dietary surveillance at the Food and Drug Administration's Center for Food Safety and Applied Nutrition, "unless in special cases when there is an illness or a physiological reason. Then a supplement might be indicated."

Generally, she adds, most people get adequate nutrients from the food supply. But if they can't or don't, she says, then

supplements taken should not be greatly in excess of the RDA for that nutrient. Or, she continues, people should pay much closer attention to what they are eating and should select the most nutritious foods possible. "People should make the proper selection from the four basics," she says, "and should place more emphasis on grains and vegetables."

Enhancing food aromas is another way to stimulate appetite. "The parts of the brain for taste and smell are also connected to hunger/satiety," says Susan Schiffman of the Duke University Medical Center, Department of Psychology. "For example, if you stop eating a meal, you do so because your sense of taste and smell are satisfied; it's not that you feel full yet," she says. . . .

She explains that seniors can intensify tastes by adding flavors and sweeteners, like herbs (not spices, which may irritate), maple syrup, bacon bits, and butter flavoring. They also can heighten the appeal of their foods by "switching from food to food while eating. That keeps up sensory interest," she says. And when preparing meals, she suggests that seniors combine different textures to make food more appetizing—for example, putting crunchy Grapenuts on smooth frozen yogurt. . . .

But perhaps the key to better eating lies not so much with the mechanics of food preparation as with the social aspects of eating. As most experts agree, mealtimes should be social occasions, spent eating in the company of others, whenever possible. If need be, senior citizens, particularly those living alone, should join a community group-dining program. . . .

Pennington adds that using a feeding service to bring meals in to homebound seniors would ensure better nutrition—and presumably provide some mealtime socialization.

Until the problem hits home, most people may not worry about how an older person eats. But research confirms that we really are—at least to a large degree—what we eat. If older people have not laid a good nutrition foundation early in life, says Blumberg, they may be at risk for various chronic diseases, including heart attacks, artherosclerosis, cancer, diabetes, and osteoporosis. And if they continue to subsist on less than wholesome foods, they jeopardize quality of life. "Nutrition," concludes Blumberg, "must be a lifelong process."

Breakfast

Waking Up To a Healthy Start

Waking up is hard to do. It's especially difficult for those "non-morning" people who'd probably like to avoid that time of day and everything that comes with it — even breakfast.

But as sure as the sun's gonna shine, breakfast always will be an important meal of the day — one that should be consumed by people of any age.

Although all three traditional meals play a significant role in supplying the daily recommended levels of essential nutrients, nutritionists often cite breakfast as the day's *most* important meal and the foundation of healthy eating habits.

Despite these recommendations, millions of Americans routinely skip breakfast. According to a 1987 report in *Cereal Foods World*, one out of four women between the ages of 25 and 34 regularly skips breakfast. Other studies show that eating habits developed during childhood have the potential to last a lifetime. Thus children who tend to omit breakfast most likely will continue this dietary habit well into adulthood.

But a review of breakfast-related research over the last 30 years may make even the tried-and-true breakfast skipper into a breakfast convert.

Studies have shown that eating breakfast is associated with improved strength and endurance in the late

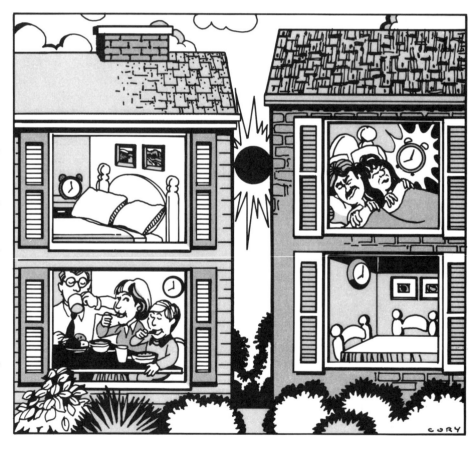

morning, along with a better attitude toward school or work.

Breakfast helps to replenish blood glucose levels, which is important since the brain itself has no reserves of glucose, its main energy source, and constantly must be replenished.

Studies show that sustained mental work requires large turnover of brain glucose and its metabolic components.

"When you consider it's been eight or nine hours since you've had a meal, it's obvious that refueling at

From *Food Insight,* March/April 1992, pp. 1, 4-5. Reproduced with permission of *Food Insight,* a publication of the International Food Information Council Foundation.

breakfast will make you feel and perform better during the day," said Diane Odland, nutritionist at the U.S. Department of Agriculture Human Nutrition Information Service.

Researchers at the University of Health Sciences/Chicago Medical School agree. They examined whether eating breakfast has any advantageous effects on late-morning mood, satiety or cognitive performance.

Forty normal-weight adults participated in the breakfast study, all of whom normally ate breakfast. Subjects fasted overnight and came to the laboratory in the early morning to perform baseline tests that measured reasoning, inference and problem-solving.

While one-third of subjects continued fasting, others ate one of two breakfasts that each contained 450-500 calories. In the high-fiber "balanced" breakfast, 59 percent of calories were supplied by carbohydrates and roughly 20 percent of calories were supplied by protein and fat each. In the low-fiber "unbalanced" breakfast, 61 percent of calories came from carbohydrates, 35 percent were supplied by fat and 4 percent were supplied by protein.

Study Results

Participants were tested for cognitive performance 30 minutes after mealtime, and then two hours and four hours later. Results confirmed that eating breakfast of either nutritional composition was beneficial. Skipping breakfast consistently caused hunger and led to performance difficulties on tasks requiring concentration.

"Eating breakfast of any kind prevented many of the adverse effects of fasting," such as irritability and fatigue, according to principal investigator, Bonnie Spring, Ph.D. Spring added that those who ate the balanced breakfast scored significantly higher on tests than those who ate the unbalanced breakfast.

In terms of suppressing hunger, the balanced breakfast also was most effective. The unbalanced breakfast

Breakfast Tips

Avoid the temptation to be a breakfast skipper by following these quick tips from USDA's Human Nutrition Information Service:

▲ **No time? Build a breakfast around foods that are ready to eat or take little preparation time. There are plenty that qualify: fresh and canned fruits, milk, yogurt, cheese, cottage cheese, ready-to-eat cold cereals and instant breakfast mixes.**

▲ **Take it to go... Try celery stuffed with peanut butter or a meat or cheese spread, dried fruits or vegetable juices.**

▲ **Perk up cereals... Top cereals with fruit or stir chopped nuts such as peanuts, pecans and walnuts into cooked cereal.**

▲ **Not hungry yet? Drink juice. Something is better than nothing. Have some bread or crackers later in the morning, then drink some milk and eat some cheese, an egg or peanut butter.**

▲ **Don't skip if you're on a diet. There's no evidence that skipping meals will help you lose weight. In fact, studies show that most people who skip breakfast tend to eat more later in the day. Some even select more calorically-dense foods than those who eat breakfast. ■**

suppressed hunger only relative to fasting; but four hours later, those who ate the unbalanced breakfast were as hungry as those who fasted.

School Breakfast Program

The potential role of breakfast in helping children perform at peak capacity in the classroom was first documented more than 30 years ago at the University of Iowa Medical College. Researchers found that children who skipped breakfast had trouble concentrating at school and became inattentive and restless by late morning. These behavior problems were linked to low blood sugar levels, which had never been replenished by a morning meal and allowed fatigue, irritability and restlessness to develop. Such behaviors are counterproductive to learning.

These and other findings helped confirm the hypothesis that children who go to school hungry cannot perform well. To address this problem, Congress enacted the school breakfast program as part of the Child Nutrition Act of 1966.

Today, nearly 37,000 schools

nationwide offer the breakfast program, reaching a total of 4 million children daily. The federal subsidy allows schools to make breakfasts that meet certain nutritional guidelines available to children on a reduced-cost basis, or free to those from low-income families.

In addition to improved cognitive functioning, breakfast has been shown to have other benefits. A 1987 study of third to sixth grade Massachusetts schoolchildren found that children participating in a school breakfast program had improved test scores as well as reduced rates of tardiness and absenteeism.

How does breakfast impact adults? Much of the breakfast research on adults has focused on this meal's overall nutritional contribution to the daily diet.

Breakfast and Nutrition

Researchers at USDA's Human Nutrition Research Center on Aging at Tufts University analyzed three-day diet records of 650 Boston area senior citizens to find what foods contributed the most calories in their

3. THROUGH THE LIFE SPAN: DIET AND DISEASE

diets. Selecting optimal diets are critical to the aged, many of whom are trying to lose or control their weight for effective disease management. Other elderly, however, are at risk for undernutrition due to social and physical problems.

Of the various eating patterns that emerged, the diet in which most of the breakfast calories were supplied by cereal, milk and fruit provided the best nutritional profile overall among those tested. According to Tufts researcher Katherine Tucker, Ph.D., the vitamin-fortified breakfast cereals, as well as the vitamins in milk, helped participants reach the recommended dietary allowances for calcium and vitamins B6, riboflavin and folate.

The nutritional benefits of breakfast cereals also were shown in a recent survey of more than 4,000 households by General Mills, Inc. Adults who ate cereal for breakfast consumed an average of 10 percent fewer calories than those who selected other breakfast foods, with only 20 percent of their calories coming from fat.

Moreover, those who ate cereal for breakfast maintained a better nutritional profile over the entire day than when they opted for other breakfast menus. For example, on days when participants ate cereal for breakfast, they ate fewer calories from fat throughout the day and 40 percent less cholesterol. They also consumed 20 percent more of essential vitamins and minerals than on non-cereal days.

Thus, for kids as well as adults, balanced breakfast choices can help provide the healthy edge needed for optimum physical and cognitive performance. For those who don't yet consume breakfast, it's never too late to wake up to a healthy start.

BENEFITS AND RISKS OF VEGETARIAN DIETS

Susan Digott, M.S., R.D.
Johanna Dwyer, ScD., R.D.

Ms. Dingott is a staff nutritionist at New England Memorial Hospital, Stoneham, Massachusetts. Dr. Dwyer is director of the Frances Stern Nutrition Center, New England Medical Center Hospitals, and professor of medicine (nutrition) and community health at Tufts University Medical School. This article was prepared with partial support from grants MCJ8241 and MCJ9120 from the MCH Service, U.S. Dept. of Health and Human Services.

The eating patterns and health practices of vegetarians are as diverse as those of nonvegetarians (omnivores). Table 1 shows how vegetarians differ in the types of animal foods they eat. Vegetarians also vary in their attitudes towards supplementation, conventional medicine, and many other matters that may affect their health. Thus there are hundreds if not thousands of ways to be vegetarian.

To be safe from a nutritional standpoint, any eating pattern, vegetarian or otherwise, must provide balance, variety, and moderation. It must meet special nutrient needs that arise during infancy, adolescence, pregnancy, lactation, and other stages of life. It must accommodate special therapeutic consid-erations that individuals with certain health problems may require. It should also reduce risks of diet-related diseases.

Considerable agreement exists among experts about the dietary patterns that lower chronic disease risks. The American Heart Association, American Cancer Society, National Cholesterol Education Program, and Committee on Diet and Health of the National Research Council all recommend that adults reduce fat consumption to 30% of calories, with no more than 10% of calories as saturated fat. Some vegetarians—especially those who eat no animal foods at all—achieve these recommended intakes better than most omnivores [Am J Clin Nutr 48:712-738, 1988]. However, vegan diets may fall short in certain nutrients unless they are carefully planned.

Table 2 summarizes some of the positive aspects of vegetarian eating. But ill-planned vegetarian diets pose substantial risks (see Table 3). Problems most commonly occur with vegan diets because vegans eliminate all animal foods and may also avoid foods that are processed or not "organically grown." Vegans often refuse to use supplements and may eschew

TABLE 1. TYPES OF VEGETARIAN DIETS

Type	Prohibited Foods	Typical Health Practices
Vegan	Meat, fish, poultry, eggs, dairy products	Vegans tend to be physically active, avoid drugs and tobacco products, and rely on unconventional rather than conventional health care. Exceptions include macrobiotics who often smoke cigarettes and Rastafarians who smoke marijuana.
Lactovegetarian Lacto-ovo-vegetarian Semivegetarian	Meat, fish, poultry, eggs Meat, fish, poultry Meat, but may include small amounts of fish and poultry in the diet	Varies from group to group. Some use vitamin and mineral products; others do not. More likely than omnivores to be physically active and not smoke or use alcohol. Links to conventional health care system tend to be stronger than those of vegans.

From *Nutrition Forum*, Vol. 8, No. 8, November/December 1991, p. 45-47. Reprinted with permission from *Nutrition Forum Newsletter,* now published by Stephen Barrett, M.D., P. O. Box 1747, Allentown, PA 18105.

3. THROUGH THE LIFE SPAN: DIET AND DISEASE

conventional medical care as well [Am J Clin Nutr 48:811-818, 1988].

One danger of vegan diets is insufficient energy intake (calories), especially during infancy and early childhood. If energy needs are not met, body proteins will be broken down for energy, and this creates additional problems [Ann Rev Nut 11:61-92, 1991]. Therefore, adequate energy intake should be the foremost consideration in vegan dietary planning.

Low protein digestibility and quality are other potential risks. Protein quality depends on both digestibility and amino acid composition. The digestibility of protein in the usual American mixed diet is good, probably 95% to 96%. But plant protein foods high in fiber or other inhibitors may have

digestibilities as low as 80% [World Health Organization Technical Report 724, 1985]. The digestibility of one vegetable protein in one child's vegan diet was found to be only 86% [Am J Clin Nutr 48:868-874, 1988]. Low protein quality is rarely seen in American vegetarian diets, except among vegans or fruitarians who eat small amounts of a single plant food (such as rice or fruit) as a staple. Single plant protein foods usually are lower in protein quality than most animal proteins because they lack significant amounts of various essential amino acids. Table 4 indicates the limiting amino acids (the essential amino acids present in shortest supply) in foods commonly consumed by vegetarians.

Plant foods low in particular amino acids can be com-

TABLE 2. POSSIBLE BENEFITS OF VEGETARIAN EATING

Characteristic	Comments/Possible Mechanisms
Leanness	Vegetarians tend to be more physically active than nonvegetarians [Am J Public Health 79:1283-1288, 1989]. Higher intakes of dietary fiber may decrease absorption of food by 2-3 % and contribute to a feeling of fullness.
Lower blood pressure	Vegans, who consume a diet very low in fat, tend to have blood pressures 10–15 mm Hg lower than nonvegetarians of similar age and gender. Much of this effect appears to be related to body weight rather than other dietary variables [Am J Clin Nutr 48:795-800, 1989].
Lower serum cholesterol	Total blood cholesterol levels are lower in vegans than in lactovegetarians or nonvegetarians. Whole-fat milk products and eggs tend to raise serum blood lipids due to their saturated fat and cholesterol content. Vegetarians often use non-fat or lowfat milk, and vegans use no milk or eggs at all [Am J Clin Nutr 48:712-738, 1988].
Less colon cancer?	Diets high in animal foods may increase the incidence of colon cancer by increasing the fecal concentration of various carcinogens [Nature 294:453-456, 1981, Br J Cancer 28:94, 1973]. A high intake of animal fat may increase the risk of colon cancer [N Engl J Med 323:1664-1672, 1990]. It also is possible that carcinogens are produced by cooking meat at very high temperatures.

TABLE 3. POSSIBLE RISKS OF VEGETARIAN EATING

Risk	Comments
Osteoporosis	There is little evidence that a vegetarian diet causes or cures osteoporosis. One recent study of 290 postmenopausal women found no differences in the measurements of bone mineralization between nonvegetarians and lacto-ovo-vegetarians [Am J Clin Nutr 50:517-523, 1989].
Rickets	Vegan children who have limited sun exposure may be at risk of developing rickets secondary to vitamin D deficiency. One study found very low intakes of calcium and vitamin D among macrobiotic infants. Only one received a daily supplement of vitamin D, and 15 (28%) were found to have rickets [Am J Clin Nutr 47:89-92, 1988]. Another study found low serum concentrations of vitamin D among lactating macrobiotic women in Boston [Obstet Gynecol 70:870-874, 1987].
Iron-deficiency anemia	In one recent study, low serum ferritin levels (a sensitive measure of iron storage status) were found in 5% of male and 27% of female lacto-ovo-vegetarians, and mean ferritin levels of omnivores were significantly higher than those of vegetarians [Am J Clin Nutr 45:785-789,1987].
Macrocytic anemia	Signs of vitamin B-12 deficiency have been observed in some breast-fed infants of women who are strict vegetarians [Am J Clin Nutr 47:89-92 1988].
Emaciation or slowed growth	Excessive leanness and/or slow growth have been noted among vegan and vegetarian infants and young children after weaning [Am J Clin Nutr 47:89-92 1988].

TABLE 4. PROTEIN COMPLEMENTATION

Proteins low in certain amino acids can be combined with others
containing them to form complete amino acid mixtures.

Food Group	Limiting Amino Acids	Combine With	Examples
Legumes (beans, peas, lentils)	Tryptophan, methionine	Grains Nuts/seeds	Lentil soup with cornbread Peanut-sesame seed mix
Grains (wheat, rice, oats, barley, corn, rye)	Lysine, isoleucine, threonine	Legumes Dairy	Kidney beans and rice Whole-grain cereal with milk
Nuts/seeds (almond, cashew, filbert, pumpkin, sesame, sunflower, walnut)	Lysine, isoleucine	Legumes	Kidney bean soup with sesame seeds
Animal foods	Not as limited	Any of above	Vegetables with yogurt dressing

bined with plant or animal foods containing them to provide a mixture containing all the essential amino acids. These combinations of "complementary" proteins compensate for the limited amounts of amino acids in the proteins of individual plants. Table 4 shows, for example, how legumes (which are low in two essential amino acids) can be combined with grains (which contain ample amounts of these two but are low in three others) to supply a mixture adequate to meet body needs.

It is not necessary to eat complementary proteins at every meal; it suffices to eat them over the course of a day. Both body protein breakdown and amino acids from recently ingested proteins provide a general body pool of amino acids that can temporarily fill any gaps.

Practical Tips

To assure adequacy with respect to energy and other nutrients, vegetarians should follow these simple principles:

• *Include foods that are calorically and nutrient dense.* Cooked legumes, whole-grain breads, enriched cereals, nuts, and nut spreads (such as peanut, cashew or tahini butter) are concentrated sources of calories, protein, vitamins, and minerals.

• *Choose foods that provide enough iron, calcium, and zinc.* Since their diets contain no animal foods, which are particularly rich in these minerals, this should be a special concern for vegans. Small amounts of animal foods, such as milk and eggs, increase the bioavailability of iron from plant foods eaten at the meal. Plant sources of iron include dried figs, prunes and raisins, pumpkin seeds, sesame seeds, and soybean nuts. Iron-fortified cereals also are excellent sources of iron. To ensure that iron intake is satisfactory, eat good sources of vitamin C, such as tomato, broccoli, melon, or orange or other

citrus juice at each meal. These foods enhance absorption of the iron in legumes and grains by making it more soluble.

Low-fat or skim milk, or milk products, such as yogurt and cheese are excellent sources of calcium for lacto-(ovo)vegetarians. Vegans can get calcium from foods such as tofu, kale, broccoli, sunflower seeds, dried figs, tortillas, calcium-fortified *Total* breakfast cereal (48 mg/1 oz serving), or *Citrus Hill Plus Calcium* orange juice (160 mg/6 oz serving). Vitamin D is also needed to increase the efficiency of calcium absorption. Fortified milk, and milk products can provide vitamin D, but vegans who lack adequate exposure to sunlight (or who use sunscreens) may need to take a vitamin D supplement.

Lacto-ovo-vegetarians can get zinc from egg products. Dried beans, peas, lentils, nuts and seeds are good plant sources of zinc. However, the zinc in fruits and vegetables is less bioavailable than the zinc from animal sources. Vegans and lacto-vegetarians may prefer to use yeast-leavened whole-grain products to increase the bioavailability of the zinc in whole grains by inactivating zinc inhibitors.

• Limit foods that are high in phytates (whole grains, bran, and soy products) and oxalates (spinach, rhubarb, and chocolate), since phytates can inhibit the absorption of iron, calcium, and zinc.

Vegetarians with special health problems may need expert help. The *Diet Manual, Including a Vegetarian Meal Plan* recently published by the Seventh-day Adventist Dietetic Association, P.O. Box 75, Loma Linda, CA 92354, is an excellent reference for health professionals.

Vegetarianism based on sound nutrition principles can be a healthful choice, but neither vegetarians nor omnivores have a monopoly on healthful eating. Vegetarians are just as diverse in their health status as are nonvegetarians. Similar health benefits can be gained from both well-selected omnivorous and vegetarian diets.

Cholesterol

Put knowledge behind your numbers to lower your confusion level

"My doctor just gave me the results of my cholesterol test. He said, 'Your good cholesterol is low—that's bad, and your bad cholesterol is high—that's bad too. You need to raise your good and lower your bad—that would be good.' "

Confusing? You bet it is.

Chances are you know your cholesterol level is important and that it shouldn't be too high. But beyond that you may be unsure exactly how cholesterol fits into the cardiovascular disease puzzle.

Maybe you're too concerned about your cholesterol. Maybe you're not concerned enough.

In the following pages, we answer common questions, such as:
■ What exactly is cholesterol?
■ How can cholesterol be both good and bad?
■ What does cholesterol do in your body?
■ What is an elevated cholesterol level?
■ When should you be concerned?
■ What can you do about your concerns?

Why all the fuss about cholesterol?

Your blood cholesterol is important. Heart and blood vessel (cardiovascular) disease is the No. 1 killer of Americans, and study after study points to elevated cholesterol as a major contributor to the problem.

In general:
■ The higher your cholesterol level, the greater your risk of cardiovascular disease.
■ The higher your cholesterol level, the greater your chances of dying of cardiovascular disease.
■ You can lower your risk of cardiovascular disease by lowering your cholesterol level.

Cholesterol and cardiovascular disease

The good news . . . Deaths from cardiovascular disease continue to fall. This encouraging trend is due to improved treatment and modification of cardiovascular disease risk factors, including cholesterol.

In 1980, heart attacks accounted for 163 deaths per 100,000 people. By 1990, this number had dropped to 112 people per 100,000.

The numbers for stroke are improving, too. In 1980, strokes claimed 41 people per 100,000. By 1990 this figure was down to 28.

The bad news . . . Far too many people still die from cardiovascular disease. The American Heart Association reports that cardiovascular disease still kills almost 1 million Americans each year. This is more than all cancer deaths combined.

Many of these deaths occur because of narrowed or blocked arteries (ath-

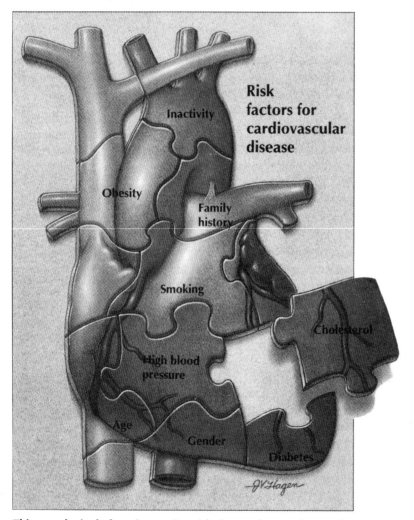

Risk factors for cardiovascular disease

Inactivity
Obesity
Family history
Smoking
Cholesterol
High blood pressure
Age
Gender
Diabetes

This puzzle includes nine major risk factors for cardiovascular disease, the nation's No. 1 killer. Cholesterol is among the most complex and important of all risk factors.

erosclerosis). Cholesterol plays a significant role in this largely preventable condition.

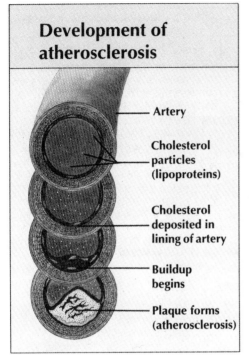

Development of atherosclerosis

— Artery

Cholesterol particles (lipoproteins)

Cholesterol deposited in lining of artery

Buildup begins

Plaque forms (atherosclerosis)

A high number of cholesterol particles (lipoproteins) in your blood increases your risk for a buildup of cholesterol within the wall of your artery. Eventually, bumps called plaques may form, narrowing or even blocking your artery.

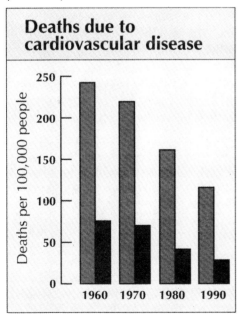

Deaths due to cardiovascular disease

Deaths per 100,000 people

250 — 200 — 150 — 100 — 50 — 0

1960   1970   1980   1990

Deaths from heart attacks (gray bars) and stroke (black bars) are declining. This encouraging trend is due to improved treatment and modification of cardiovascular disease risk factors, including cholesterol.

(*Sources: National Center for Health Statistics and American Heart Association.*)

Atherosclerosis (ATH-ro-scler-OH-sis) is a silent, painless process in which cholesterol-containing fatty deposits accumulate in the walls of your arteries. These accumulations occur as bumps called plaques. (See illustration.)

As plaque builds up, the interior of your artery narrows. This reduces the flow of blood. If reduced flow occurs in your coronary (heart) arteries, it can lead to a type of chest pain called angina pectoris.

As a plaque enlarges, the inner lining of your artery becomes roughened. A tear or rupture in the plaque may cause a blood clot to form. Such a clot can block the flow of blood or break free and plug an artery downstream.

If the flow of blood to a part of your heart is stopped, you'll have a heart attack. If blood flow to a part of your brain stops, you'll have a stroke.

Many factors influence the clogging of arteries. Cholesterol is important in the process, but it's not the only piece of the puzzle.

What is cholesterol?

Cholesterol is a waxy, fat-like substance (lipid). Although it's often discussed as if it were a poison, you can't live without it. Cholesterol is essential to your body's cell membranes, to the insulation of your nerves and to the production of certain hormones. It's used by your liver to make bile acids, which help digest your food.

The confusion that clouds cholesterol is partly due to the way some people use the word. "Cholesterol" is often a catch-all term for both the cholesterol you eat and the cholesterol in your blood.

■ *Your dietary cholesterol*—Cholesterol exists in your food as a dietary lipid. You'll find cholesterol only in animal products, such as meat and dairy foods.

■ *Your blood cholesterol*—Cholesterol also exists in a different way as a natural component of your blood lipids.

The cholesterol in your blood comes both from your liver and from the foods you eat. Your liver makes about 80 percent of your blood cholesterol. Only about 20 percent comes from your diet.

The amount of fat and cholesterol you eat may influence all levels of your blood lipids, including your blood cholesterol levels.

Blood cholesterol—the good, the bad and the ugly

To be carried in your blood, your body coats cholesterol with proteins called apoproteins (AP-oh-PRO-teens). Once

coated, they form a package called lipoproteins (LIP-oh-PRO-teens).

Lipoproteins carry both cholesterol and triglycerides (another blood lipid) in your blood.

Some of your lipoproteins are called low-density lipoproteins (LDLs). They contain lots of cholesterol. Others are called high-density lipoproteins (HDLs). They contain mostly protein.

A third type of lipoprotein is called a very-low-density lipoprotein (VLDL). This type contains cholesterol, triglycerides and protein.

Some people call LDL "bad cholesterol" and HDL "good cholesterol." Here's why:

Cholesterol serves as a building material in cells throughout your body. LDL particles, which carry cholesterol, attach themselves to receptors on cell surfaces and are then received into your cells.

If there are too many LDL particles in your blood, if your liver cells (LDL receptors) do not receive LDL particles normally, or, if there are too few LDL receptors in your liver, your body's cells become saturated with cholesterol from the LDL particles. Cholesterol is then deposited in your artery walls.

At this point your high-density lipoproteins (HDLs) play their "good" role. They actually pick up cholesterol deposited in your artery walls and transport it to your liver for disposal.

The situation can turn ugly if too much cholesterol from LDL particles remains deposited in your artery walls. Your arteries will develop plaques and begin to narrow. This is atherosclerosis.

This is why a high HDL level relative to an LDL level is good. It can help protect you from developing atherosclerosis.

What's to blame?

Why do some people have high cholesterol? High levels result from genetic makeup or lifestyle choices, or both. Your genes can give you cells that don't remove LDL cholesterol from your blood efficiently, or a liver that produces too much cholesterol as VLDL particles, or too few HDL particles.

Lifestyle choices such as smoking, diet and inactivity can also cause or contribute to high cholesterol levels, leaving you at risk for atherosclerosis.

The cholesterol test

The only way to find out if your blood lipids are in a desirable range is to have them tested. The test is done by taking a blood sample after you have fasted overnight. You should have this test every three to five years—more often if you have a problem with your cholesterol level.

How much fat is that?

Limit fat to "30 percent of daily calories." Good advice. But what does it really mean?

This table converts this recommended guideline into the actual amount of fat you should limit yourself to daily.

If you eat . . .	Allow yourself this much fat daily . . .
1,400 calories	47 grams
1,600 calories	53 grams
1,800 calories	60 grams
2,000 calories	67 grams
2,200 calories	73 grams
2,400 calories	80 grams
2,600 calories	87 grams
2,800 calories	93 grams

Note: 1,400 calories is the minimum you should eat if you're trying to lose weight. 1,600 calories is about right for many inactive women and some older adults. 2,200 calories is about right for many sedentary men, most children, teenage girls and active women. 2,800 is about right for teenage boys, many active men and some very active women.

Calorie allowances are based on recommendations of the National Academy of Sciences and on calorie intakes reported by people in national food consumption surveys.

The test should measure your total cholesterol, HDL cholesterol and triglycerides. (Total cholesterol is made up of your LDL, HDL and other blood cholesterol particles.)

Some laboratories measure LDL directly, as part of the blood test. However, if your triglycerides are normal, your doctor can calculate your LDL level using the following formula:

$$\text{Total cholesterol} - \left(\text{HDL} + \frac{\text{triglycerides}}{5}\right) = \text{LDL}$$

In addition to your LDL level, your doctor might calculate the ratios between your LDL and HDL cholesterol, or between your total cholesterol and HDL.

Today, physicians pay more attention to your HDL number. Studies show that even with a desirable total cholesterol level, if you have a low HDL level, you may be at risk for cardiovascular disease.

It's critical to realize that numbers in the table on this page are only guidelines. If your numbers stray from the desirable ranges, your physician will counsel you.

Remember this too: Each number takes on greater meaning when you look at it in relation to the other numbers on your test and in relation to your other cardiovascular disease risk factors.

Other cardiovascular risk factors— the remaining puzzle pieces

To make the picture of your cardiovascular health more complete, you must consider your other risk factors for cardiovascular disease. (See illustration.) Each risk factor may influence your lipid levels.

The more risk factors you have, in combination with undesirable lipid levels, the greater your risk of developing cardiovascular disease. If you have several risk factors, their effects don't simply add up, they amplify each other.

For example, if you have high total cholesterol and you smoke, you're at much greater risk than a nonsmoker with the same cholesterol level.

However, you can make this amplifying effect work for you. Eating a diet low in fat, combined with exercise, can help you lose weight. At the same time, you can reduce your risk of high blood pressure, heart attack and stroke.

Risk factors for cardiovascular disease are divided into those you can change and those you can't. Consider

Your blood test: What do those numbers mean?

Your lipid levels can tell your doctor whether you're a candidate for cardiovascular disease. As you compare your numbers with these, remember: Numbers alone don't tell the whole story. Rely on your physician to interpret your test results.

Test	Your level (in mg/dl) *		
	Desirable	*Borderline*	*Undesirable*
Total cholesterol	Below 200	200-240	Above 240
HDL cholesterol	Above 45	35-45	Below 35
Triglycerides	Below 200	200-400	Above 400
LDL cholesterol	Below 130	130-160	Above 160
Cholesterol/HDL	Below 4.5	4.5-5.5	Above 5.5
LDL/HDL	Below 3	3-5	Above 5

* For people without known heart disease

Note: The numbers in this table represent a compilation of informed medical opinions from a variety of sources.

how each risk factor affects your blood cholesterol and triglycerides.

Here are factors you can change:

■ *Smoking*—Smoking cigarettes damages the walls of your blood vessels, making them prone to accumulate fatty deposits. Smoking may also lower your HDL by as much as 15 percent. If you stop smoking, your HDL may return to its higher level.

■ *High blood pressure*—By damaging the walls of your arteries, high blood pressure can accelerate the development of atherosclerosis. Some medications for high blood pressure increase LDL and triglyceride levels and decrease HDL levels. Other medications don't.

■ *Inactivity*—Lack of physical exercise is associated with a decrease in HDL. Aerobic exercise is one way to increase your HDL. Aerobic activity is any exercise that requires continuous movement of your arms and legs and increases your breathing. Even 30 to 45 minutes of brisk walking every other day helps protect your cardiovascular system.

■ *Obesity*—Excess weight increases your triglycerides. It also lowers your HDL and increases your VLDL cholesterol. Losing just five or 10 pounds can improve your triglyceride and cholesterol levels.

■ *Diabetes*—Diabetes can increase triglycerides and decrease HDL in many people. Diabetes accelerates the development of atherosclerosis which, in turn, increases the risk for heart attack, stroke and reduced circulation to your feet.

If you have diabetes, have your total cholesterol, triglycerides and HDL tested at least annually. Keep your weight and blood sugar under control. Still, complications may develop. Diabetes is not a risk factor you can always change. (See *Mayo Clinic Health Letter* Medical Essay on diabetes, June 1992.)

These are risk factors you can't change:

■ *Age*—As you age, your level of LDL cholesterol usually increases. Researchers aren't sure why. The increase could be caused by aging or by an increase in your body fat.

■ *Gender*—Until age 45, men generally have higher total cholesterol levels than women. Also, up to about this age, women tend to have higher HDL levels. However, after menopause, women's total cholesterol rises and the protective HDL drops.

Caution: Don't think of cardiovascular disease as mainly a man's disease. Cardiovascular disease is also the No. 1 killer of women, claiming almost 500,000 women each year. Cancer kills fewer than 220,000 women. Women get cardiovascular disease as often as men; it just happens later in life.

■ *Family history*—If members of your family have undesirable lipid levels and cardiovascular problems, your risks for these problems are increased.

Your first lines of defense against high cholesterol

Diet and exercise are your first lines of defense against undesirable lipid levels. Changes in your diet, along with exercise, can reduce your blood cholesterol level by up to 15 percent. However, some people have genetically determined lipid problems (especially LDL) that don't respond to diet and require medication.

Making diet changes to improve your blood cholesterol levels involves three steps:

■ *Reduce your weight by reducing your total fat*—Limit all types of fat, saturated, polyunsaturated and mono-unsaturated, to no more than 30 percent of your total daily calories. Because all foods with fats contain a combination of these fats, it's important to reduce total fat.

Don't assume each food you eat must have less than 30 percent of its calories from fat. Use the guideline as a daily average. By balancing occasional high-fat foods with low-fat choices, your fat intake should average 30 percent of your daily calories.

■ *Reduce saturated fat*—No more than one-third of the fat you eat should be saturated. Major sources of saturated fat are butter, cheese, whole milk, cream, meat, poultry, chocolate, coconut, palm and palm kernel oil, lard and solid shortenings.

■ *Reduce dietary cholesterol*—Your daily limit for dietary cholesterol is 300 milligrams. A good way to accomplish this goal is to avoid dairy products made with whole milk and cream, and organ meats such as liver and tongue.

These limits on fat and cholesterol can also help you lose weight, which can improve your blood lipid levels. . . .

Exercise enhances the benefits of diet

A low-fat, low-cholesterol diet can improve your VLDL cholesterol level. If you also exercise and lose excess weight, you may see even greater improvements in your triglyceride and cholesterol levels.

Exercise helps you lose excess weight and reduces your chances of gaining weight as you get older.

For these benefits, set up your program using these guidelines and your doctor's advice:

■ *Choose aerobic activity*—Get involved in brisk walking, jogging, bicycling or cross-country skiing.

■ *Build up time and frequency*—Gradually work up to exercising for 30 to 45 minutes at least three times a week. If you're severely overweight or have been inactive for many years, take several months to gradually work up to this level. The higher the level of your activity, the greater your rate of weight loss.

■ *Keep it up*—Schedule a regular time for exercise. Make exercise fun. If it's not enjoyable you'll have difficulty exercising regularly, year in and year out.

Find a friend, or join an exercise group, to keep you motivated and committed to exercise. Or take up an activity that keeps you active.

Unless you stay with your program, you may not be able to keep off the pounds exercise helped you lose. Staying active also may prevent a gain in weight that often accompanies age. This, in turn, may help maintain lower levels of blood fats.

When are medications necessary?

Often changes in diet, exercise and smoking habits will improve your VLDL cholesterol and triglyceride levels. But if you've carried out these important lifestyle changes and your total cholesterol, especially your LDL level, remains high, your doctor may recommend a medication.

Before recommending a medication, your doctor will use careful judgment and weigh many variables—your changeable risk factors, your age, your current health, and the drug's side effects. If you need a medication to lower your cholesterol, chances are you will need it for many years.

Your LDL cholesterol level is usually the deciding factor. If you have no risk factors for cardiovascular disease, an LDL level over 190 generally requires medication. With two or more risk factors, an LDL level over 160 may require medication.

And remember . . .

The issue of cholesterol and cardiovascular health is important, but by no means simple. Just knowing your total cholesterol level is not enough. Understanding how your other blood fat levels and your cardiovascular disease risk factors influence this number is essential.

Only with this knowledge can cholesterol assume its proper place in the cardiovascular disease puzzle.

A lifelong program to build strong bones

Osteoporosis is a word that's come into common usage fairly recently, but the condition is by no means a recent discovery. Meaning "porous bones" in Latin, osteoporosis literally is a thinning of the bones that makes them fragile and brittle, so that they fracture easily. It's about eight times more common in women than men. For both men and women, however, the chief risk factor is age: the disease usually becomes detectable in people in their sixties, seventies, and beyond. About 1.3 million older people suffer fractures each year in this country due to osteoporosis. It can also result in a decrease in height because of the compression of the vertebrae in the spine, and causes the stooped posture known as "dowager's hump." It's a major cause of disability among older women.

There's no cure for osteoporosis, though there are treatments. Like hypertension, osteoporosis has been called a "silent disease." Thus you may not be aware of it until you actually fracture a bone. Prevention is the best line of defense.

Unfortunately, many women think they don't have to start worrying about osteoporosis until menopause. This a myth. Recent research shows that certain lifelong habits are the best preventive against osteoporosis. About 45% of a person's bone mass is formed during the teen years, and indeed young adulthood or even the teen years are the right time to form the health habits that help prevent osteoporosis. Still, it's never too late to begin. Bones, like skin, deserve special care.

How bones gain—and lose—mass

Bones, many people think, are solid and unchanging, comparable to the inner structure of a building. Nothing could be further from the truth. Hard like ivory on the surface, but spongy and pliable inside, bone is living, dynamic tissue—a combination of collagen and minerals. Bone is about 50% water—not "dry bones" at all, the old song notwithstanding. Bone has two main functions: first to act as a support system, rigid enough to withstand strong forces and flexible enough to permit movement; and second, to store calcium. Bone consists of two kinds of cells: one builds tissue and lays down calcium and other minerals, which it derives from the bloodstream; the other type removes calcium and releases it, so that it can be used for other essential bodily functions.

Your bones continue to evolve and change throughout your life. Bone tissue constantly "remodels" itself (lays down, releases, and then replaces calcium), but for most of adult life there is equilibrium—calcium is laid down and released without apparent change in bone density. However, at about age 35 for women and slightly later for men, bone density begins to decrease.

Many factors influence the processes carried on by bone tissue. The sex hormones (testosterone in men, estrogen in women) are a major influence on calcium uptake by bone tissue and thus skeletal strength. Other hormones aid in the release of calcium and the breakdown of bone mass.

Second, certain nutritional factors—your intake of calcium and vitamin D, for instance, as well as other nutrients whose function in bone building is not fully understood—play an important role in bone formation and maintenance, too.

Third, there is physical activity. Bones respond to mechanical stress by becoming denser and stronger. This stress comes primarily from weight-bearing activity, in which your legs support your body, and from strength-building activity such as weight lifting. If you walk a lot, for example, your leg bones will respond by increasing their mass. If you regularly use your arms to lift weights or swing a tennis racket, the bones in your arms will grow stronger. Perhaps the most dramatic demonstration of the influence of weight-bearing exercise is found in astronauts who spend several weeks in space. In this weightless environment, even these healthy young people lose significant amounts of bone mass.

Another influence on bone is genetics. Asian and Caucasian women tend to be small-boned, which makes them susceptible to osteoporosis. African and many African-American women tend to have more bone mass throughout life (a protective genetic trait), though that doesn't mean they never get osteoporosis.

Gender may be the most important factor in the bone-maintenance game, and women are at a disadvantage. They begin life with less bone mass, on average, than men. Then at menopause, usually around 50, a woman's supply of estrogen decreases, and her bone loss is more rapid than a man's. That's why, after age 65, so many women suffer from osteoporosis.

Osteoporosis does not mean that the bone is diseased or

Calcium supplements: the new news is good news

It's better to get the calcium you need from food than from pills because food also contains other nutrients you need—including those, such as vitamin D, magnesium, and boron, that are important in building bone. But many women, especially older women who tend not to eat dairy products, just don't get enough calcium.

Until recently, there have been serious questions about whether calcium supplements do any good. The *Wellness Letter* at first recommended them, then backed off in 1988. But research since then has made it clear that supplements can help—even in women well past menopause who are not on hormone replacement therapy. A well-designed study from Australia, published in October 1991 in the *New England Journal of Medicine*, showed that postmenopausal women who exercised regularly and took calcium supplements were able to increase bone density significantly. And in February 1993 in the same journal, a study from New Zealand provided strong corroborating evidence that supplements slow bone loss and reverse osteoporosis in postmenopausal women.

How much calcium is enough? The minimal healthy intake of calcium for postmenopausal women is 1,500 milligrams daily, and more would be even better. The best plan seems to be to get *at least* 750 milligrams of calcium from your diet. Skim milk and nonfat yogurt are excellent sources because they also contain vitamin D, which is necessary for calcium absorption. A pint of milk together with a cup of broccoli or some other leafy green vegetable would supply this much calcium. Then bring the total to 1,750 milligrams by taking a 1,000-milligram supplement. There's no convincing evidence so far that one kind of calcium supplement is significantly better than another.

abnormal. It just means there's less of it—that is, when new bone forms, it's less dense. The body continues to remove calcium from the bone storehouse, but in older people some of this calcium is not replaced.

Prevention: when and how

If hereditary factors or a small frame size puts you at risk for osteoporosis, you can't do much about it—but that's all the more reason to take preventive steps. The best time to begin a program of prevention is in childhood and then continue it throughout your life. In your twenties and early thirties, bone density is on the increase. The more bone you build early in life, the better you will be able to withstand bone loss later. But even if you've waited until your forties, fifties, or sixties, there's still plenty of reason to follow this preventive program:

■ **Make weight-bearing exercise part of your daily life.** That means walking, running, cycling, dancing, or weight-lifting—or activities such as housework or mowing the grass. Swimming and yoga are not weight-bearing exercises, and thus don't build bones, though they have other benefits. Exercise should be part of your life at all stages, but a high level of physical activity is particularly important as you grow older.

■ **Consume enough calcium.** Besides building strong bones and maintaining bone density and strength, calcium also plays a role in regulating your heartbeat and other vital functions. The daily recommended dietary allowance, or RDA, is 800 milligrams daily, except for adolescents and young adults (aged 11 to 24) and pregnant or lactating women, who are advised to consume 1,200 milligrams daily; many experts recommend that postmenopausal women consume at least 1,500 milligrams. A cup of milk provides 300 milligrams of calcium; 8 ounces of yogurt, 300 to 450 milligrams. Cottage cheese, by the way, has little calcium. Most hard cheeses have about 200 milligrams per ounce, but are also high in sodium, cholesterol, and saturated fat. The vitamin D added to milk and the lactose naturally in milk and dairy products are thought to aid in the absorption of calcium.

Many dark green leafy vegetables are rich in calcium. A half-cup serving of cooked broccoli, beet greens, or kale has about 90 milligrams. Herring, salmon, and sardines—if eaten with the small bones—are also good calcium sources. Tofu (soybean curd) often contains a fair amount of calcium, too. But the best sources of calcium for most Americans, who usually don't eat much kale, beet greens, or fish bones, remain low-fat or nonfat dairy products.

■ **If you smoke, stop.** Not only for the strength of your bones, but for your general health and well-being.

What puts you at risk: a checklist
■ **Increasing age.**

■ **Being female.** By age 65, the average man still has 91% of his bone mass, but the average woman has only about 74%.

■ **Being chronically underweight** or having a slight frame.

■ **Being Caucasian or Asian** (usually small-boned).

■ **Having osteoporosis in the family.**

■ **A poor diet**, low in vitamins and minerals, especially calcium.

■ **Being sedentary** and lack of weight-bearing exercise.

■ **Smoking.** In women this lowers the estrogen content of the blood, thus weakening the bones. Smoking is particularly dangerous for women who have other risk factors for osteoporosis.

■ **Heavy drinking.** It's not known why heavy drinking weakens the bones—perhaps because heavy drinkers often eat a poor diet.

■ **Long-term use of certain medications.** Some people with asthma and rheumatoid arthritis take cortisone for long periods, which can diminish bone strength. So can long-term use of thyroid hormones, which are sometimes used to treat obesity, although most physicians do not recommend them for this purpose.

■ **If you drink, drink only lightly or moderately.** Light to moderate drinking is defined as an average of no more than two drinks a day. A drink is defined as five ounces of wine, 12 ounces of beer, or 1.5 ounces of 80-proof liquor (all contain about half an ounce of pure alcohol).

■ **Consider hormone replacement therapy (HRT)** if you are menopausal. This consists of low-dose estrogen and progesterone treatments that can unquestionably slow bone loss and prevent fractures as well as reduce hot flashes and other common menopausal symptoms. The added progesterone also reduces the risk of endometrial cancer. HRT probably protects against heart disease, though the evidence remains controversial. (It's estrogen, not the combination of estrogen with progesterone, that's known to be protective.) HRT, if used to prevent osteoporosis, should be started at menopause for maximum effect.

But menopause is not a medical condition that automatically requires drugs. Some women do very well without HRT, which has its downside, too. It may increase the risk of breast cancer, though the evidence isn't yet clear. Still, women who have had breast cancer should not undergo HRT. Those with migraine headaches, diabetes, and other disorders are sometimes advised against it. All women should be informed about HRT and, at menopause, should discuss the pros and cons with their physicians.

In particular, if you have additional risk factors for osteoporosis (see box), you should consider HRT. But whether you take it or not, you should address the risk factors that you can modify: begin an exercise program if you're sedentary, increase your calcium intake, don't smoke, and limit your alcohol intake.

If you are taking oral contraceptives, you'll be pleased to learn that recent studies have shown that their use has a notable positive effect on bone density, independent of other beneficial factors such as calcium intake and exercise.

HYPERTENSION: ROLE OF SELECT NUTRIENTS

Hypertension, or high blood pressure, is a serious disease affecting nearly 60 million Americans, or one in every three adults (1–4). Uncontrolled high blood pressure increases the risk of developing stroke, heart disease, and several types of kidney disease. Developing strategies to lower the prevalence of hypertension in the general population is an important public health objective (3).

Blood pressure generally is presented as two numbers, such as "120 over 80." The numerator is the systolic (contracting) pressure and the denominator is the diastolic (resting) pressure. Hypertension often is defined as a systolic blood pressure greater than or equal to 140 millimeters of mercury (mm Hg), and/or a diastolic blood pressure greater than or equal to 90 mm Hg (4). Risk of hypertension is greater in older than in younger adults, in males than in females, and in blacks than in whites (4, 5). The majority of hypertensive patients have mild elevations in blood pressure (4).

In about 95 percent of patients with hypertension (i.e., so-called "essential" hypertension), the cause of the disease is unknown (6). Essential hypertension is thought to be the end result of a variety of factors, both genetic and environmental. Among environmental factors, improved nutrition is an important intervention in the prevention and treatment of hypertension (1, 4–13).

This *Digest* reviews recent findings regarding the effect of weight control, and intake of sodium, potassium, calcium, and magnesium on blood pressure. Readers are referred to other reviews for information on the blood pressure effects of additional dietary factors such as fat, carbohydrate, caffeine, and alcohol (4, 6, 11, 12).

Recently, non pharmacologic interventions, or lifestyle modifications, have gained acceptance both as the sole treatment of hypertension or as an adjunct to drug therapy (4, 7–13). At present, nondrug therapies such as tobacco avoidance, weight reduction in overweight patients, increased physical activity, and moderation of dietary sodium and alcohol intake are widely advocated as initial treatment for most mildly hypertensive patients (4, 6–12).

Changes in life style, including diet, are recommended by many health professionals to treat and lower risk of hypertension (2, 4, 11)

Several studies support the effectiveness of lifestyle changes in lowering blood pressure or reducing risk of hypertension (7–13). However, health professionals do not know which individuals would benefit most from specific lifestyle changes (14). Recent studies suggest that plasma renin activity might be a marker for the blood pressure response to nonpharmacologic treatments (15).

Weight Control. Obesity is a major risk factor for hypertension, and reducing excess body weight is a key strategy for the prevention and treatment of high blood pressure (6–14, 16).

Findings from epidemiological studies suggest a direct association between body weight or adiposity and blood pressure (4, 6, 11). Moreover, in longitudinal studies, there is a positive correlation between change in weight and blood pressure over time (6). Centrally located or upper body fat is associated with a higher level of blood pressure than peripherally located body fat (6, 11).

The blood pressure-lowering effect of weight reduction is supported by several recent studies (7–10, 17, 18). Some findings indicate that weight loss lowers blood pressure more than does reducing sodium intake (8, 10).

According to observations from the Trial of Antihypertensive Interventions and Management (TAIM) (17), a controlled clinical intervention of diet and drug therapy in 787 mildly hypertensive patients, the blood pressure-lowering effect of weight loss (at least 4.5 kg) was similar to that achieved with low dose drug therapy. Moreover, when combined with drug treatment, weight loss showed an additive hypotensive effect (17).

Even a modest weight loss of 10 pounds can lower blood pressure in obese hypertensive patients (18). Weight loss in overweight patients also may diminish salt sensitivity (19). Nonobese individuals have been shown to be less sensitive to salt-induced increases in blood pressure than obese individuals (19).

Weight loss, achieved by decreasing calorie intake and increasing physical activity, is recommended for overweight patients, particularly those with hypertension (2–4, 6, 8–12, 16–18). For other individuals, avoidance of obesity or age-related weight gain helps to reduce risk of hypertension. Regular aerobic exercise not only contributes to weight loss, but also may help prevent and treat hypertension (11, 12).

Dietary Sodium. Findings from experimental animal studies and epidemiologic and clinical trials in humans suggest an association between sodium intake and blood pressure (5, 6, 19). Severe restriction in salt (sodium chloride) intake (less than 1 g/day) tends to lower blood pressure, while an increase in salt consumption aggravates hypertension (5).

There is wide variability in genetic susceptibility to salt-induced hypertention, with some individuals being more salt-sensitive than others.

Population studies suggest a positive, but weak, association between sodium intake and blood pressure (19–21). This finding was supported by Intersalt (20), an international epidemiological study involving over 10,000 adults aged 20 to 59 years at 52 centers from 32 countries.

Intersalt investigators estimated that lowering average sodium intake by 100 mmol per day (2300 mg sodium) would reduce systolic and diastolic blood pressures by 2.2 mm Hg and 0.1 mm Hg, respectively (20). An important finding of the Intersalt study was the positive association between sodium intake and an age-related increase in blood pressure. This observation led the researchers to suggest that consuming a high sodium intake throughout life may contribute in part to the age-

related increase in blood pressure in Western cultures.

A number of clinical interventions indicate that restricting dietary sodium decreases blood pressure (10, 19, 22, 23). In general, reducing sodium intake lowers blood pressure more in hypertensive than in normotensive individuals and lowers systolic more than diastolic blood pressure (1, 22).

A recent analysis of the results of 23 published short-term trials (22) revealed that moderate sodium restriction lowered systolic blood pressure and diastolic pressure in hypertensive patients by 4.9 mm Hg and 2.6 mm Hg, respectively. In normotensive individuals, sodium restriction decreased systolic and diastolic blood pressures by 1.7 mm Hg and 1.0 mm Hg, respectively.

Not all studies support a positive association between sodium intake and blood pressure, however (1, 19, 20). Several factors may explain the inconsistent findings regarding the impact of sodium on blood pressure. First, the effect of dietary sodium on blood pressure depends on providing sodium as the chloride salt (1, 6, 19).

Second, individuals vary in their blood pressure response to changes in dietary sodium (1, 6, 19, 24). An estimated 30 to 60 percent of hypertensives and 15 to 45 percent of normotensives are salt-sensitive (1, 19).

Unfortunately, reliable means to identify individuals in the population who would benefit most from sodium reduction are unavailable. However, blacks, obese individuals, older adults, and hypertensive patients appear to be especially sensitive to changes in dietary sodium chloride (19, 24). Other markers for salt sensitivity include low plasma renin levels, disturbances in calcium metabolism, an exaggerated natriuretic response to volume expansion, and increased sympathetic nervous system activity (6, 11, 15, 19). Research is focusing on identifying physiologic or genetic markers to distinguish individuals who would benefit from salt reduction.

Third, other nutrients and their interactions may influence the relationship between sodium intake and blood pressure (6, 19, 25, 26). Po-

tassium, calcium, and magnesium not only influence blood pressure on their own, but also may modify the blood pressure response to dietary salt (19). When calcium intake is adequate, the hypertensive response to dietary sodium appears to be reduced (26). Further, the hypertensive response of salt may be influenced more by the sodium-to-potassium ratio than by sodium alone (26). Fourth, errors in measuring both sodium intake and blood pressure could obscure true underlying relationships between sodium (or other nutrients) and blood pressure.

Most Americans can reduce their intake of salt and sodium by choosing foods with less salt, and using salt sparingly, if at all, in food preparation and at the table (2, 29). Reading food labels for the amount of sodium per serving also is helpful.

Several health professional organizations recommend that Americans reduce or moderate their sodium intake (2, 27–30). The estimated minimum requirement for sodium is 500 mg/day (27). In the U.S., dietary sodium intake ranges from 3,000 to 6,000 mg/day (1, 29), an amount well above this minimum. Therefore, the general population is advised to reduce sodium intake to 2400 mg/day (6 g salt) (2728).

Lowering dietary sodium may be especially beneficial for individuals whose blood pressure levels are high, who are salt-sensitive, or who are at high risk of hypertension (1). Moderate salt restriction also can enhance the effectiveness of antihypertensive medication (1, 19). Moreover, there is no evidence that moderately lowering salt intake poses any serious health risk (1, 29).

Consumers soon may see health claims regarding sodium and hypertension on food labels 1). The Food and Drug Administration (1), following an extensive review of the scientific literature regarding the relationship between sodium intake and hypertension, is proposing to authorize health claims on some food labels that would state that a low sodium intake is associated with lower blood pressure in some people.

Potassium. A number of studies suggest that increasing potassium intake has a modest blood pressure lowering effect (4, 5, 20, 28, 30, 31). In several animal models of hypertension, high potassium intake reduces blood pressure, often by attenuating a salt-induced rise in blood pressure (5, 19). Animal studies also indicate that a diet high in potassium may protect against vascular damage or stroke (30).

Epidemiological investigations, such as the Intersalt study, point to an inverse relation between potassium intake and blood pressure (4, 6, 20, 32, 33). Findings of a recent longitudinal study in the Netherlands involving 233 children aged 5 to 17 years suggest that a sufficient intake of potassium or a reduction in the dietary sodium to potassium ratio may be beneficial in the early prevention of hypertension (33). However, not all population studies support a hypotensive effect of potassium (16, 34).

Findings of clinical trials, although not consistent, indicate a modest blood pressure-lowering effect of increased potassium intake (6, 31, 35, 36). According to a recent meta-analysis of 19 clinical trials of potassium involving 586 subjects (both normotensives and hypertensives), increased potassium intake lowered systolic and diastolic blood pressure of the overall group by 5.9 mm Hg and 3.4 mm Hg, respectively (31).

In general, the hypotensive effect of potassium is more pronounced in hypertensive than in normotensive individuals and increases with the duration of the study (6, 31). Furthermore, most studies that have demonstrated an antihypertensive effect of potassium have involved subjects consuming a diet high in sodium chloride (5, 6, 11, 19, 35, 37). Increasing

potassium intake is thought to lower blood pressure by increasing sodium excretion (6, 19, 35).

Consuming foods high in potassium may reduce the need for antihypertensive medication (38). The minimum requirement for potassium is approximately 1,600 to 2,000 mg per day, and adults probably consume about 3,500 mg a day (27). Diet is the preferred means to meet potassium needs (12, 31, 38–40). Major sources of potassium in the food supply include vegetables, dairy products, meat, poultry, fish, and fruits (27, 41). Although potassium supplements may be useful to treat diuretic-induced hypokalemia, their routine use is costly and potentially hazardous, especially for patients at risk of high blood potassium levels (12, 40).

Calcium. Evidence accumulated over the past decade suggests that calcium intake favorably affects blood pressure levels, at least in some individuals (5, 6, 42).

Several epidemiological studies indicate an inverse association between dietary calcium and blood pressure (34,42–44). A prospective study of over 58,000 female registered nurses noted an independent and significant inverse association between dietary calcium and hypertension (34). Similarly, a recent study involving over 1,900 Japanese men found an inverse association between total calcium intake, particularly from dairy foods, and systolic blood pressure (44).

Clinical intervention trials reveal a small, but variable, hypotensive effect of calcium (42, 45, 46). According to a recent review of 19 randomized, controlled clinical trials, calcium supplementation reduced systolic and diastolic blood pressures by 1.8 mm Hg and 0.7 mm Hg, respectively (42).

In general, calcium's effect on blood pressure is greater in hypertensive than in normotensive subjects (10). However, a recent double blind trial observed a small blood pressure lowering effect of milk in young normotensive women (47). The authors attributed the hypotensive effect of

milk to its content of calcium, potassium, and magnesium.

Several studies suggest that increasing calcium intake reduces the risk of hypertension during pregnancy (48–51). One investigation found that women who developed preeclampsia or gestational hypertension had a lower calcium intake from dairy foods during the first 20 weeks of pregnancy than normotensive controls (48).

Increasing calcium intake potentially may benefit individuals at risk of hypertension. However, data are insufficient to recommend increasing calcium intakes beyond RDA levels to prevent or treat hypertension (11, 12, 52, 53).

Although these findings are promising, a large study presently being sponsored by the National Institutes of Health should provide more definitive conclusions regarding the role of calcium in preventing hypertension during pregnancy (52). In the meantime, pregnant women are encouraged to consume at least the RDA for calcium from their diets (50, 52).

The finding that not all individuals respond to increased calcium intake with a reduction in blood pressure may explain the failure of some studies to support a beneficial effect of calcium on blood pressure (6, 10, 45). Calcium lowers blood pressure in about one-third of patients with essential hypertension (5). In general, patients with low renin and salt-sensitive hypertension (i .e., blacks, the elderly) appear to be responsive to increased calcium intake (6, 10). At present, there is no way to identify individuals who would benefit most from increased calcium intake. A threshold effect of calcium intake, above which additional calcium does not lower blood pressure further, also may explain in part the variable influence of calcium on blood pressure (26, 53–55).

The mechanism by which calcium lowers blood pressure is unknown, although a variety of possibilities have been proposed (5, 6, 19, 50, 56–58). Calcium affects circulating levels of parathyroid hormone and renin, which in turn may modulate intracellular ionized calcium, resulting in smooth muscle relaxation (50). Calcium also may blunt the blood pressure enhancing effect of a high salt intake (26, 56–58). The protective effect of calcium appears to be most pronounced in the presence of a high sodium intake (56, 57).

Magnesium. There is suggestive, but not consistent, evidence that magnesium lowers blood pressure (34, 59, 60). When the relation of various nutritional factors to hypertension was examined prospectively among more than 58,000 female registered nurses, those who consumed at least the RDA for magnesium had a one-third less chance of developing hypertension than the nurses who consumed lower intakes of magnesium (34).

Despite epidemiological studies that associate magnesium intake with a downward trend in blood pressure, clinical trials in hypertensive patients neither prove nor refute an antihypertensive effect of magnesium (61). The hypotensive effect of magnesium may be restricted to magnesium-deficient individuals (62). Possible interactions of magnesium with other nutrients also may explain magnesium's inconsistent effects on blood pressure (59, 63).

There is no convincing evidence to justify an increase in magnesium intake beyond the RDA to prevent or treat hypertension (4). Adequate magnesium intake can be obtained from usual intakes of dietary sources such as dairy products, grain products, vegetables, meat, poultry and fish, legumes, nuts, and soy (41). More rigorous long-term studies are necessary before increasing magnesium can be considered to be a useful, nonpharmacologic approach to blood pressure reduction.

REFERENCES

1. Food and Drug Administration, Department of Health and Human Services. Fed. Regist. *56* (Nov.27): 60825, 1991.

2. U.S. Department of Agriculture and U.S. Department of Health and Human Services. *Nutrition and Your Health: Dietary Guidelines for Americans.* 3rd edition. Home & Garden Bulletin No. 232. Washington, DC: USDA/DHHS, 1990.

3. U.S. Department of Health and Human Services, Public Health Service. *Healthy People 2000. National Health Promotion and Disease Prevention Objectives.* DHHS Publ. No. (PHS) 91–50212. Washington, DC: Superintendent of Documents, U.S. Government Printing Office, September 1990.

4. Joint National Committee on Detection, Evaluation, and Treatment of High Blood Pressure. Arch. Intern. Med. *148*: 1023, 1988.

5. Haddy, F. H. Hypertension *18* (suppl III): III–179, 1991.

6. Kotchen, T. A., J. M. Kotchen, and M. A. Boegehold. Hypertension *18* (suppl I): I–115, 1991.

7. Stamler, R., J. Stamler, F. C. Gosch, et. al. JAMA *262*: 1801, 1989.

8. Hypertension Prevention Trial Research Group. Arch. Intern. Med. *150*: 153, 1990.

9. Treatment of Mild Hypertension Research Group. Arch. Intern. Med. *151*: 1413, 1991.

10. Trials of Hypertension Prevention Collaborative Research Group. JAMA *267*: 1213, 1992.

11. Kaplan, N. M. Hypertension *18* (suppl I): I-153, 1991.

12. Kaplan, N. M. Nonpharmacologic treatment of hypertension. Curr. Opin. Nephrol. Hypertens. In press, 1992.

13. Applegate, W. B., S. T. Miller, J. T. Elam, et. al. Arch. Intern. Med. *152*: 1162, 1992.

14. Pickering, T. G. JAMA *267*: 1256, 1992.

15. Blaufox, M. D., H. B. Lee, B. Davis, et. al. JAMA *267*: 1221, 1992.

16. Ford, E. S., and R. S. Cooper. Hypertension *18*: 598, 1991.

17. Wassertheil-Smoller, S., M. D. Blaufox, A. S. Oberman, et. al. Arch. Intern. Med. *152*: 131, 1992.

18. Schotte, D. E., and A. J. Stunkard. Arch. Intern. Med. *150*: 1701, 1990.

19. Muntzel, M., and T. Drueke. Am. J. Hypertens. *5* (suppl I): 1S, 1992.

20. The INTERSALT Cooperative Research Group. Br. Med. J. 297: 319, 1988.

21. Law, M. R., C. D. Frost, and N. J. Wald. Br. Med. J. *302*: 811, 1991.

22. Cutler, J. A., D. Follman, P. Elliot, et. al. Hypertension *17* (suppl I): I–27, 1991.

23. Law, M. R., C. D. Frost, and N. J. Wald. Br. Med. J. *302*: 819, 1991.

24. Weinberger, M. H., and N. S. Fineberg. Hypertension *18*: 67, 1991.

25. Kurtz, T. W., and R. C. Morris, Jr. Am. J. Hypertens. *3*: 152S, 1990.

26. Gruchow, H. W., K. A. Sobocinski, and J. J. Barboriak. Am. J. Clin. Nutr. *48*: 1463, 1988.

27. Food and Nutrition Board, Subcommittee on the Tenth Edition of the RDAs. *Recommended Dietary Allowances, 10th Edition.* Washington, DC: National Academy Press, 1989.

28. Food and Nutrition Board, Committee on Diet and Health, Commission of Life Sciences, National Research Council. *Diet and Health. Implications for Reducing Chronic Disease Risk.* Washington, DC: National Academy Press, 1989.

29. U.S. Department of Health and Human Services. *The Surgeon General's Report on Nutrition and Health.* DHHS (PHS) Pub. No. 88–50210 (GPO Stock No. 017-001-11465) Washington, DC: U. S. Government Printing Office, 1988.

30. Joint World Health Organization/ International Society of Hypertension Guidelines Committee. J. Hypertens. *10*: 97, 1992.

31. Cappuccio, F. P., and G. A. MacGregor. J. Hypertens. *9*: 465, 1991.

32. Krishna, G. G. J. Am. Soc. Nephrol. *1*: 43, 1990.

33. Geleijnse, J. M., D. E. Grobbee, and A. Hofman. Br. Med. J. *300*: 899, 1990.

34. Witteman, J. C. M., W. C. Willett, M. J. Stampfer, et al. Circulation *80*: 1320, 1989.

35. Krishna, G. G., E. Miller, and S. Kapoor. N. Engl. J. Med. *320*: 1177, 1989.

36. Krishna, G. G., and S. C. Kappor. Ann. Intern. Med. *115*: 77, 1991.

37. Grimm, R. H., Jr., J. D. Neaton, P. J. Elmer, et. al. N. Engl. J. Med. *322*: 569, 1990.

38. Siani, A., P. Strazzullo, A. Giacco, et al. Ann. Intern. Med. *115*: 753, 1991.

39. Kaplan, N. M., and C. V. S. Ram. N. Engl. J. Med. *322*: 623, 1990.

40. Swales, J. D. Br. Med. J. *303*: 1084, 1991.

41. Life Sciences Research Office, Federation of American Societies for Experimental Biology. *Nutrition Monitoring in the United States—An Update Report on Nutrition Monitoring.* Prepared for the U. S. Department of Agriculture and the U. S. Department of Health and Human Services. DHHS Publ. No. (PHS) 89-1255. Public Health Service. Washington, DC: U.S. Government Printing Office, September 1989.

42. Cutler, J. A., and E. Brittain. Am. J. Hypertens. *3(8, pt 2)*: 137S, 1990.

43. Gillman, M. W., S. A. Oliveria, L. L. Moore, et al. JAMA *267*: 2340, 1992.

44. Iso, H., A. Terao, A. Kitamura, et. al. Am. J. Epidemiol. *133*: 776, 1991.

45. Mikami, H., T. Ogihara, and Y. Tabuchi. Am. J. Hypertens. *3*: 147S, 1990.

46. Grobbee, D. E., and A. Hofman. Lancet 2: 703, 1986.

47. Van Beresteijn, E. C. H., M. Van Schaik, and G. Schaafsma. J. Intern. Med. *228*: 477, 1990.

48. Marcoux, S., J. Brisson, and J. Fabia. Am. J. Epidemiol. *133*: 1266, 1991.

49. Belizan, J. M., J. Villar, L. Gonzalez, et. al. N. Engl. J. Med. *325*: 1399, 1991.

50. Repke, J. T., and J. Villar. Am. J. Clin. Nutr. *54*: 237S, 1991.

51. Knight, K. B., and R. E. Keith. Am. J. Clin. Nutr. *55*: 891, 1992.

52. Ferris, T. F. N. Engl. J. Med. *325*: 1439, 1991.

53. McCarron, D. A., C. D. Morris, E. Young, et. al. Am. J. clin. Nutr. *54*: 215S, 1991.

54. Sowers, J. R., M. B. Zemel, P. C. Zemel, et. al. Am. J. Hypertens. *4*: 577, 1991.

55. Orwoll, E. S., and S. Oviatt. Am. J. Clin. Nutr. *52*: 717, 1990.

56. Hamet, P., M. Daignault-Gelinas, J. Lambert, et. al. Am. J. Hypertens. *5*: 378, 1992.

57. Hamet, P., E. Mongeau, J. Lambert, et. al. Hypertension *17(suppl I)*: I-150, 1991.

58. Oparil, S., Y. F. Chen, H. Jin, et. al. Am. J. Clin. Nutr. *54*: 227S, 1991.

59. Evans, G. H., C. M. Weaver, D. D. Harrington, et. al. J. Hypertens. *8*: 327, 1990.

60. Joffres, M. R., D. M. Reed, and K. Yano. Am. J. Clin. Nutr. *45*: 469, 1987.

61. Welton, P. K., and M. J. Klag. A. J. Cardiol. *63(suppl G)*: 26G, 1989.

62. Zemel, P. C., M. B. Zemel, M. Urberg, et. al. Am. J. Clin. Nutr. *51*: 665, 1990.

63. Shingu, T., H. Matsuura, M. Kusaka, et. al. J. Hypertens. *9*: 1021, 1991.

ACKNOWLEDGMENTS

National Dairy Council® assumes the responsibility for this publication. However, we would like to acknowledge the help and suggestions of the following reviewers in its preparation:

■ M. W. Gillman, M. D.
Assistant Professor of Medicine & Pediatrics
Evans Section of Preventive Medicine & Epidemiology
Boston University School of Medicine
Boston, MA

■ H. M. Gruchow, Ph. D.
Professor and Head, Public Health Education
University of North Carolina at Greensboro
Greensboro, North Carolina

■ N. M. Kaplan, M. D.
Professor of Internal Medicine
Department of Medicine
University of Texas
Southwestern Medical Center at Dallas
Dallas, Texas

The *Dairy Council Digest®* is written and edited by Lois D. McBean, M.S., R.D.

THE DIET/CANCER CONNECTION

Experts estimate that dietary factors contribute to fully one-third of the 500,000 cancer deaths that occur each year. Fortunately, research on food and cancer has shown that you *can* take dietary steps to lessen your chances of developing cancer. But, though questionable marketing campaigns would have you believe otherwise, there is no evidence as yet that you can prevent cancer by taking megadoses of vitamins A or E, or taking fiber supplements. As one expert put it, "As far as diet and cancer are concerned, we are where we were with diet and heart disease 20 years ago: We knew heart disease was related to fat, but did not yet know the specifics about saturated fats or cholesterol."

Two substances have emerged as the most powerful dietary influences on cancer: Fat, as a promoter, and fiber, as a protector. Certain micronutrients knows as antioxidants, such as vitamins A, C, and E, and beta-carotene (which gives carrots their orange color, and is converted by the body to vitamin A) may also play a protective role. (In the body, antioxidants sweep up the cancer-promoting, unstable oxygen molecules known as free radicals.) Other elements of the diet—as well as dyes, preservatives, and other food additives—appear less likely to have a strong effect.

IS IT THE CHICKEN OR THE EGG?

Fat and fiber are at odds with one another in the diet. That is, if you eat a lot of fiber, you probably don't eat too much fat, and vice versa. A high-fiber diet has been associated with a reduction in colon cancer in many population studies (see Different diets; different cancers), although some studies have found no effect. Fat, on the other hand, has been implicated as a contributing cause of colon, breast, and prostate cancers—three of the most common types of cancer in the developed world.

The most compelling evidence is for colon cancer: A recent study of over 88,000 nurses found that a high intake of animal fat—specifically red meat—increases the risk of colon cancer. During the six years that the women were followed, 150 developed colon cancer; those women who ate beef, pork, or lamb as a main dish every day had two-and-a-half times the risk of developing colon cancer as women who consumed these meats less than once a month. However, critics have noted that the study compared only unusual levels of red meat consumption: daily (by most standards a very high intake of animal fat), versus once a month (by most standards an unusually low intake). The Nurses Study did not find an association between high-fat diets and breast cancer, although numerous other population studies have suggested a connection.

Despite such evidence, there is not an open-and-shut case for fat: It may in fact be calories that count (fat contains nine calories per gram, compared with four calories per gram of carbohydrate or protein). Animal studies have consistently shown that cutting calories leads to fewer tumors, even if fat intake is not reduced. Rats who were fed 25% fewer calories but five times the fat as controls had significantly fewer tumors. (Granted, such a diet would be hard for people to sustain.) Animal studies have also shown that even late in life, restricting calories can be an effective tumor preventive.

In humans, being overweight is a proven risk factor for cancer. A large-scale 12-year study conducted by the American Cancer Society found that women who were 40% over ideal weight had up to a 55% greater risk of dying from cancer than normal-weight women, while obese men had up to 33% more deaths from cancer than normal-weight men. Likewise, exercise may play a role: Men in sedentary jobs have a higher risk of developing colon cancer than more-active men. Having participated in college athletics is also correlated with a reduced risk of cancer.

Possibly an even more significant risk for cancer is what a high-fat (or high-calorie) diet lacks: sufficient fiber. Fiber is that portion of foods that remains intact during the digestive process. Vegetables, fruits, and whole grain foods are all high in fiber. Fiber absorbs water, so that stools stay softer. Researchers hypothesize that by diluting stool, fiber limits contact between any carcinogens in the stool and the lining of the colon. Laboratory studies of some components of fiber have found they have a separate anticarcinogenic effect. Also, many fiber-rich vegetables such as broccoli are also high in antioxidant nutrients, which may further lower the risk of some cancers.

However, different types of fiber have been shown to affect cancer risk differently. In animal studies, wheat bran has proven to be the most effective, while some other fibers, such as corn bran, actually appear to increase tumor formation. Until more is known about specific fibers and their role in cancer, taking fiber supplements to prevent cancer doesn't seem wise. What does make sense is to cut back on fats and include a wide variety of fiber-rich foods in your diet.

BEYOND FAT AND FIBER

Even in the case of fat and fiber, it is hard to pin down quantifiable amounts of a particular nutrient to take or avoid. In fact, in 1984, when the American Cancer Society issued its first dietary guidelines for cancer prevention, it noted that firm scientific evidence pointing to specific connections between diet and cancer was lacking. And while hundreds of studies have been undertaken on the subject since then, the current cancer-preventive guidelines (summarized in "Cancer-proofing your eating") are called "directional"—that is, they are based on general eating habits. Despite the "breakthroughs" commonly reported in newspapers—selenium prevents cancer X; nitrates cause cancer—evidence as to just which foods cause cancer and which protect against it is still sketchy, for the reasons outlined below:

Cancer is more than one disease. At its simplest, cancer may be defined as the disordered growth of misbehaving cells in the body. However, there are many different types of cancer. Just as treatments differ among cancers, what causes one type of cancer is often different from what causes another. In some cases, a substance that prevents one cancer may contribute to another kind of cancer. For example, some studies have associated vitamin A with reduced rates of oral, lung, and bladder cancer—but with increases in prostate cancer. So, at best, specific foods can be said to protect or promote specific cancer, not cancer in general.

The sum of the parts may be greater than the whole. Studies have tended to look at large elements in the diet, such as fat or fiber. But as heart-disease research has proven, components of a single dietary element may have different effects on disease: Cholesterol blood levels are raised by saturated (animal) fat, but are relatively unaffected by polyunsaturated fats, or even lowered by monounsaturated fats, such as olive oil. It is entirely possible that, for instance, insoluble fiber (the type of fiber found in whole grains, such as breads and rice) will affect cancer risk differently from soluble fiber, which is found mostly in vegetables and fruits. For example, carcinogen expert Dr. Paul Talalay of Johns Hopkins recently isolated a substance in broccoli called sulphoaphane, which is a potent anticarcinogen.

Different diets; different cancers

What we know about diet and cancer comes primarily by way of large population, or *epidemiologic*, studies. Some epidemiologic studies compare cancer rates in different countries with disparate diets. Such *correlation* studies, as they are known, establish trends. For example, rates of colon cancer are lower in Japan, where a low-fat diet is the norm, than in America, where we eat a high-fat diet. However, correlation studies cannot sufficiently establish a cause-and-effect relationship, because lifestyle differences other than diet may be responsible for the variations in cancer in different cultures.

Further proof may come from so-called *migration* studies, which observe cancer rates in groups such as immigrants whose diets are undergoing change. To go back to the Japanese example, researchers following Japanese immigrants to this country have found that rates of colon cancer increase in the immigrants as they adopt the higher-fat American diet.

Laboratory studies may duplicate these findings in cells or in animals. However, because different animal species respond to carcinogens in different ways, the results of these studies cannot be directly applied to humans. Only controlled *intervention* trials in humans—giving one group a specific quantity of a nutrient and another matched group a placebo, and following cancer trends in both groups—can firmly establish cause and effect. Of course, such trials are unethical if the substance being tested is even suspected of causing cancer, so in many cases the evidence will remain circumstantial.

There may be a fine line between protection and harm. Some micronutrients, in particular the antioxidant vitamins A, C, and E and beta-carotene, may be cancer protective. However, it is possible that antioxidants in high doses may interfere with other beneficial elements in the diet. For example, there is some evidence that taking daily beta carotene for six months will deplete your skin cells of vitamin E. Also, megadoses of some vitamins can cause very serious adverse effects—although unscrupulous salespeople are marketing cancer-protective supplements based on preliminary evidence.

THE BOTTOM LINE

The delicate work of teasing out the connections between fat, fiber, and cancer provides a good example of why it is hard to isolate the impact of a solitary nutrient on cancer. Rather, there seems to be a synergistic effect between foods and even exercise that affects your cancer risk. Says Dr. Peter Greenwald, director of cancer prevention and control at the National Cancer Institute: "The fact is that

3. THROUGH THE LIFE SPAN: DIET AND DISEASE

Cancer-proofing your eating

In 1991, the American Cancer Society updated its guidelines on dietary measures that may lower cancer risk. In the seven years since the first guidelines were released, there has been a plethora of new research on diet and cancer. Findings from that research have been incorporated into the new recommendations—but very few specific changes have resulted. The new guidelines only further affirm the old, since more evidence backs them up now than when they were first published in 1984. In addition, they have proven to be heart-healthy and to help prevent diabetes. As noted in the guidelines, "The dietary advice in this report can be epitomized in two words—variety and moderation. A varied diet, eaten in moderation, offers the best hope for lowering the risk of a disease that yearly claims a half-million lives in this country, together with untold pain and grief."

Substance	Associated cancers	Comments	Steps to take
Fiber	May **decrease** risk of colorectal cancer.	Different types of fiber may affect cancer risk differently. Benefits may also be due to lower fat intakes usually associated with high-fiber diets.	Eat 4 to 5 servings a day of a variety of vegetables, fruits, whole-grain cereals, and legumes. Maximize fiber in vegetables and fruits by eating them unpeeled.
Fruits and vegetables	May **decrease** risk of colorectal and breast cancers.	Good sources of fiber (see above). Cruciferous vegetables, such as broccoli, cabbage, and Brussels sprouts, also contain indoles—nitrogen compounds which, in some studies, have knocked out carcinogens that can lead to breast cancer.	To maximize indole intake, eat vegetables raw, steamed, or microwaved—boiling leaches up to half the indoles.
Fat	May **increase** risk of breast, colon, and prostate cancers.	Lowering fat intake will almost automatically lower caloric intake and boost fiber intake—steps that will also lower cancer risk.	Decrease calories from fat to 25 to 30% of total daily calories. (Current average intake is 40% of total calories.)
Alcohol	Heavy use **increases** risk of cancers of the oral cavity, larynx, and esophagus; moderate use may **increase** breast cancer risk.	Cigarette smoking in conjunction with alcohol drinking greatly increases cancer risk. Alcohol use also can cause liver cirrhosis, which may lead to liver cancer.	Drink only occasionally and sparingly.
Salt-cured, smoked, barbecued and nitrite-preserved foods	May **increase** risk of stomach, esophageal, and lung cancers.	Smoking and charcoal-grilling foods produces tars that are similar to those in cigarette smoke, and are absorbed by the food. Manufacturers have substantially decreased nitrites used in meat preservation.	Opt for other cooking methods; limit intake of salt-cured and nitrite preserved foods.
Beta carotene and antioxidant vitamins (A, C, and E)	Inconclusive	Vitamin E and beta carotene have been associated with lower rates of cancer in humans; a lesser effect has been noted with the other antioxidant nutrients. More research is needed.	Eat a balanced and varied diet to insure you get the RDA for all vitamins; do not take megadose vitamin supplements.
Selenium	Inconclusive	Limited evidence shows this trace element may protect against breast and colon cancers—however, it is very toxic in high doses.	Taking selenium supplements can be very dangerous; you get all the selenium you need from a varied diet.
Artificial sweeteners	Inconclusive	High levels of saccharin cause bladder cancer in rats, but no evidence of this in humans. Long-term effects of aspartame are unknown.	Moderate use poses no risk.
Coffee and caffeine	None	Both coffee and caffeine have received a clean bill of health.	Moderate use of coffee and caffeine is fine.
Food additives	None	Chemical additives found to be carcinogenic in animals have been banned; insufficient evidence that additives currently in use have any cancer risk or benefit.	None

Designer foods

The National Cancer Institute is sponsoring a $20.5 million research project on so-called designer foods. Rather than focusing on the "big" foodstuffs associated with cancer, such as fats and fiber, the project aims at identifying the chemical components in foods—particularly fruits, vegetables, and grains—that confer cancer protection. Called phytochemicals, these elements can be incorporated in extra doses into foods that naturally contain low levels. (Calcium-enriched orange juice, which has been available for a few years and is targeted at preventing osteoporosis, is a type of designer food.)

Beta-carotene is one example of a phytochemical, but there are hundreds more with decidedly futuristic names: terpenoids, flavonoids, coumarins, phenolic acids, and liminoids, for starters. These substances are found in abundance in foods such as garlic, licorice root, soybeans, citrus fruits, flaxseed, and umbelliferous vegetables such as parsley, carrots, and celery. It will be some time before they can be loaded into foodstuffs, then pass the clinical trials and FDA safety tests necessary to put them on the supermarket shelf. But someday, you may be asking for seconds of flavonoid-enriched yogurt or sulfur-laced bread (a sulfur-containing compound is the active ingredient in garlic). . . .

with all the evidence we have, we cannot tell precisely how much of a benefit a person who is, say middle-aged, would get from changing his or her diet, and how long it would take to get the benefit. We think [dietary changes are] useful based on migration studies and so forth, but we don't have specific quantitative data. That requires a trial."

Some such trials are under way. However, until results are in, it is impossible to say "take this amount of nutrient X, and cut this amount of nutrient Y from your diet and you will lower your risk of Z type of cancer by X%." Until then, the conclusions of research to date can be applied in their broadest sense to the diet. For example, it is safe and prudent to say that eating more fiber and less fat is wise. And as Hopkins oncological epidemiologist Dr. Kathy Helzlsouer says, "As long as you get the cancer protection, to a large degree it really doesn't matter whether it's the decreased fat or increased fiber that's providing it."

In the future, as research continues, specific nutrients might be prescribed as chemopreventives—drugs or supplements taken to prevent cancer. Beta-carotene is currently being tested on the 22,000 doctors who are part of the ongoing Physicians' Health Study, conducted by Dr. Charles Hennekens of Harvard Medical School. Half of the participating physicians are taking a 50 mg beta-carotene pill every other day to determine whether this lowers cancer risk; the rest take a placebo. The study, which began in 1982, is scheduled to run until 1995. (This is the same study that found that taking an aspirin every other day lowers risk of heart attack. See the February 1992 issue of *Health After 50.*)

Another possibility is that foods might be designed and grown to maximize cancer protection (see "designer foods" box). For now, eating the type of diet described in the guidelines on the preceding page incorporates the knowledge on diet and cancer to date, and gives you the best assurance of cutting your cancer risk.

Fat and Weight Control

A round man cannot be expected to fit in a square hole right away. He must have time to modify his shape.
—Mark Twain in *More Tramps Abroad*

There have been times and places in history when fat was considered beautiful. Harry Golden, writing in *Only in America* (Cleveland, Ohio: The World Publishing Company, 1958), describes how it was in the Lower East Side of New York when he was a boy. For 2 cents and accompanied by lots of fanfare, the salesman would guess a person's weight and weigh him or her in public. It was a big social event on Saturday nights in a society where a women bragged about gaining 5 pounds and practiced ways to simulate a double chin. Harry and his mother, however, had differing views:

> When I weigh myself I do not look at the results. I just listen to the gears grind and, when everything quiets down, I simply step off the scales and walk away. By this system I have won the battle, leaving the machine frustrated, if not useless. I was always a fat kid and once when I complained about it my mother said, "Nothing at all to worry about; in America the fat man is always the boss and the skinny man is always the bookkeeper."

Society today does not view fat pounds with pride. Thin is in. It is the willowy person who is seen as beautiful, socially acceptable, and appealing to the opposite sex. Those of us with bulges and bumps will knead and pound, use saunas and starve—anything to lose a pound.

Entrepreneurs make nearly $30 billion a year from Americans' desire to be thin. Publish a book about a catchy new diet that promises quick weight loss, and you are an overnight success! Never mind that the weight loss scheme is unsafe or unproven. Many of the millions preoccupied with weight control will be unable to resist any product or method that guarantees a quick result. And thus the dieters are off on the next plunge down the roller coaster of weight loss and gain.

In 1980 we believed that within 10 years the overweight problem in the United States could easily be reduced to 10 percent of men and 17 percent of women. It was disheartening, then, in 1990, to discover that at least 26 percent of the adult population was still overweight. A recent analysis of 30-year data by the National Center for Health Statistics shows a trend of increasing obesity, particularly among young adults and black males. This is not good news for the Year 2000 goal that calls for reducing overweight to no more than 20 percent of adults.

Nor is there complete agreement on when one has achieved the right weight. The term "healthy weight" has replaced "ideal or desirable weight" to emphasize the connection to health. In some circles, the concept of "wellness" is preferred because it is perceived as being more dynamic and inclusive of personal responsibility. Recent revisions of weight tables show significant changes such as acceptable weight gain with age and lack of gender differentiation. Other methods for determining appropriate weight include waist to hip ratios, skinfold thickness at specified points, and body mass index.

Mounting evidence points to increasing morbidity and mortality as weights exceed healthy ranges, especially when they are more than 20 percent higher (see "Health Risks of Obesity"). Linkages seem clear to hyperlipidemia and coronary heart disease, high blood pressure, noninsulin-dependent diabetes, and various cancers. Excess weight also aggravates osteoarthritis, especially in the knees. Still, concern is greater about *where* the fat is; abdominal fat is more predictive of some chronic diseases than is fat on hips and thighs.

Does it follow, then, that weight loss will lower mortality rates? Unfortunately the evidence appears quite to the contrary (article 34). Of equal interest and concern are the possible negative effects of weight gain and loss cycles (article 35). Certainly this information does not prove that one should never lose weight. It does show that there is much detective work yet to be done and that here, too, risks and benefits must be carefully considered.

What is known as the nondiet movement is described in "Nondiet Movement Gains Strength." This movement responds to the increasing interest in total wellness and to concern that weight obsession in America is creating a crisis situation. Extremes of this obsession were found by medical researchers at the University of South Carolina, where children as young as 9 years evidenced severe eating disorders, including bulimia and anorexia. Over 40 percent of the fifth graders studied believed themselves to be fat and wanted to lose weight, even though 80 percent were not overweight.

For the person who does decide to lose weight and who is serious about keeping it off, good news is still hard to find. No magic bullet that is both effective and safe has yet been discovered. Although weight loss is possible, the level of commitment must be high, and the probability of long-term reduction is not encouraging. Repeated weight gain and loss, a pattern established by many Americans, is often accompanied by reduced self-esteem and other problems. A weight reduction plan cannot be called successful unless the weight loss can be maintained, and herein lies one of the problems associated with many popular plans (see article 40). It remains true that *effective* methods program a slow weight loss of one-half to one pound per week and include behavior modification so that life-styles change on a permanent basis.

Manufacturers and food establishments have responded to the many people wishing to reduce fat and sugar and thus, presumably, calories. Increasing numbers of fast-food chains offer lower-fat items, and some provide salad bars as well. Even restaurants offering haute cuisine feature gourmet foods without the calorie-laden sauces. In the grocery store, too, more and more lower-calorie items are available, such as candy bars and fat-free cakes and cookies. Many new products contain fat (see article 6 in unit 1) and sugar substitutes. Although it is too soon to know if these products will be useful in weight control, early evidence is not convincing (articles 38 and 39).

No doubt science will yet produce other ways of controlling weight. Most people hope that any innovations or new strategies will permit appetite satisfaction and an occasional strawberry shortcake.

Looking Ahead: Challenge Questions

Find a description of a new trendy diet and evaluate it for effectiveness and safety.

At what times is food the most important to you? How would you have to change your life-style to lose weight and maintain that loss?

How many products with fat and sugar substitutes have you tried? What was your purpose in using them? Did you reduce total calories or compensate with something else?

What strategies do you think would be effective in achieving national weight-reduction goals for the year 2000?

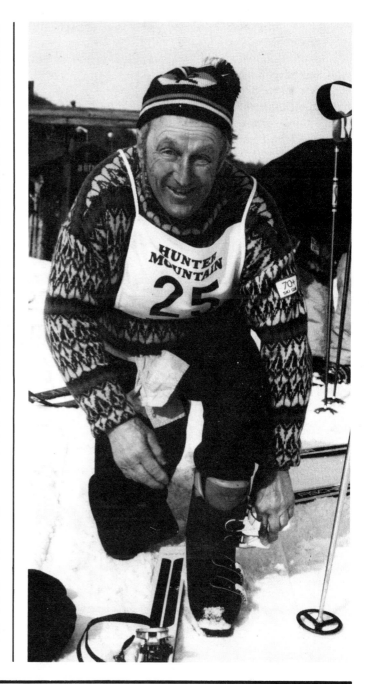

Health risks of obesity

Kendra Rosencrans

Kendra Rosencrans, M.S., Associate editor of Obesity & Health, has a masters degree from Columbia University in journalism with an emphasis on health and science.

The chain binding obesity to major health problems has been forged link by link over the past several years by researchers around the globe.

Obesity and fat distribution have been established as major contributors to:

- Heart disease
- Diabetes
- Hypertension
- Some types of cancer
- Stroke

All are leading causes of death in the United States.

Nearly 40 years ago the National Institutes of Health declared obesity to be the nation's No. 1 health problem. A Congressional subcommittee estimates that obesity contributes to health costs of $140 billion per year that could be avoided.

Yet, "obesity continues to humble the scientific community by eluding effective understanding and intervention in many important respects," said Shiriki Kumanyika, associate professor of nutrition epidemiology at Pennsylvania State University.

But one thing remains clear when recent scientific evidence is reviewed – obesity still means health risk.

A number of studies, including the Build and Blood Pressure studies, the American Cancer Society study, and the Framingham study, when controlled for smoking, find the lowest mortality for ostensibly healthy persons at weights 5-15 percent below average for both sexes. Significant risks are reached at a weight about 20 percent or more above optimal, by height/weight tables *(see Fig. 1)*.

With age, the risks of obesity appear to decrease *(Fig. 2)*, according to findings from the 1979 Build Study *(Am J Clin Nutr 1991;53:1595S-1603S)*.

Heart disease

One of the most recent studies to reiterate the connec-

Fig. 1

Mortality rates by weight

Percent of desirable wt.	Relative risk of death (percent)					
	Build & Blood Pressure Study 1959		American Cancer Society study		Build & Blood Pressure Study 1979	
	Male	Female	Male	Female	Male	Female
80	95	87	110	100	105	110
90	90	89	100	95	94	97
110	113	109	107	108	111	107
120	125	121	121	123	120	110
130	142	130	137	138	135	125
140	167	—	162	163	153	136
150	200	—	210	—	177	149
160	250	—	—	—	210	167

Mortality rates tend to be lowest at about 90 percent of desirable weight and increase with increasing weight, according to three major national studies.

OBESITY & HEALTH (REF: AM J CLIN NUTR 1991;53:1596S)

Fig. 2

Mortality by weight and age

Percent of desirable wt.		Relative risk of death (percent)				
	Age:	20-29	30-39	40-49	50-59	60-69
Men						
>75		102	105	112	128	135
75 - 85		94	93	98	113	120
85 - 95		95	92	93	100	100
95 - 105		98	95	96	94	95
105 - 115		103	112	109	100	101
115 - 125		125	128	118	109	101
Women						
>75		—	—	117	146	134
75 - 85		118	124	110	105	106
85 - 95		88	101	92	93	90
95 - 105		112	86	96	97	101
105 - 115		90	99	103	99	102
115 - 125		118	110	115	103	103

Mortality rates with increasing degree of overweight are higher for younger men and women (ages 20-49) than for older men and women (ages 50-69) in the Build Study 1979. With age, risks of obesity appear to decrease.

OBESITY & HEALTH (REF: AM J CLIN NUTR 1991;53:1596S)

Reprinted from *Obesity & Health,* Journal of Research, News and Contemporary Issues, Vol. 6, No. 2, May/June 1992, pp. 45-47, 51. Copyright © 1992 by Health Living Institute, Hettinger, ND.

tion between weight and heart disease comes from an analysis of the Framingham Heart Study.

Findings published in the New England Journal of Medicine say that a lifetime of losing and regaining weight, known as weight cycling or yo-yo dieting, may mean greater risks for coronary heart disease and other severe health problems.

The study, which followed 3,130 men and women for 32 years, showed that individuals with high weight variability – many weight changes or large changes – were 25 to 100 percent more likely to be victims of heart disease and premature death than those whose weight remained stable. *(NEMJ 1991;324:1839-44.)*

The increased mortality and morbidity due to coronary heart disease and increased total mortality seemed to hold true regardless of the initial weight, long-term weight trend and/or cardiovascular risk factors such as blood pressure, cholesterol level, glucose tolerance, smoking and physical activity.

Being overweight is associated with about 40 percent of all heart disease in U.S. women.

Another study in the same journal established a link between obesity and heart disease in women *(NEMJ 1990;322:882-889).*

Researchers based at Brigham and Women's Hospital in Boston found that being overweight is associated with about 40 percent of all heart disease in U.S. women, and gaining 20 extra pounds during adulthood doubles the risk.

The findings are part of the Nurses' Health Study, an eight-year review of 115,886 healthy women ages 30 to 55. The women were grouped into five categories and the numbers of women who developed chest pains or had heart attacks were tabulated for each group.

The relationship between obesity and heart disease was clear. After controlling for smoking, the leanest one-fifth of the women, who weighed 5 percent or more below desirable weight, had the lowest number of incidents. Women 15 to 29 percent above desirable weight had 80 percent more heart disease, and women 30 percent or more over desirable weight had more than three times the lean women's risk.

According to the American Heart Association, about 500,000 people will die from heart attacks in 1992, making it the No.1 cause of death in the United States. Cancer and stroke rank second and third.

Cancer

National Institutes of Health researchers link abdominal fat distribution to breast cancer for women *(J Natl Cancer Inst 1990;82:286-290).*

A total of 2,201 women ages 30 to 62 were followed for 28 years in the Framingham Heart Study. After the fourth examination 106 had developed breast cancer. When those cases were looked at according to fat distribution, women who fell in the quartile with highest centralized fat were at an increased risk for breast cancer.

Researchers found no association between breast cancer and degree of obesity by either skinfold or body mass index. Older women were more likely to be in the fourth, or highest quartile.

Studies have shown that central adiposity increases as women age and that abdominal fat cells increase in size with menopause. Fat distribution may change with menopause for some women.

The researchers suggest that although obese women of every build have increased estrogen, women with abdominal obesity may have more of an increase in biologically significant estrogen, contributing to an increased risk of breast cancer.

Upper body obesity is also a risk factor in uterine or endometrial cancer, even when cross-referenced according to age and body ass index, say researchers at the H. Lee Moffitt Cancer Center and Research Institute at the University of South Florida, Tampa *(JAMA 1991;266:1808-1811).*

The increased risk is attributed to increased endogenous estrogen production, particularly non-protein-bound estrogen, unopposed by progesterone.

They also confirmed that women with uterine cancer and upper body obesity have an increased incidence of diabetes and hypertension.

A 12-year study by the American Cancer Society also associates obesity with increased death from uterine cancer, and cancers of the gallbladder, kidney, stomach, colon and breast *(Nutr and Cancer, Nov/Dec 1991;335, Am Cancer Society).*

In the study, women who were 40 percent above desirable weight had up to 55 percent greater mortality. Similarly obese

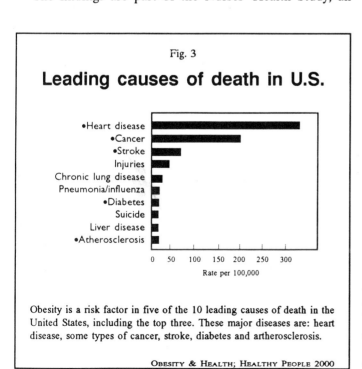

Fig. 3

Leading causes of death in U.S.

- •Heart disease
- •Cancer
- •Stroke
- Injuries
- Chronic lung disease
- Pneumonia/influenza
- •Diabetes
- Suicide
- Liver disease
- •Atherosclerosis

Rate per 100,000

Obesity is a risk factor in five of the 10 leading causes of death in the United States, including the top three. These major diseases are: heart disease, some types of cancer, stroke, diabetes and artherosclerosis.

OBESITY & HEALTH; HEALTHY PEOPLE 2000

men had up to 33 percent greater mortality from cancer than normal weight men.

A Harvard researcher is studying the effect of body fat on puberty. Rose Frisch, PhD, says that girls are reaching menarche three to four years earlier, at 12.8 years instead of age 15, than they did 100 years ago because they are heavier. Menarche is more related to size, weight and percent body fat than chronological age, she says.

Since estrogen has been linked to breast cancer and cancers of the reproductive system, and since girls who reach puberty early are exposed to higher levels of estrogen longer, Frisch suggests that these girls are at a higher risk for cancer.

Her study of 5,398 former college athletes and non-athletes showed that former athletes had a "significantly lower lifetime occurrence of breast cancer and other cancers of the reproductive system, compared to non-athletes." *(Adipose Tissue and Reproduction, edited by Frisch, 1990 Karger, Basel, Switzerland.)*

Non-athletes showed a risk for reproductive cancer that was 2.53 times higher than the athletes. Their risk for breast cancer was also 1.86 times greater than for the athletes. The analysis controlled for potential confounders, including age, age of menarche, age of first birth, smoking, and family cancer history.

Other health problems

While many studies establish a relationship between obesity and health risk, that risk seems to increase with degree of obesity and begins "to reach significance at a weight greater than 20 percent above ideal, using life insurance height-weight tables or body mass index greater than 27," says F. Xavier Pi-Sunyer, MD, director of the NIH-funded New York Obesity Center, professor of medicine at Columbia University, and director of endocrinology, diabetes and nutrition at St. Lukes-Roosevelt Hospital in New York.

In the Nov/Dec 1991 issue of *Obesity and Health*, Pi-Sunyer said that obesity increases health risks not only to heart disease and cancer, but also hypertension, insulin resistance, in some studies, high total and LDL cholesterol.

"As obesity becomes more severe, there is a greater incidence of stroke, menstrual irregularities, reduced fertility, chronic hypoxia with cyanosis and hypercapnia, sleep apnea, gout, degenerative joint disease of the hips and knees, fatty liver, and fungal and yeast infections of the skin," Pi-Sunyer said.

He also said venous circulatory disease is common in obese people and is manifested by varicose veins and venous stasis. In addition, thrombophlebitis and pulmonary embolus is higher among obese people, particularly after major surgery.

Gallbadder disease has been reported as affecting 28 to 45 percent of severely obese individuals, and occurs three to four times more often in obese than in nonobese individuals, according to Pi-Sunyer. The combination of increased age with increased weight further enhances the risk. In addition, weight-reduction diets can cause added problems. About 25 percent of persons on very low calorie diets develop gallstones, he said.

Fig. 4

Mortality by weight and disease

	Women		Men	
	120-129%	140% +	120-129%	140% +
Diabetes	3.34	7.90	2.56	5.19
Digestive diseases	1.61	2.29	1.88	3.99
Coronary heart disease	1.39	2.07	1.32	1.95
Cerebral vascular lesions	1.16	1.52	1.17	2.27
Cancer, all sites	1.19	1.55	1.09	1.33
All causes	1.29	1.89	1.27	1.87

Risk by degree of overweight

Mortality rates increase with degree of overweight for both women and men. Rates for 130-139%, omitted here, were generally less than midway between the rates given.

OBESITY & HEALTH; AMERICAN CANCER SOCIETY

Women with a history of adult obesity, especially black women, may be at higher risk for osteoarthritis – degenerative arthritis of the knees in which the cushioning cartilage of the joint wears away and the bones slowly grow together.

Researchers from the Boston University Multipurpose Arthritis Center found in two studies that being obese, female and/or black increases the risk of developing osteoarthritis *(Am J Epidimiol 1988;128:1:179-189, Ann Intern Med 1988;109:18-24).*

The researchers looked at data from two previous health studies – the first National Health and Nutrition Examination Survey (NHANES I) which ran from 1971-75, and the Framingham Heart Study.

An analysis of both showed that women who had been obese throughout their adult lives – 20 to 25 years – had a higher rate of the disease, although the same was not true of men.

Fig. 5

Disease risks for black Americans
(Per 100, not adjusted)

	Obese	Non-obese
Age 18 to 30		
Hypertension	9.3	3.6
Diabetes	2.5	0.9
T Chol 200 mg/dl	31	22
Age 45 to 64		
Hypertension	62	55
Diabetes	21	10
T Chol 200 mg/dl	30	24

Overweight increases risk factors and accounts for a substantial portion of the diabetes, hypercholesterolemia and hypertension in young and middle-aged black Americans.

OBESITY & HEALTH (REF: NIH MINORITY CONF., AUG 1990)

The rate of osteoarthritis also increased among both men and women who steadily gained weight as adults, with an especially high rate among the very obese. African-Americans also tended to have a higher rate of osteoarthritis than whites.

High-risk populations

Two recent studies suggest obesity rates may be increasing faster for African-Americans than white Americans. In addition, they are at higher risk for many health problems in which obesity is a contributor – diabetes, hypertension, stroke, and coronary heart disease.

The Bogalusa Heart Study found that school children in the study, ages 5 to 14, gained an average of 2.5 kg between 1973 and 1984. However, black males averaged a 3.2 kg gain and black females gained an average of 2.8 kg (*O&H Nov 1988:1*).

Other researchers report that obesity among black teenagers has increased 53 percent in the past 15 to 20 years, compared with a 35 percent increase for white teens (*Am J Dis Child 1987;141:535-540*).

According to data from the 1976-1980 NHANES II study, 44 percent of black women over age 20 are obese, compared with 26 percent of white women. Between the ages of 45 and 74, 60 percent of the black women in the study were obese, with nearly 17 percent at the level of the 95th percentile. The study showed that 30 percent of black men are obese, compared to 25 percent white men.

African-Americans also tend to have a more dangerous body fat distribution than whites, with more centralized obesity. A University of Texas study found black children ages 1 to 17 have more centralized fat than white children (*O&H Dec 1988:5*).

Coronary heart disease is the leading cause of death among African-Americans. A report on the National Heart, Lung and Blood Institute CARDIA and ARIC studies which examined coronary artery and atherosclerosis risks, says risk factors among African-Americans increase with obesity, with little gender difference.

Hypertension and diabetes are also serious health conditions with a high incidence among African-Americans, according to the National Center for Health Statistics.

Diabetes is the third leading cause of death among African-Americans, with rates twice as high as for whites ages 45 to 65, and nearly three times as high over age 65. Type II – non-insulin dependent diabetes – is 33 percent higher than for whites, with the highest rates among obese black women.

The NHANES II study found critical hypertension levels in 40 percent of black women and 28 percent of black men, compared with 20 percent for white women and 21 percent for white men. At age 65-74, prevalence among black women was 60 percent.

Obesity and related health problems are also high among Native Americans.

Adult-onset diabetes is now a major cause of death and morbidity in most American Indian populations. Diabetes-related mortality for Indians is more than twice as high as for all races in the United States, according to the Department of Health and Human Services Task Force on Black and Minority health.

Fat patterns

"The distribution of body fat is directly related to health risks," said New York Obesity Center director Pi-Sunyer. "Abdominal or central obesity is more dangerous than gluteal femoral or peripheral obesity. The amount of intraabdominal fat seems to determine increased peril.

"The risk of coronary heart disease, stroke, hypertension and diabetes increases for men and women with increased central obesity, even independent of total fat mass."

Abdominal obesity is currently measured by the waist-hip ratio (WHR), also known as the abdominal-gluteal ratio, found by dividing the waist measurement by the hip measure. A rule of thumb is the higher the WHR, the greater the risk. Ratios above 0.95 for men and 0.80 for women are associated with greater risk, according to the Dietary Guidelines for Americans from the U.S. Department of Agriculture, Human Nutrition Information Service. (*O&H Jan/Feb 1992:5; Jan/Feb 1991:1-4; Nov 1987:1-4.*)

Weight Loss Escalates Risk of Death

Frances M. Berg

The National Institutes of Health panel, Methods for Voluntary Weight Loss and Control, March 30-April 1, 1992, received a startling answer when it asked the question: "What are the benefits and adverse effects of weight loss?"

Scientists at federal research centers told the panel there is little evidence weight loss lowers mortality rates. On the contrary, most studies show weight loss in the general population is associated with increased risk of death.

The evidence is reported below:

Framingham Heart Study

Men and women who lost weight through 10 years had the highest death rates during 18 years of follow-up in an NIH study based on the Framingham data, reported Millicent Higgins, MD, Associate Director of the Epidemiology and Biometry Program at the National Heart, Lung and Blood Institute, NIH, in Bethesda, Md.

In younger men, death rates were lowest in the weight stable group. In older men death rates were lowest in the weight gain group (which was also lower in weight than the other two).

In younger women, death rates were similar in all groups for the first 6 years; after that they were lowest in the weight gain group. In older women, mortality rates were similar for the weight stable and weight gain groups.

Subjects were measured at 2-year intervals for 10 years. Deaths the next 4 years were excluded. Age and initial weights, but not smoking, were adjusted.

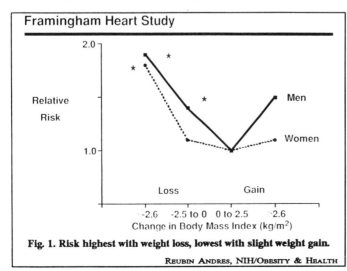

Fig. 1. Risk highest with weight loss, lowest with slight weight gain.

REUBIN ANDRES, NIH/OBESITY & HEALTH

More of the weight loss group were smokers at the final exam, and fewer had quit smoking.

CARDIA

Higgins also reported to the panel on the CARDIA study (Coronary Artery Risk Development in Young Adults). Again, weight loss was associated with increased morbidity and mortality as well as, paradoxically, improvements in blood pressure and lipid factors.

This study included 3,593 young men and women, ages 18 to 30, examined initially, then at 2 and 5 years. Three groups were defined by their first two exams: weight loss of 5 or more pounds; weight stable; weight gain of 5 or more pounds. They were subdivided by whether their weight at 5 years was above or below the median for gain.

Women in the weight loss group were initially heavier and had higher rates of smoking.

Higgins said smoking was associated with leanness and weight loss, and may account in part for these results. More of the weight gain group had quit smoking (nearly 20 percent of women smokers in the weight gain group had quit, compared with about 8 percent in the other two; about 23 percent of men smokers had quit in the weight gain group compared with 4 to 6 percent in the other two).

Reprinted from *Obesity & Health*, Journal of Research, News and Contemporary Issues, Vol. 6, No. 4, July/August 1992, pp. 64-65, 74. Copyright © 1992 by Health Living Institute, Hettinger, ND.

NHANES I Follow-up, CDC
Risks of weight loss

All causes maximum weight lost	Maximum BMI		
Men	**<26**	**26-<29**	**29+**
<5%	1.0	0.9	1.5
5-<15%	1.1	1.3	1.2
15%+	1.8	2.1	2.0
Women			
<5%	1.0	0.8	1.5
5-<15%	1.5	1.4	1.8
15%+	2.7	1.9	2.8

Fig. 2. CDC study compares effects of weight loss at three weight levels. Higher mortality is associated with higher weight loss for all levels, except that moderate weight loss appears beneficial in very overweight men.

OBESITY & HEALTH

Ten Studies
Risks of weight loss

	Loss in BMI (adj. to 10 yr)		Relative risk of death Men	Women
Framingham	2.5 - 0	1.4	1.1	
		>2.5	1.9	1.8
Dutch Elderly		5+	1.45	1.05
Alameda County		0.5	1.56	
Baltimore Aging	2.8 - 0.4		1.25	
		>2.8	1.33	
Honolulu Heart		>0.4	1.45	
Lipid Research		0.6	1.27	
British Heart		5-2	1.6	
		>5	2.0	

Fig. 3. Loss of weight is associated with mortality in these studies. Two other studies reporting only gains (Paris Prospective and Harvard Alumni) found highest risk in the lowest gain group. In another study mortality was unrelated to weight loss or gain, Andres.

OBESITY & HEALTH

NHANES I Follow-up

The Centers of Disease Control NHANES I Follow-up study, reported by Elsie Pamuk, PhD, Epidemiologist at CDC in Atlanta, found weight loss associated with increased risk of death for both men and women, also for cardiovascular and noncardiovascular diseases. The more weight lost, the higher the risk (see fig. 2).

Maintaining a stable weight meant no increased risk for moderately overweight men and women (BMI 26 – <29). But a weight loss of 15 percent or more (of maximum weight) was associated with higher death rates, regardless of their weight.

For women in all three weight groups, any amount of weight loss increased their mortality rate. This was true of men, also, except for men in the highest weight group (BMI 29 or higher) for whom a moderate weight loss (between 5 and 15 percent) seemed beneficial. Losing more weight, however, again increased their risk.

This study used NHANES I data of 2,140 men and 2,550 women, age 45–74, based on measurements in 1971–75 and their recall of the heaviest weight they had ever been. They were followed for about 10 years (through 1987), with deaths in the first 5 years excluded. Adjustments were also made for previously diagnosed illness.

Subjects were divided into three groups by their maximum weight, then subdivided into three categories by percent of maximum weigh lost. Nearly two-thirds had lost 5 percent or more.

The study was adjusted for age, race, parity for women and baseline smoking.

Numerous analyses were performed to control for preexisting illness. However, the results still held. They were even intensified, for example, when cardiovascular disease, not believed to be related to weight loss, was looked at separately.

Similarly, attempts were made to control for smoking by isolating three baseline categories: never smoked, former smoker and current smoker. Current analysis is now being performed separately with the never smoked group.

Ten studies

A "surprising consistency" in results from 10 widely varying studies indicates that weight loss is invariably and usually progressively associated with high mortality, reported Reubin Andres, MD, Clinical Director of the National Institute on Aging Gerontology Research Center, NIH, Baltimore.

The studies varied widely in design, technique, initial "cleanup" for disease and smoking issues, periods of follow-up (8 to 22 years), age of subjects and populations (see figs. 1, 3, 4, 5, 6).

Andres concludes that, while for certain conditions weight loss may be a benefit, "For the general population, the results of the 10 studies do not support the idea that losing weight will increase longevity . . . (but) the opposite conclusion.

"If body weight for optimal survival increases with age, then weight gain with the passage of time is permissible and can even be recommended."

MRFIT

Two studies in progress, MRFIT (Multiple Risk Factor Intervention Trial) and the Harvard Alumni Study, suggest higher rates of morbidity and mortality for men with higher levels of weight fluctuation, reported Steven Blair, PED, Director of Epidemiology, Cooper Institute for Aerobics Research, Dallas. In addition to weight cycling effects, he said, MRFIT also shows highest death rates for men who lose weight, lowest risk with stable weight, and slightly elevated risk with weight gain.

4. FAT AND WEIGHT CONTROL

The MRFIT prevention study followed for 10 years 10,534 men who were initially in the upper 10 to 15 percent of risk for coronary heart disease, but with no clinical evidence of it. Men with severe obesity (over 1.5 times ideal weight) were excluded, as were deaths in the first year of follow-up. A randomly assigned special intervention group of 5,323 were examined every 4 months; the others had annual exams.

Results show progressively higher mortality for coronary heart disease, cardiovascular disease and all causes: with higher incidence of weight fluctuation; with weight cycling once or more; and with weight loss. With weight gain there was slightly increased risk. In general, the effects were heightened for the special intervention group.

The study is controlled for age, race, cholesterol levels, weight, smoking, alcohol consumption and physical activity and also for changes in smoking, alcohol consumption and physical activity.

Harvard alumni

The Harvard Alumni Study findings, given by Blair, are consistent with MRFIT in that men with the highest weight fluctuation had the highest disease rates, and men with the lowest fluctuation the lowest disease rates.

Weight fluctuation in the ongoing study, which began in 1962 and includes 11,140 men, was assessed by two methods in the 1988 questionnaire.

From nine body drawings the men checked those that best matched their shape at present, at college entrance, and at ages 25, 40, 50 and 60. They also reported the number of times they had lost some weight (under 5 pounds, 5, 10, 20, and 50 or more pounds) and this was calculated as total lifetime pounds loss.

Defining three groups by degree of weight fluctuation, the Harvard study finds these progressively higher rates of nonfatal diseases with higher weight fluctuation:

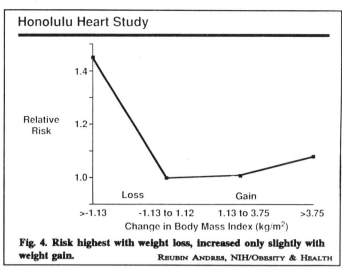

Fig. 4. Risk highest with weight loss, increased only slightly with weight gain.   Reubin Andres, NIH/Obesity & Health

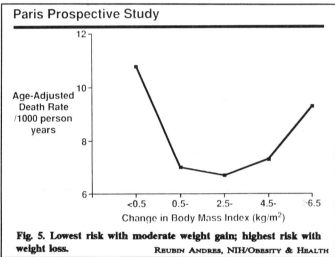

Fig. 5. Lowest risk with moderate weight gain; highest risk with weight loss.   Reubin Andres, NIH/Obesity & Health

a. Coronary heart disease (1.00, 1.15, 1.30)
b. Myocardial infarction (1.00, 1.12, 1.29)
c. Hypertension (1.00, 1.07, 1.11)
d. Diabetes Type II (1.00, 1.09, 1.42)

Defining three categories by total pounds lost, the study finds progressively higher rates of the above conditions with more pounds lost.

Opposing findings

David Williamson, PhD, Epidemiologist, Centers for Disease Control, Atlanta reported studies which showed opposite results, but says these were seriously flawed. A Metropolitan Life Insurance Company study found that moderately overweight men who reduced weight decreased their mortality rate to 20 percent lower than men who did not reduce; for

women the reduction in mortality was 37 percent. In the more severely overweight group, men who lost weight decreased mortality rate 39 percent, women 16 percent.

Summary

In these studies, which find higher mortality with weight loss, two possibly confounding issues are preexisting illness and smoking. However, the researchers say they believe these factors would not change the results.

Special analyses were conducted on various factors in attempts to control for the effects of diseases associated with weight loss which could lead to early death. The researchers looked at cardiovascular disease, which is not a wasting disease, separately from other diseases, and found an even stronger relationship.

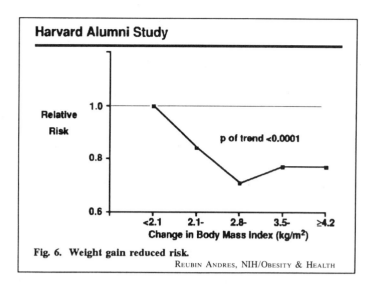

Fig. 6. Weight gain reduced risk.

REUBIN ANDRES, NIH/OBESITY & HEALTH

They excluded all deaths for a period of years.

Blair says in interview, that he has been examining this effect of higher mortality with weight loss and weight fluctuation for three years, doing "all sorts of analysis—and can't make it go away." He says there appears to be no separate effect with cancer which, as a wasting disease, one might expect.

Furthermore, Blair says, "I do not believe this can be explained by changes in smoking. When we look at smokers, never smokers or intermittent smokers, we don't see any difference. Results are in the same direction."

The NHANES I Follow-up study at CDC is now looking separately at non-smokers. Pamuk says she doesn't think the results will be much different, because, "the study shows the same effects in older women, and not many were smokers."

Since these findings are preliminary, the NIH panel statement did not recommend treatment changes: "While the data are provocative, they are sufficiently inconclusive and should not dictate clinical practice. Specific research efforts addressing

this question are urgently needed.

"The fact that many people who stop smoking gain weight makes comparisons of weight gainers and weight losers more dIfficult. Also that most of the studies cannot distinguish purposeful weight loss from that associated with illness, psychosocial distress, or other reasons. We need to know much more about the individuals who have lost weight and why they, unlike participants in programs, appear to keep weight off."

The evidence on weight cycling was found similarly controversial: "Data presented on the health effects of repeated weight gains and losses, or weight cycling, also are inconclusive. Cycling appears to affect energy metabolism and may result in faster regains of weight, but the evidence that weight cycling has longer term negative effects on psychological and physical health needs further confirmation."

Pamuk suggests these findings may be showing that losing weight, by itself, does not always improve health, or that some types of voluntary weight loss may be harmful.

More attention needs to be paid to how the weight is lost and whether it is sustained, she says.

It is difficult to work with data which was collected for other purposes, as in the NHANES follow-up, she notes. Needed information may not be available. There are "just not enough facts out there," and research money is tight.

However, Pamuk suggests that health recommendations may need to be reconsidered. "The general assumption has been that weight loss is helpful . . . but perhaps maintaining stable weight will be found to be the best course."

From the public health view, Williamson says he feels we "should focus less on loss of weight, and more on maintaining healthy behaviors, especially for people who are moderately overweight."

Both assert that a primary health objective should be the prevention of obesity, through early establishment of a healthy diet and regular physical activity.

Despite these findings, the reports confirmed an improvement of cardiovascular risk factors with weight loss. Higher mortality was generally associated with obesity.

In addition to this research, the panel was given an overview of other obesity research, treatment and concerns. A summary of the final statement was published in the May/June 1992 issue of *Obesity & Health* (page 42).

Abstracts and Statement, Methods for Voluntary Weight Loss and Control, NIH Technology Assessment Conference, March 30-Apil 1, 1992. National Institutes of Health. Research papers to be published in a special issue of the Annals of Internal Medicine.

Yo-Yo dieting threatens heart

Gain-lose-gain cycle may be as risky as staying obese

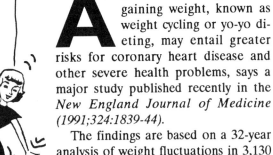

A lifetime of losing and regaining weight, known as weight cycling or yo-yo dieting, may entail greater risks for coronary heart disease and other severe health problems, says a major study published recently in the *New England Journal of Medicine* (1991;324:1839-44).

The findings are based on a 32-year analysis of weight fluctuations in 3,130 men and women in the Framingham Heart Study.

Individuals with a high weight variability – many weight changes or large changes – were 25 to 100 percent more likely to be victims of heart disease and premature death than those whose weight remained stable. They had increased mortality and morbidity due to coronary heart disease and increased total mortality.

These results seemed to hold true regardless of the individual's initial weight, long-term weight trend and/or cardiovascular risk factors such as blood pressure, cholesterol level, glucose tolerance, smoking and physical activity.

Kelly Brownell, PhD, a psychologist and weight specialist at Yale University who directed the study, says the harmful effects of yo-yo dieting may be equal to the risks of remaining obese.

Weight cycling has been under investigation since 1986 at several institutions following studies that indicated weight loss and regain on the very low calorie diet made subsequent weight loss on the same diet more difficult. Researchers from Goteborg, Sweden, and Boston University are involved in the current study.

The report cites their research in Sweden which found large fluctuations in body weight, measured at three intervals, was associated with heart disease in men and total mortality in both men and women.

In view of their findings, they suggest it may be important to look at public health implications of current weight loss practices. They note that about half of American women and one-fourth of men are dieting at any one time, with many of these efforts unsuccessful. Weight is commonly regained and the cycle repeated.

"The pressure in this society to be thin at all costs may be exacting a serious toll," Brownell says. The study's findings indicate that weight cycling is "potentially a very serious public health issue because it affects such large numbers of people."

Even though nearly 50 percent of women who diet are not overweight, the weight cycling risks are seen at all weight

---

Individuals with high weight variability were 25 to 100 percent more likely to be victims of heart disease and premature death than those whose weight remained stable

---

categories, whether thin or obese.

"It may be equally bad to lose the same five pounds 10 times as to lose 50 pounds and regain it once," said Brownell.

High weight variability
Relative risk

The relative risk for a high degree of weight variability compared with a low degree of variability is as follows:

Men

Total mortality	1.30
Mortality due to CHD	1.48
Morbidity due to CHD	1.48
Morbidity due to cancer	1.04

Women

Total mortality	1.27
Mortality due to CHD	1.47
Morbidity due to CHD	1.42
Morbidity due to cancer	1.16

This age-adjusted analysis compares the highest one-third of the group in weight variability with the lowest one-third, or least variability. CHD denotes coronary heart disease. All variables except cancer were significantly related to weight variability.

Variability vs stability

The researchers calculated variability by dividing the standard deviation of each person's nine body mass index values (BMI) through the 32 years by his or her average BMI. This showed how much weight fluctuated around the average. A high degree of variability indicates many changes or large changes; a low value indicates weight stability. Weight change direction was also determined as to whether a general weight gain or loss occurred over time.

In an effort to exclude weight changes that may have been caused by illness, the diseases and deaths were not counted unless they occurred at least four years after weight was measured.

The degree of weight variability was evaluated in relation to total mortality, mortality from coronary heart disease, morbidity due to coronary heart disease and morbidity due to cancer. Risks were considerably increased for all except cancer, which did not differ significantly.

When age groups were considered separately, weight fluctuation was most strongly associated with adverse health outcomes in the youngest group (age 30-40). This is also the group seen as most likely to diet.

The researchers found that a person's weight at age 25 makes an important contribution to whether there will be great variability.

Both men and women gained weight at an average rate of .11 kg per square meter per year. (People tend to gain percent body fat as they age and gain fat in the abdomen.)

The researchers say weight cycling may account for the observed increase in deaths in these ways:

1. Factors that influence coronary risk (such as cholesterol levels) may change with fluctuating weight and end up worse than before.
2. The amount and distribution of body fat as weight is lost and regained may change. During weight loss, a person loses both fat and lean body mass, but may regain mostly fat. This fat tends to settle in the abdomen, a location linked to increased heart disease risk.
3. People may increasingly prefer high-fat diets when they lose and regain weight. Studies have shown that weight-cycling laboratory animals tend to eat more fat.

Findings stir controversy

These findings are likely to be controversial and to further fuel the weight cycling debate among scientists, says Claude Bouchard, PhD, of Laval University, Quebec, in an editorial in the same issue of the *New England Journal of Medicine*

Bouchard notes that a recent review of 18 studies of weight cycling in rodents found no clear evidence that weight cycling makes future weight loss harder and weight gain easier. They found no evidence that it increases total body fat or central adiposity, increases subsequent caloric intake, increases food efficiency, decreases energy expenditure, or increases blood pressure, insulin resistance, or cholesterol levels. Bouchard suggests there may be a preference for dietary fat in refeeding and that the observed risks could result from a higher fat intake.

Human populations are not easily investigated, as he points out, because researchers must obtain measurements over a long period of time, assess many risk factors, and control for numerous variables.

Bouchard stresses the need for more and better-designed animal research which will control for diet composition across the cycles of weight gain and loss, and measure changes in fat location.

Frances Berg

Does dieting cause more harm than good?

It is difficult to find any scientific justification for the continued use of dietary treatments for obesity, David M. Garner, PhD, of the Department of Psychiatry, Michigan State University, East Lansing, told dietitians at the 74th Annual Meeting of the American Dietetic Association Oct. 28-31 in Dallas. Most weight lost is regained, he said, a fact often obscured by follow-up periods too short to capture the later phases.

Besides inefficacy as a reason to abandon dietary treatments, Garner advanced other arguments.

Treating obesity is usually justified by its apparent adverse effects on health and longevity, but there is evidence that a stable weight may be safer than weight fluctuation or even weight reduction, he charged.

Further, Garner contended dieting may precipitate binge eating, eating disorders and untoward psychological effects such as depression, anxiety, social withdrawal and personality changes. It may also contribute to repeated weight cycles, provide patients with failure experiences, expose them to professionals who hold them in low regard, cause them to see themselves as deviant and flawed, confuse their perceptions of hunger and satiety, and divert their attention away from other problems.

Garner said such negative consequences do not occur all the time nor to all people, but they need to be given more serious consideration than they have in the past.

Garner served as a special consultant to the Michigan Health Council Task Force to Establish Weight Loss Guidelines, which set recommendations for weight loss programs in Michigan and produced the 1990 publication Toward Safe Weight Loss. (J Am Diet Assoc 1991 Suppl 91:9:A-152)

QUIT WATCHING THE SCALES?

For decades, public-health scientists have joined the fashion and diet industries in pressuring Americans to lose weight. Now mounting evidence has raised doubts about the health benefits of this national obsession with getting slim. The "ideal" weights, defined by insurance companies decades ago and promulgated by health authorities ever since, may actually be too low for people over 40. And people of any age may do themselves more harm than good if they continually struggle to keep weight at some "ideal" level.

Study after study has shown that the ideal weight for middle-aged and older people is considerably higher than those insurance figures have indicated. An as-yet-unpublished review from the National Institute on Aging evaluated 13 major studies and concluded that people actually live longer if they put on a few pounds as they get older. The researchers, led by gerontologist Reubin Andres, M.D., noted that trying to prevent that natural weight gain may be not only futile but hazardous. Some people, of course, do have medical reasons to try to lose weight. But even for them, the numbers on the scale may be less important than such other factors as the distribution of fat on the body and the person's susceptibility to coronary heart disease.

Weight and health: The big picture

Outright obesity usually does pose a threat to health. Obesity—generally defined as weight at least 25 to 30 percent over what's desirable for one's height—is commonly associated with high blood pressure and high cholesterol levels, two major risk factors for coronary heart disease. Obesity is also associated with the most common kind of diabetes and raises the risk of gallstones, gout, and cancer of the gallbladder, uterus, and ovaries. For all those reasons, it's not surprising that people who are obese die younger, on average, than people of normal weight.

The link between weight and life expectancy was systematically studied by researchers at the Metropolitan Life Insurance Company. Their familiar height-and-weight tables show the range of weights for each height that was statistically associated with the longest life. People with weights much above those ranges, the Metropolitan Life figures showed, had a shorter life expectancy.

But the actuaries who constructed those tables oversimplified the data. They ignored the interaction between weight and other factors, like high blood pressure, that could be harmful to health. And they ignored the age of their insurance holders: They assumed that a 55-year-old should weigh no more than a 25-year-old, and lumped together people from all age categories.

Now there is good evidence that the weight associated with the lowest mortality actually increases as you age. In one large-scale study, Norwegian researchers followed 1.7 million people—more than half of all Norwegians older than age 14—for 16 years. Moderately lean young people did indeed have a lower death rate than heavier young people. But the optimal weights for middle-aged and older people were an average of 10 pounds higher than even the most liberal insurance tables had indicated.

Those findings led Andres to reexamine the insurance data. Sure enough, when he took age into account, the figures showed that the optimal weight for long life crept up by several pounds each decade. People lived longest if they weighed even less in their 20s or 30s than the insurance tables had suggested. But they did best at weights higher than the recommended limits when they were older.

Andres's upcoming review of 13 studies, all prospective and all lasting 12 years or more, strengthens the case for modest weight gain with age. There are two caveats: People who are already overweight as teenagers or young adults should try to lose weight, not gain more; and no one should gain too much weight over time. (Researchers disagree on precisely how much weight a person can safely gain, with estimates ranging from 2 to 10 pounds per decade.)

It's still not clear just why middle-aged and older people who are slightly plump live longer than thin people do. According to one theory, thinness might reflect another underlying health problem, such as cigarette smoking or an undetected cancer, that shortened life. However, several studies have controlled for that possibility, and the advantage of mild plumpness still holds.

It is possible, however, that extra body fat could help people survive the impact of a wasting illness, such as cancer or lung disease, which consumes body tissue. Indeed, studies consistently show that thin people have a higher death rate from lung ailments and certain tumors than other people do. In the Norwegian study, for example, very thin people had just as high a death rate as very fat people did—and the diseases most likely to kill the lean included chronic bronchitis and emphysema, lung cancer, stomach cancer, and tuberculosis.

Where's the fat?

In addition to age, the distribution of fat on the body makes a major difference in how that fat affects health. Many studies have shown that fat concentrated around the belly increases the risk of many of the same problems that are associated with obesity—high blood pressure, high cholesterol, coronary disease, and diabetes. (Indeed, abdominal fat seems to raise the risk of developing those conditions even more than obesity does. In contrast, fat stored mostly around the hips and thighs seems to have little if any effect on that risk.)

Swedish studies have long indicated that apple-shaped (pot-bellied) people tend to die sooner than pear-shaped (broad-hipped) people. In January, Minnesota researchers strengthened that finding when they published a report based on the Iowa Women's Health Study, which involved more than 40,000 older women. The researchers found that the higher the ratio of a woman's waistline to her hip circumference—and thus the more apple-shaped her body—the higher her risk of death during the five-year study.

Researchers believe that abdominal fat is dangerous partly because it readily migrates into the bloodstream and on to the liver, which converts the fat into substances that can raise blood-cholesterol levels. In addition, abdominal fat cells tend to be larger than other fat cells. And studies have linked large fat cells with complex metabolic changes that can raise blood-sugar levels and blood pressure. However, there's a positive side to abdominal fat, at least for men: They shed fat more readily from the waist than from the hips when they lose weight.

The dangers of dieting

While moderate increases in weight aren't as dangerous as researchers once thought, strenuous dieting to lose or maintain weight may be more of a hazard than anyone realized.

It's certainly clear that dieting is usually futile in the long run. The body responds to a strict low-calorie diet as it would to starvation, by lowering its metabolic rate, the speed at which the body burns

calories to provide energy. In addition, much of the weight you do lose on a low-calorie diet often comes from muscle tissue. Losing muscle tissue, which burns lots of energy, further lowers the body's metabolic rate.

As a result, when you stop dieting, you tend to regain the weight you lost, and often more. More ominously, the regained pounds are mostly fat. And that fat tends to settle in the worst possible place—around the belly.

Dropping just 10 to 15 pounds might substantially improve your condition, possibly reducing or even eliminating the need for drugs.

"Yo-yo dieting"—repeatedly losing and regaining weight—is especially undesirable. The ongoing Framingham Heart Study has shown that people whose weight fluctuated the most over the course of about 20 years had a higher overall death rate than those whose weight fluctuated the least. The researchers checked the records of the 40 patients whose weight varied the most, and found that at least half of them, probably more, had indeed been chronic dieters.

Last October, researchers from Harvard and Stanford Universities reported the results of a 12-year study of nearly 12,000 middle-aged and older Harvard alumni. Men who gained up to 11 pounds over a dozen years had roughly the same death rate as those whose weight remained stable during that time. Men who gained more than that did have a higher-than-average death rate. But men who lost more than a few pounds also had a higher death rate, particularly from coronary disease—apparently because the net weight loss usually came after several cycles of yo-yo dieting.

Do you need to lose?

To answer that question, start by checking the table (see box) which incorporates the latest findings on weight and health. The table, endorsed by the U.S. Department of Agriculture and the Department of Health and Human Services, allows for some weight gain after a person's mid-30s. It makes no distinction between men and women, since studies have shown surprisingly little difference between the optimal weight ranges for each sex. But the table offers broad ranges of acceptable weights—up to 52 pounds for each height—in part to allow for differences in how much of that weight represents fat rather than muscle.

But weight alone does not provide a complete picture of how extra body fat will actually affect your health. First, you need to consider whether you have any of the conditions that excess fat may aggravate: primarily high blood pressure, high blood cholesterol, coronary heart disease, and diabetes. If so, dropping just 10 to 15 pounds might substantially improve your condition, sometimes reducing or eliminating the need for medications. People with a family history of coronary heart disease or diabetes are

> *The regained pounds are mostly fat, and that fat tends to settle in the worst possible place—around the dieter's abdomen.*

also likely to benefit from losing weight. In addition, weight loss can ease the pain of low-back problems or arthritic joints.

Next, check your waist-to-hip ratio. To do that, measure your waist at the narrowest point between the bottom of your rib cage and the top of your pelvis. Then divide that figure by the size of your hips at the widest protrusion of your buttocks, to arrive at the waist-to-hip ratio. For women, who are usually pear-shaped, a ratio that exceeds 0.8 signals a shift towards abdominal fat and an increase in the risk of disease. For men, any ratio of 1.0 or more, indicating a waist at least as big as the hips, is similarly undesirable. Losing weight tends to shrink the waistline, particularly in men, and theoretically that should reduce the risk of disease.

How to lose weight safely

Even if you're sure that you would indeed benefit from losing weight, you need to go about it safely. Forget about going on a temporary, aggressive diet, and instead make a permanent commitment to maintaining healthy, weight-managing habits.

Regular exercise is a crucial part of any successful weight-control program. Working out burns calories and helps maintain or build the muscle tissue that can keep your metabolic rate from slowing down. If you need to lose only 10 pounds or less, exercise alone may be enough. To shed more weight than that, try combining exercise with a low-fat diet. Try eating smaller portions, too, since many people routinely underestimate the amount of food they actually eat. But don't cut back dramatically on your calorie intake: That increases the likelihood of regaining any lost weight.

Lose weight in stages. Lose a few pounds, then ease up for a while; be certain you can maintain that loss before you resume a more rigorous regimen. Make sure you can keep up your exercise program, and make sure that the dietary changes you've made are changes you can maintain.

Whether or not you lose much weight, following a low-fat diet and working out regularly will improve your overall health. In particular, those steps can improve your blood pressure and cholesterol levels—the same improvements you would expect to see if you lost weight.

Acceptable weights for adults [1]		
Height	**Weight (lbs)**	
	19 to 34 years	**35 years and over**
5'0"	97-128	108-138
5'1"	101-132	111-143
5'2"	104-137	115-148
5'3"	107-141	119-152
5'4"	111-146	122-157
5'5"	114-150	126-162
5'6"	118-155	130-167
5'7"	121-160	134-172
5'8"	125-164	138-178
5'9"	129-169	142-183
5'10"	132-174	146-188
5'11"	136-179	151-194
6'0"	140-184	155-199
6'1"	144-189	159-205
6'2"	148-195	164-210
6'3"	152-200	168-216
6'4"	156-205	173-222
6'5"	160-211	177-228
6'6"	164-216	182-234

1. Values in this table are for height without shoes and weight without clothes.
Source: Dietary Guidelines for Americans.

Nondiet movement gains strength

Frances M. Berg, M.S.

Frances M. Berg, MS, editor and publisher of Obesity & Health, is an adjunct professor, University of North Dakota School of Medicine, Grand Forks, and a licensed nutritionist with a graduate degree in family social science from the University of Minnesota.

A new movement is rising from the turmoil of widespread frustration with diets that don't work, pressures to be thin, and the crises in eating disorders that grips America.

This nondiet health-enhancing paradigm focuses on wellness solutions and rejects weight loss dieting and food restraint. Spurred by eating disorder specialists, it is gaining momentum in Canada through national health policy and in the U.S. in Congressional hearings and through a major National Institutes of Health conference.

Treatment programs using the new approach usually focus on the following three factors:

1) feeling good about oneself;
2) eating well in a natural, relaxed way; and
3) being comfortably active.

This calls for wellness, not weight loss. It encourages pleasure in eating, not restraint. The new paradigm says "listen to your body, be kind to your body," not "your body is wrong, it needs fixing." It teaches an awareness of hunger and how to respond to internal signals, not eating prescribed foods at specified times.

This approach offers a journey of self-discovery, not tests of will power. It celebrates self-esteem, diversity and accepting people as they are, not judging and putting others in molds. It encourages women to get on with living and stop putting their lives on hold while waiting to be thin.

The new paradigm calls for wellness, not weight loss . . . for pleasure in eating, not restraint.

The new approach says "trust yourself, be good to yourself, enjoy life." It challenges old rules for weight loss, as well as the current direction taken by fitness and wellness programs. It is a way of making peace with one's body, and making peace with food.

The anti-diet movement grows out of a concern by educators, health care providers and nutritionists that America's weight obsession is causing a major crisis.

It differs from other "nondiet" approaches which limit fat or sugar intake.

"We are still on the fringe," says Susan Kano, author of *Making Peace with Food.* "The general population is not ready for this, but it will be."

'Epidemic' in fat fears

Weight obsession is strongly linked to eating disorders.

Among high school and college students, the prevalence of anorexia nervosa is about .5 percent, and of bulimia nervosa, 2 percent, 90 percent of them female, according to Laura Hill, PhD, Director of the National Anorexic Aid Society. The student rate of eating disorders, including all clinical variations, is about 10 percent.

"We are not seeing a drop yet," says Hill. The incidence of clinical cases continues to increase, along with an "epidemic" rise in such symptoms as fear of fat, body shape distortions and bingeing.

Of patients with anorexia nervosa who remain chronic, one study found 7 percent had died within 10 years. An-

other found a death rate of 20 percent in 30 years, says Hill.

"How easily weight obsession is dismissed as an inevitable phase of female development," charge Susan Wooley, PhD, and O. Wayne Wooley, PhD, clinical psychologists at the University of Cincinnati Medical Center. "Would things be different if our hospitals and clinics were filled with young men whose educations and careers were arrested by the onset of anorexia nervosa, bulimia, or the need to make dieting and body shaping exercise a full-time pursuit?"

"Would things be different if our hospitals and clinics were filled with young men whose educations and careers were arrested by the need to make dieting and body shaping exercise a full-time pursuit?"

Increasing pressures on women to be thin are vividly illustrated by a 30-year survey of Miss America contestants and Playboy magazine centerfold girls.

Both have become thinner, year by year, and are now at an anorectic level of 13 to 19 percent below their expected weight. Miss America entries today have thinner hips than ever before, yet are not as thin as Playboy centerfolds. For both, weight has leveled off because, the researchers suggest, they can go no lower without risk of death *(O&HSep/Oct92:83).*

Pressure to be thin

From a feminist perspective, the selling of thinness is seen as a manipulative tool to prevent women from gaining power in the work force.

In a searing account, Naomi Wolf, author of *The Beauty Myth,* charges that the political and corporate power structure, the media, and women's magazines and their advertisers unite to force women into a competition of continual striving for thinness and beauty. It's a cruel struggle they can't win, she says. Every woman is made to feel a failure, no matter her successes. She is ever an inadequate object on display.

Further, Wolf points out that simple starvation, in the quest of weight loss, effectively keeps women weak, preoccupied and passive, off track from any career ambitions.

The woman-as-object theme is also explored by Kano. Women are dehumanized, she writes, by beauty contests, body-building contests and pornography, as well as by advertisers and the fashion industry, all of which show women as thin mannequins. Women's clothing, which is often tight and has an ornamental purpose with little regard for comfort or movement, is part of this.

Another explanation for pressures to be thin, given by Susan Wooley and David Garner, PhD, eating disorder specialist at Michigan State University, is that as women have moved into previously male-dominated activities, the maternal shape has developed negative connotations, while the masculine shape has come to symbolize self-discipline and competency (*Clin Psych Rev 1991;11:729-780*).

Negative stereotypes are widely associated with being overweight, particularly for women. The prejudice and discrimination that comes from weightism, or fatism, is well documented – in social relationships, employment, education and the medical community (*O&H Jan89:5-6*).

Dieting failures

In response to these pressures to be thin, is a rise in dieting and restrained eating, not only for women, but for men as well.

Research shows 40 percent of U.S. women are currently dieting, nearly two-thirds of them not overweight; that 61 percent of adolescent girls and 28 percent of boys have been on a weight loss diet in the past year; and that as many as 50 percent of 9-year-old girls and 80 percent of 10-year-olds in a California school have dieted, only 15 percent of

them overweight (*O&H May/Jun92:48; Jul/Aug92:69-72*). Americans spend more than $30 billion annually on weight loss, plus investing a great deal of time and emotional energy.

But is the effort successful? Hardly.

"It is difficult to find any scientific justification for the continued use of dietary treatments of obesity," write Garner and Wooley.

"Regardless of the specific techniques used, most participants regain the weight lost. There is remarkable consistency in the pattern of regain across behavioral, dietary and very low calorie diet approaches to obesity. Most approaches lead to weight loss during active treatment, however, most participants ultimately regain to levels that approximate their pre-treatment weight."

Garner and Wooley say the inevitability of this result is often obscured by studies which claim success after a follow-up that is too short to show what really happens in later phases.

They charge that, contrary to scientific tradition which assumes there are no treatment effects until demonstrated, weight loss interventions are presumed effective until there is explicit evidence to the contrary. But "the reality is that we do not have effective treatment to offer, and we should be candid about this until there is reliable evidence to the contrary."

Dieting can kill

Regain is not the only outcome of failed diets. Proponents of the new paradigm say dieting itself does great harm.

"Dieting is not just about eating," says Janet Polivy, PhD, a professor of psychology and psychiatry at the University of Toronto, who has researched dieting and its effects for over 16 years. "It is an entire way of life. Life has a different meaning for people when they become dieters. Their self-image and self-esteem is all tied up in this."

The dangers of dieting, says Polivy, include medical and psychological harm, eating disorders, financial cost, and diminished lifestyle.

Medical disorders and conditions that she documents as being directly attributed to weight loss include: gallstones, cardiac disorders, fainting, weakness, fatigue, both slowed and increased heart rate, anemia, gouty arthritis, edema, headache, nausea, hair loss and thinning hair, elevated cholesterol, hypotension, diarrhea, aching muscles, abdominal pain, elevated uric acid levels, cold intolerance, increased pulse rate, muscle weakness, loss of lean tissue, changes in liver function, constipation, dry skin, muscle cramps, amenorrhea and decreased libido, refeeding risks from fasting diets such as edema, potassium deficiencies, biliary tract disorders and pancreatic complications, and death.

"We don't know how many are dying," adds Polivy. Ironically, most deaths are blamed on the victims' overweight, she says, rather than the true culprit – radical attempts to lose weight.

Dieting deaths are not recorded as such in the U.S., according to the Centers for Disease Control. Most appear to be listed as heart disease deaths.

Chronic dieters also respond differently than non-dieters in a variety of situations, Polivy explains. They are easily upset, emotional, have mood swings, are more likely to eat when anxious, have trouble concentrating on the task at hand with any kind of distraction, can go longer without food and eat less under "ideal" circumstances, but binge or eat more once started and then experience guilt, are compliant and willing to please, have lower self-esteem, are preoccupied with weight and body dissatisfaction, have a need for perfection, have lost touch with internal signals of hunger and satiety and rely on cognitive cues for eating, salivate more

> "Starvation keeps women weak, preoccupied and passive, off track from career ambitions"

when faced with attractive food, and have higher levels of digestive hormones and elevated levels of free fatty acids in their blood.

A chronic dieter focuses on food, eating and weight both for herself and in her perception of others, has low self-esteem, and is eager to please and do what others ask of her. Polivy argues that dieting is causal to these factors.

Dieting also promotes weight cycling, which may increase health risk. A study based on 32 years of weight fluctuations for 3,230 persons in the Framingham Heart Study found those with many weight changes or large changes were 25 to 100 percent more likely to die from heart disease or die prematurely than persons with stable weight (O&H Nov/Dec91:93).

Ellyn Satter, RD, a childhood eating specialist in Wisconsin, says it's time to define the problem of childhood obesity in ways it can be solved. "Diets are not an option. Restricting food intake, even in indirect ways, profoundly distorts developmental needs."

An industry based on false hope

Weight loss products and programs are largely unregulated and not held accountable for harm resulting from their use. Evidence of safety and efficacy are seldom required, and U.S. regulatory agencies have been permissive in allowing exploitive, false and misleading advertising.

"The diet industry is now built on a foundation of false promises and false hopes," charges Rep. Ron Wyden, D., Ore, chairman of the Congressional hearings investigating the weight loss industry.

Even when maintained, weight loss may not increase longevity, as has been assumed.

On the contrary, federal studies reported at a recent National Institutes of Health conference show increased mortality. Reubin Andres, clinical director of the National Institute on Aging Research center, presented 10 studies showing weight loss consistently associated with higher death rates.

A study based on the Framingham data showed mortality for women at

"If you cannot help, at least do no harm"

nearly all ages and weight levels was highest with weight loss and lowest with moderate weight gain. For older men, mortality rates were also lower in the weight gain group. A CDC study found weight loss associated with increased risk of death for both men and women, and also for cardiovascular and noncardiovascular diseases. The more weight lost, the higher the risk.

Although these findings are still tentative, they "do not support the idea that losing weight will increase longevity (but) the opposite conclusion," says Andres. He suggests that some weight gain over time is permissible and may even be recommended (O&H Jul/Aug92:64-65).

This is not to minimize the health risks of obesity. Obesity and abdominal fat distribution have been established as major contributors to heart disease, diabetes, hypertension, stroke and some types of cancer (O&H92:45-51).

Federal support

Not surprisingly, official support for the anti-dieting movement comes most readily from Canada, led by the research of Canadian eating disorder specialists such as Janet Polivy and Peter Herman, PhD, at the University of Toronto.

In 1988 Health and Welfare Canada initiated a policy advocating the acceptance of a broad range of healthy weights. It issued challenges to both consumers and professionals to make healthy changes in five areas (attitudes, lifestyle, treatment, environment, knowledge) in dealing more effectively with weightism and the problems of obesity (O&H Mar89:17-24).

Health care workers in Canada were issued a clear warning: *If you cannot help, at least do no harm.*

At that time, the U.S. was still turning up the pressure through its public health directive that 50 percent of overweight Americans should be on weight loss regimens by 1990 (O&H Jan88:1-5).

However, the nondieting movement was energized by 1990 U.S. Congressional hearings which began to look clearly, for the first time, at what was going on in the dieting industry and whether consumers were being treated fairly. The hearings revealed widespread abuse and forced regulatory agencies to take action against fraud and false advertising (O&HJun90:41-46; Jan/Feb91:9-12).

This was followed by a major National Institutes of Health Technology Assessment Conference in March 1992 on *Methods for Voluntary Weight Loss and Control.* After hearing evidence, the conference panel issued a critical statement concluding that weight loss strategies have caused harm, most often the weight lost is regained, dropout rates are high, repeated lose/gain cycles may have adverse effects, trying to achieve body weights and shapes presented in the media is not an appropriate goal for most people, unrealistically thin ideals create problems, many Americans who are not overweight are trying to lose – which may have significant physical and psychological health consequences, and that most major studies suggest increased mortality is associated with weight loss.

This was a landmark statement in the obesity field in that it showed a readiness to question long-held assumptions in the health community.

It was a shocking question in 1984, when the Wooleys asked, "Should obesity be treated at all?" in *Eating and Its Disorders*, edited by Stunkard and Steller. Their conclusion – that it would be hard to construct a rational case for treating any but massive, life-endangering obesity – was largely ignored.

"It has been over a decade since two major reviews questioned the effectiveness and social appropriateness of behavioral treatments for obesity," said Garn and Wooley, recently. "Other papers and books have since appeared challenging the basic precepts which underlie dietary treatments for obesity. Their arguments, however, have not been embraced, accepted, or in many cases, even addressed by the mainstream of behavioral scientists and health care professionals who treat obesity."

The question is asked more frequently now. It was addressed briefly at the 1991 American Dietetic Association annual meeting in Dallas, and with a major panel discussion at the 1992 meeting of the North American Association for the Study of Obesity in Atlanta.

New positive approach

AHELP

To bring together professionals with similar concerns, to help strengthen the new anti-diet health-based paradigm, and to develop and research new ways large people can be helped without a focus on weight loss, is a new organization. Joe McVoy, PhD, director of the Eating Disorders Program at Saint Albans Psychiatric Hospital in Radford, Va., convened the first conference of the Association for the Health Enrichment of Large Persons (AHELP) in Virginia in 1991 and the second in May 1992. A 1993 conference will be in California.

"We want to alter the thinking of those who stigmatize large people into dieting, forcing their patients into unhealthy practices and promoting self-hate," says McVoy.

He expresses concern that therapists and doctors often do damage to the emotional and physical health of large patients through their treatment of them, and warns that "health professionals have the greatest potential for harm, but they also have the greatest potential for change."

"We want to tap the creative people out there who have unique and successful programs and ask them to share their ideas," says McVoy.

His goals for AHELP are to develop a new theoretical foundation. "It must be more broad based and multidisciplinary with more creative options to help move obese persons into the direction of self-acceptance and health restoration rather than merely counting pounds lost as an indicator of self-esteem and treatment success.

> ## "Trust your body to want what is good for you. Your body is meant to feel good"

"We believe that large men and women are entitled to healthy, fulfilled lives, and are dedicated to providing them with support, education, therapy, and medical care to achieve this. We feel that the societal prejudice against fat people and weight loss through dieting have the most harmful effects. Consequently, we actively oppose fatism within both our profession and our society, and oppose food restriction for weight loss."

Vitality

Vitality is a new nation-wide Canadian program designed by Health and Welfare Canada which combines the three components of the nondiet, health-based paradigm: feeling good about oneself, eating well, and being active.

According to Vitality: "These three elements help you enjoy life to the fullest. They work together to make you feel healthy and energetic. When these three aspects are in balance in our lives, we can move more smoothly and with less effort – we'll be 'in synch' with ourselves and our environment."

Vitality de-emphasizes body weight, and fosters self-empowerment within the social environment.

It encourages people to take charge of how they eat, how active they are, how they think about themselves. "Being proud of how your body looks and moves and believing in your own self-worth are more important than social pressures to be perfect."

The focus is on preventing weight problems, not on treating them. The new program will focus first on young adults, ages 25 to 44, as the group with broad family influence and also that has high risk of developing heart disease, cancer and diabetes.

Nondieting treatment programs developed and taught in Canada by Janet Polivy, Donna Ciliska and Linda Omichinski, are designed to work with Vitality, and with the earlier Canadian guidelines calling for acceptance of a wide range of sizes and shapes. Indeed, Polivy was instrumental in helping form national policy; she serves on the Canadian health department's Task Force on the Treatment of Obesity.

Polivy, who co-authored the book Breaking the Diet Habit: The Natural Weight Alternative., with Herman, has developed Stop Dieting, a 10-session program to help people break patterns of restrained eating, based on their extensive research on dieting and its effects. Participants learn to substitute normal eating behavior for current eating patterns. They schedule meals to recondition hunger, eating only when hungry, and eliminate dieting behavior and mentality.

Stop Dieting, a program by Donna Ciliska, PhD, associate professor of nursing at McMaster University, Ontario, sets the goal of re-establishing normal eating, improving self-esteem, learning self-acceptance and how to deal with negative messages about body shape.

Her 12-week program is specifically for large women who have been chronic dieters. It covers cultural pressures to be thin, the effects of dieting on mood, behavior and eating patterns, and learning normal eating, which she defines as the eating of three meals a day, with snacks between if meals are more than three or four hours apart.

Ciliska is researching the results of her program with 160 women in a randomized test, comparing differences between the Stop Dieting program and a more traditional behavioral program.

HUGS, another Canadian program, by Linda Omichinski, RD, author of You Count, Calories Don't, is a 10-week skills training program based on "deprogramming individuals from the diet mentality and reprogramming them onto a healthy lifestyle.

"It's about freeing yourself from the preoccupation with food and weight, " says Omichinski.

Based on the three components of self-acceptance, healthy eating and active living, the focus is on overall health, with the caution that a healthy lifestyle may not necessarily result in a change in weight or body shape.

Focus inside

Going even farther along the road to breaking up compulsive eating patterns and replacing them with freedom to choose is *Overcoming Overeating*, by Jane Hirschmann and Carol Munter. This program is strongly focused on going to the inside self, not the outside, to determine when to eat, what food, and how much. It's a three-part plan of: "freeing yourself, feeding yourself and finding yourself."

Initial steps include legalizing all foods, eating as much as desired of formerly forbidden foods, while getting acquainted with one's body in an accepting way. The scale is out, a full-length mirror is in, and the closet gets cleaned of any clothes that don't fit or don't feel right. Negative thoughts are put aside and replaced with nonjudgmental ones.

In the second phase, the individual seeks to distinguish "stomach" hunger from "mouth" hunger. She responds to the first and looks for causes of anxiety that may trigger the latter, while being accepting and even compassionate of any binge-type behavior. Response to internal signals must be prompt and accurate as to type of food and quantity eaten. This entails carrying a "food bag" – an ample supply of a variety of foods.

"Grazing" may replace eating meals either temporarily or long-term.

The "finding yourself" phase strengthens self-assertion and self-esteem. It breaks apart the symbolic power of food, as well as entrenched ritual patterns of anxiety, eating, self-hate, recrimination and resolve.

The Hirschmann and Munter plan is used in the worksite wellness program of Conoco Oil Company. Senior coordinator of the *Pleasure Principle Wellness* Conoco program, Karen Carrier, MEd, and dietitian Mary Tierney, RD, say participants ask themselves, "How much longer do I want to go on obsessing about weight."

In a three-year follow-up study, they report significantly lower stress, less restrained eating, less preoccupation with food, and increased self-esteem and self-acceptance.

"Trust your body to want what is good for it. Your body is meant to feel good," says Carrier. "Each eating experience is an opportunity to 'caretake' yourself and begin eating your way out of the trouble you've been in with your body size and food."

A fitness vision

Much of what people are learning in the health and fitness movement could actually be making them less healthy by causing them to take a negative view of themselves, charges Carrier. "Lives often become very rigid, almost as if the eating and exercise behaviors drive them, instead of the person driving them. Many who keep themselves slim do so only with rigidity and self-control, unable ever to relax or let down."

A broader vision of exercise is a part of the new approach.

Instead of viewing exercise as a religion, which glorifies muscles and sweat, and appeals to few, Gail Johnston, a health and fitness consultant in California, says a better approach focuses on exercise as a pleasurable experience, as an activity everyone can enjoy, succeed in, and work into their daily life.

It's not necessary to lose weight to achieve the benefits of exercise, she says. Nor is it necessary to count heart rate or work up to training levels.

"Imagine being able to enjoy physical activity just for the sheer joy, without worry about doing enough, being competent or losing weight," says Johnston.

"Trendsetters in health promotion are beginning to use visions such as these as the basis for re-evaluating how they can do a better job helping people become more active."

Pleasure Principle Wellness

Eating and Body talk – Internal Cue
1. Free yourself up from restrictive eating plans!
2. Eat in rhythm with your stomach.
3. Create an abundant supply of food.
4. Learn about and add new foods to your diet.
5. Choose not to weigh yourself.
6. Talk about your eating and your body in kinder terms.
7. Work at realistic self-acceptance.

Exercise – Internal Cue
1. Stay away from highly structured exercise plans.
2. Respect variability in your body's need for movement.
3. Choose not to take your heart rate.
4. Explore your range of options for movement.

5. Leave the feedback panels on exercise equipment off!
6. Opt out of fitness tests.
7. Think of exercise as a way to add pleasure to your life.

In the employee wellness program of Conoco Oil Company, men and women are urged to accept their bodies in a respectful, nonjudgmental way, to make peace with their bodies, to pay attention to how the body feels, to "love your body just the way it is." A key is learning to understand and respond to the different types of hunger in a nurturing way.

Wellness materials available from Conoco Wellness, 600 N. Dairy Ashford, Box 2197, Houston, TX 77252 (713-293-5050).

Low Calorie Sweeteners and Dieting

Kathleen Meister

Kathleen Meister, M.S., is a freelance writer, associate editor of the Nutrition Research Newsletter *and a former ACSH research associate.*

Could drinking diet sodas cause you to gain weight? This disconcerting idea has been suggested repeatedly in the popular press. Every year or two, a new batch of newspaper and magazine articles announces that low-calorie sweeteners make people feel hungrier or that users of these sweeteners are more likely than non-users to gain weight.

Such reports have aroused understandable concern among the 100 million Americans who use low-calorie sweeteners such as aspartame and saccharin. They do not, however, represent an up-to-date, balanced view of the scientific evidence. As is often the case, some segments of the news media have taken isolated research findings out of context, with the emphasis on sensationalism rather than common sense. Let's take a look at the whole picture.

The Case Against Sweeteners

Claims that low-calorie sweeteners are the dieter's worst friend have been based primarily on two pieces of scientific evidence. One was a large survey conducted by the American Cancer Society (ACS). The other was a series of short-term tests performed at Leeds University in England.

In the ACS survey, researchers examined weight change over a one-year period in 78,000 women between the ages of 50 and 69 who were participating in a study of lifestyle and cancer death rates. The study was not designed to assess the relationship between low-calorie sweeteners and weight change and was not well suited to this purpose.

The popularity of low-calorie sweeteners has soared in the past three decades, but Americans have not become thinner.

The women filled out a questionnaire which asked whether they used artificial sweeteners and whether they drank diet sodas. Since the survey was conducted in 1982, before aspartame was widely available, the principal sweetener used by these women was saccharin. Before analyzing the data, the researchers excluded from consideration certain groups of women who were in special situations that might have influenced their weight. One of these groups included women who said that their eating habits had undergone a major change in the past ten years. This group would include most serious dieters.

Do Sweetener Users Gain Weight?

The researchers then examined the data and found that among women who gained weight, users of low-calorie sweeteners gained more than non-users, although the difference between the two groups was small. Some observers have interpreted this to mean that low-calorie sweeteners will not help people to lose weight and may even hamper their dieting efforts. But let's take a closer look at the ACS findings.

- First, the difference in weight change between users and non-users was about half a pound. This difference was statistically significant (because the population studied was very large), but so small that it was clinically irrelevant.
- Second, most evaluations of this study have ignored the fact that among the most overweight women, low-calorie sweetener users lost more weight than non-users. So there is actually some evidence of a possible beneficial effect.
- Third, and most important, the findings of this study don't say anything about the role of low-calorie sweeteners in dieting, because individuals who made serious efforts to diet were excluded from consideration. The women examined here were casual users of low-calorie sweeteners. This type of sweetener use, in and of itself, does not cause weight loss.

Findings like those in the ACS study are not new. More than 35 years ago, a group of 347 obese people, 100 of whom were diabetics, were asked about their use of low-calorie sweeteners (saccharin and cyclamate) and then observed over a three-year period. There was no difference in weight loss between sweetener users and non-users. The general experience of the American public is consistent with the findings of this classic study. The popularity of low-calorie sweeteners has soared in the past three decades, but Americans have not become thinner.

Low-calorie sweeteners are not magic potions. Many dieters believe, however, that sweeteners can be a helpful part of a comprehensive weight-loss strategy.

Now let's take a close look at the Leeds studies. In these tests, volunteers drank a solution of sugar in water, a low-calorie sweetener in water or plain water. Aspartame was the sweetener tested in the first study; a later test involved aspartame, saccharin and acesulfame-K. At several time intervals after consuming the drinks, the subjects filled out self-rating forms that assessed feelings of fullness and desire to eat. The results indicated that people who consumed low-calorie sweeteners became hungrier than those who consumed plain water or sugar water.

The "Residual Hunger" Hypothesis

The researchers who conducted these studies suggested that low-calorie sweeteners may have the "paradoxical effect" of causing "residual hunger." They speculated that, "these sweeteners uncouple the sensory dimension (sweet taste) of foods from their calorific properties and so may distort the information used by the regulatory mechanisms involved in

the control of food intake . . . This confusion of psychobiological information may lead to a loss of control over appetite, particularly in vulnerable individuals of normal weight who are dieting and who may be consuming large amounts of dietary aids for weight control."

This hypothesis may seem plausible and potentially alarming. However, the Leeds studies do not prove it to be true, for three reasons.
- First, the studies used an unrealistic experimental situation in which people consumed unflavored sweetener solutions. These are unfamiliar, and many people find them unpalatable.
- Second, the apparent effects were based on hunger ratings which are not always a good predictor of how much people will eat. Food intake, considered more important than hunger because it is the actual factor that affects body weight, was not measured in one study and was unaffected by sweetener consumption in the other.
- Third, and most important, the Leeds studies constitute only a small part of a large body of scientific evidence on sweeteners and food intake. Most of this evidence does not support the hypothesis of a "paradoxical effect."

Aspartame

The scientific evidence on aspartame and food intake was comprehensively reviewed by Dr. Barbara J. Rolls of The Johns Hopkins University School of Medicine in a recent issue of the *American Journal of Clinical Nutrition*. In her review, Dr. Rolls described 18 published experiments which measured the effects of aspartame consumption on hunger ratings and food intake in human subjects.

In three of these studies (including the two conducted at Leeds), hunger ratings increased after aspartame consumption. In the 15 others, aspartame consumption either had no effect on hunger or decreased it. The

variability in these findings may reflect differences among the studies in the types of people who participated (normal vs. overweight, adults vs. children), the vehicles in which aspartame was administered (capsules, unflavored drinks, flavored drinks, chewing gum, solid foods) and the types of substances with which aspartame was compared (other low-calorie sweeteners, sugars, plain water).

If the individual isn't making a real effort to diet or if he or she uses a diet soda as an excuse to eat a high-calorie treat, low-calorie sweeteners will not have any impact on body weight.

More important and consistent, however, was the finding that aspartame consumption was never associated with an increase in food intake. Despite the wide variety of test protocols, none of the 16 studies that measured food intake found an increase after consumption of aspartame. Most showed no effect, and two showed a decrease. Dr. Rolls concluded that, "Even if aspartame increases ratings of hunger in some situations, there is no evidence that it has any impact on the controls of food intake and body weight." This is a sound conclusion based on a substantial amount of experimental evidence.

There have also been a few longer-term studies in which aspartame-sweetened foods or drinks were covertly substituted for sugar-sweetened ones for a period of days or weeks. In some instances, people ate enough other foods to make up for the calorie deficit caused by the use of aspartame; in others, there was only partial compensation. In all of these studies, however, aspartame consumption was never associated with an increase in food intake or body weight.

Saccharin

There has been much less research on saccharin than on aspartame. One series of studies in rats did indicate that drinking a saccharin solution increased the animals' food intake. Whether these results have any relevance to the human situation is uncertain. It is difficult to extrapolate experimental findings from one species to another even when the issue in question is purely physiological. When behavior is involved, as it is in this instance, it is even more problematic to assume that humans follow the same patterns as rodents.

In one human study (conducted at Leeds), subjects who had consumed saccharin-sweetened yogurt ate more of a test meal than subjects who had consumed unsweetened yogurt (both yogurts had the same calorie content). Some observers have interpreted this to mean that saccharin increases food intake. However, it is also possible that the differences in sweetness and palatability of the two yogurts, rather than the saccharin content, may have been the key factor. In the same study, subjects who consumed yogurt containing saccharin plus starch (added to bring the calorie content up to that of sugar-sweetened yogurt) did not eat more food than those who consumed sugar-sweetened yogurt.

A more recent study conducted at New York University compared hunger levels and food intakes in adult volunteers who drank either plain water or a noncarbonated soft drink sweetened with sugar or saccharin. Hunger ratings were generally highest after water, lower after saccharin and lowest after sugar was consumed. There were no differences in food intake.

The inconsistencies in these study findings can only be resolved through further research. Even though saccharin use has decreased since the introduction of aspartame, saccharin is still an important food additive. The current evidence is insufficient to allow conclusions to be drawn about the relationship of saccharin to food intake in humans.

If these products are used as part of a well-planned diet rather than as a substitute for a diet, they may help to make weight loss efforts more rewarding.

Acesulfame-K

It would be worthwhile to include the new low-calorie sweetener, acesulfame-K, in future studies. The findings on one sweetener do not necessarily apply to other sweeteners. It is conceivable that sweeteners might influence food intake through some physiological mechanism rather than through their sweet taste, and different sweeteners could have different physiological effects.

The Role of Sweeteners in Dieting

Common sense tells us that in the absence of some mysterious effect on appetite, the effects of low-calorie sweeteners on food intake depend on the person who uses them. If the individual isn't making a real effort to diet, or if he or she uses a diet soda as an excuse to eat a highly caloric treat, low-calorie sweeteners will not have any impact on body weight. However, if low-calorie sweeteners are used to increase the palatability and variety of a well-planned low-calorie diet, they could be helpful.

There are only a few scientific studies on the role of low-calorie sweeteners in serious dieting efforts. In one of these studies, male dieters assigned to use sweeteners showed better weight loss and maintenance than a comparison group that was instructed to avoid them. However, similar beneficial effects were not seen in female dieters. Another study suggested that aspartame may be beneficial in weight maintenance among formerly obese women, and that dietary control may be more difficult if use of the sweetener is prohibited.

In a trial of a multidisciplinary weight-control program, obese women who were encouraged to use aspartame (in conjunction with a low-calorie diet, exercise and behavior modification training) showed greater weight loss than women following the same program who were asked to avoid aspartame. The aspartame users were also more successful than the non-users during a later weight-maintenance portion of the same program.

When it comes to dieting, there is no free lunch. A lasting weight loss can only be achieved through a sustained change in eating and exercise habits. Low-calorie sweeteners are not magic potions. Many dieters believe, however, that sweeteners can be a helpful part of a comprehensive weight-loss strategy. Research is needed to confirm these findings. If these products are used as part of a well-planned diet rather than as a substitute for a diet, they may help to make weight loss efforts more rewarding.

Dietary Compensation for Fat Reduction and Fat Substitutes

David J. Shide PhD • Research Scientist • Program in Biobehavioral Health • Pennsylvania State University • University Park, Pennsylvania
Barbara J. Rolls PhD • Shibley Professor of Biobehavioral Health • Pennsylvania State University

Americans consume nearly 40% of their daily energy as fat, despite federal and health organization recommendations that fat intake be reduced to 30%. In spite of public awareness of risks associated with high-fat diets (heart disease, cancer, and obesity, to name but a few), most individuals have great difficulty reducing their fat intake. Most also find it difficult to comply with lower-fat diets.

Eating habits and food preferences are extremely difficult to change, partly because taste is a primary determinant of food selection. Fats endow foods with many sensory and textural characteristics, contributing to the richness of flavor and overall palatability. The desire to eat fat is so strong that it operates even in the face of death. One good example of this is patients with cardiovascular disease, who should be highly motivated to reduce their fat intake, but who are often non-compliant because they do not like the taste of low-fat foods as much as that of high-fat foods.

Poor compliance is a problem in all programs that attempt to modify the diet. Individuals typically rate low-fat diets as bland and less satisfying than regular diets. This is one reason that manufacturers are working to produce reduced-fat, low-fat, or nonfat foods that preserve the desirable sensory qualities usually associated with fat. Although information on intakes of newly introduced fat substitutes is not yet available, studies calculating the potential impact of substituting these products for dietary fat indicate they will help reduce the percentage of energy consumed in the form of fat (*J Nutr* 122:211, 1992).

Why do people consistently prefer high-fat foods? Studies by Birch and colleagues indicate that preference for fat develops at an early age (*Physiol Behav* 50:1245, 1991). Young children learn to prefer energy-dense, high-fat foods, probably through an association with the satisfaction of hunger, and these preferences persist through adulthood. This critical early experience may be one reason why preferences for high-fat foods are so resistant to change. In addition, obese and dieting individuals have a particularly strong preference for dietary fat (*Physiol Behav* 35:617, 1985). Thus, those who most need to reduce fat intake may have the greatest difficulty doing so.

Metabolic influences of fat intake

Recent research indicates fat calories may promote fat deposition and adiposity more effectively than carbohydrate calories. In overfeeding studies in Vermont, naturally lean men had difficulty gaining weight when overfed a diet primarily made up of carbohydrates, compared with a similar group of lean subjects who gained weight relatively easily when calories were supplied as fat (*Am J Clin Nutr* 41:1132, 1985). Differences in response to fat or carbohydrate calories appear to be related to differences in the ways the two macronutrients are processed. Metabolically, it costs much less to store fat as body fat than to store carbohydrate as fat, whereas eating a high-carbohydrate diet stimulates the sympathetic nervous system and metabolism.

Fat replacement and fat substitutes

How do humans respond to reductions in dietary fat? Since reducing fat intake will mean a proportional increase in carbohydrate intake, a key question is whether fat and carbohydrate have similar effects on hunger and satiety. Most short-term studies have found no differences between fat and carbohydrate in relation to hunger, satiety, or energy intake. When the fat or carbohydrate content of meals was covertly reduced by 400 to 1600 kcal, subjects made up for this so that daily energy intake remained constant (*Am J Clin Nutr*

4. FAT AND WEIGHT CONTROL

52:969,1990; *Am J Clin Nutr* 55:331, 1992). In addition, there was no evidence that individuals compensated for fat reduction by increasing subsequent intake of fatty foods (they had no fat-specific appetite).

Two studies using olestra, a noncaloric fat substitute with physical and orosensory properties that closely mimic regular fat, have yielded comparable results (*Am J Clin Nutr* 56:84, 1992; *Int J Obes* 15:1,1991). When olestra was substituted for fat at breakfast, there was a dose-related reduction in fat intake, with a reciprocal increase in carbohydrate intake in healthy lean young males. In a study that examined 2-to 5-year-olds, ingestion of olestra rather than fat was associated with a significant reduction in overall fat, but not energy, intake. (Olestra, produced by Procter and Gamble, is not yet available commercially.)

Studies of dietary fat reduction carried out at Cornell University appear to suggest that habitual, unrestricted consumption of low-fat diets may be an effective approach to weight loss (*Am J Clin Nutr* 53:1124, 1991). However, this conclusion must be considered preliminary, as subjects in these studies had access only to low-fat foods; as mentioned earlier, compliance with low-fat diets may be difficult when individuals are surrounded by palatable high-fat foods.

In the short-term studies reviewed above, where a wide variety of low- and high-fat foods were available, subjects made up the calories removed from the diet. Nevertheless, two recent longer-term studies indicate that a shift in diet composition could affect body weight, even when daily energy intake is not significantly altered. In one study (*Am J Clin Nutr* 54:304, 1991), higher energy intakes were required to maintain body weight on a very low-fat diet (20% of energy derived from fat) than on a high-fat diet (37%). In another study (*Am J Clin Nutr* 54:821, 1991), decreases in the proportion of fat in the diet were associated with weight loss.

Some unanswered questions about fat substitutes

While the assumption is that fat substitutes will help to lower fat intake and could possibly lower energy intake, a number of questions remain. For example, as large quantities of reduced-fat products become available, will individuals discover that these foods do not satisfy hunger as effectively as the full-fat versions of the foods?

Recall that children learn to prefer foods that are energy-dense, through repeated association of sensory cues with the physiological consequences of ingestion. Presumably, the same mechanisms mediating changes in preferences are operating in adults as well. If this is true, the desirability of reduced-fat foods may fall, so that they are no longer selected. Alternatively, consumption of these foods or other foods may increase in order to satisfy hunger.

Will preferences for fat be influenced by use of fat substitutes? It has been suggested that eating a low-fat diet can lead to a decrease in the preferred level of fat in some foods. It is possible that fat substitutes could reduce or prevent this change, undermining long-term compliance with low-fat diets (*Int J Obes* 15:7, 1991). It should be stressed that most of the studies reviewed here were conducted in normal-weight, nondieting individuals, and the results may differ in dieting and overweight people.

Clinical significance: Consumption of low-fat foods should be of benefit in reducing the daily percentage of calories from fat, as there is no indication that a fat-specific appetite develops following consumption of low-fat foods. It seems likely that the reduction in fat intake will be the most important and reliable health benefit associated with low-fat foods.

Suggested reading

Drewnowski A: The new fat replacements: A strategy for reducing fat consumption. *Postgrad Med* 8:111, 1990.

Rolls BJ: The impact of low-fat foods on energy and nutrient intakes. *Trends in Food Science and Technology* 2:235, 1991.

Rolls BJ, Shide DJ: The influence of dietary fat on food intake and body weight. *Nutrition Reviews* 50:283, 1992.

RATING THE DIETS

or years, dieters frustrated by cycles of losing and regaining weight have bounced from one diet fad to the next, from one commercial program to another, wondering if any of them will work. Now the Federal Trade Commission is wondering too. In March, the FTC announced that it is looking into the advertising practices of several commercial diet companies, including the nation's five largest: *Diet Center, Jenny Craig, Nutri/System, Physicians Weight Loss Centers,* and *Weight Watchers.* The FTC has asked for evidence to back up the advertised promises these companies make that their programs will bring lasting weight loss.

Diet companies have been notorious for their failure to present any solid data on their programs' results. Americans now spend more than $3-billion a year on these programs, but they have had no solid information on their benefits, if any.

We decided to conduct a survey to help fill the gap by including a section on weight loss in our 1992 Annual Questionnaire. Readers who had tried to lose weight at least once during the previous three years were invited to tell us about their experience, and 95,000 of them did. Most of them had tried to lose weight on their own, but almost 19,000—one in five—had joined professionally managed weight-loss programs. We asked them to tell us about their weight history—before using the program, at the time they finished it, six months later, and at the time they filled out the questionnaire—and asked them several questions about the dieting experience. Using their responses, we were able to compare the same five diet programs that are the chief targets of the FTC probe. We also sent staffers undercover to outlets of those five companies to experience their sales pitches first-hand.

In addition, our survey gave us information about three other programs—*Health Management Resources, Medifast,* and *Optifast*—which are designed for seriously overweight people. Unlike regular diet programs, these entail giving up food for a time and following a very-low-calorie liquid diet under a doctor's supervision.

We invited each of the eight companies we evaluated to send us any materials they thought would help us assess their programs. Only *Optifast* and *Jenny Craig* provided any information on their clients' success. The *Optifast* study was designed well enough for us to consider it scientifically valid; *Jenny Craig's* was not.

Ours is the first major scientific survey of the commercial diet industry. Among our chief findings:

■ For most people, commercial weight-loss programs are temporary palliatives at best. On average, our respondents reported that they stayed on the programs for about half a year and lost about 10 to 20 percent of their starting weight. But the average dieter gained back almost half of that weight just six months after ending the program, and more than two-thirds of it after two years (see "How Weight Returns Over Time," below).

■ None of the top five diet programs were better than the others in helping people lose weight during the program or keep it off six months later. As a group, people on the three liquid-fast programs did lose weight more rapidly than those on regular diet programs—but they gained it back at roughly the same rate.

■ Many people who went on these eight commercial programs had no clear reason to try to lose weight. More than a quarter of them did not meet the medical criteria for even moderate overweight when

How our readers lost weight on diet plans— and how most of them gained it back.

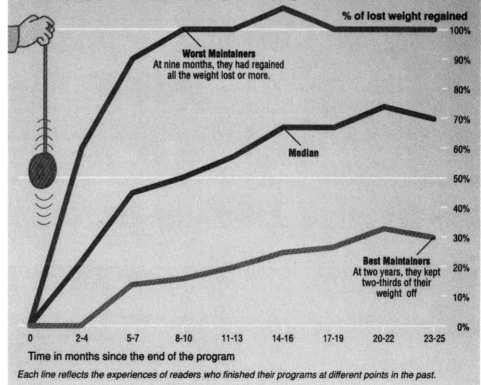

HOW LOST WEIGHT RETURNS OVER TIME

Winners and losers at weight loss Readers who went through a commercial diet program typically regained half their lost weight in a year and much of the rest in another year (a pattern shown here as the "median" line). But experience varies. When we looked at the one-quarter of our sample who regained the most weight, we found these "worst maintainers" typically regained all their weight, or more, within nine months. In contrast, the quarter of our sample who were the "best maintainers" had kept off more than two-thirds of their weight, on average, after two years. These figures are for people on the five commercial diet programs; the pattern for liquid-fast programs was similar.

% of lost weight regained

Worst Maintainers
At nine months, they had regained all the weight lost or more.

Median

Best Maintainers
At two years, they kept two-thirds of their weight off

100%
90%
80%
70%
60%
50%
40%
30%
20%
10%
0%

0   2-4   5-7   8-10   11-13   14-16   17-19   20-22   23-25

Time in months since the end of the program

Each line reflects the experiences of readers who finished their programs at different points in the past.

Diet veterans

Dieters can have good or bad experiences on any program. Here and on the following pages are some reports from CU staffers who tried diet programs on their own.

A typical diet cycle

Name: Rana Arons
Program: Nutri/System
Experience: Lost 12 pounds late last year; has gained it all back.
Comment: "I found it really difficult to stay on the program, since I go out to lunch and dinner a lot and the program is based on prepared foods. I also didn't learn anything to help me change my lifelong eating habits."

they started the program. That group of normal-weight people included a significant fraction of those who went on liquid-fast programs, which can be especially hazardous for people who are not obese.

■ Overall dissatisfaction with weight-loss programs was higher than that for all other consumer services we have evaluated in reader surveys over the years. (That dissatisfaction, however, may partly reflect the fact that diet programs make more demands on the consumer than most of the other services do.)

Despite all this, a significant minority of our respondents—about a quarter of them—did get some apparent benefit from their weight-loss regiment. Two years after finishing their program, they had kept off most of the weight they had lost. That's a better success rate than the often-quoted statistic, based largely on people in hospital clinics, that 95 percent of all diets eventually fail. But it's a far more modest success rate than many dieters are led to expect.

The four major options

Most people who want to lose weight would do well to try the least costly and difficult strategies first, and consider more elaborate programs only if those fail. Here are the major options:

Self-help. Our survey showed that going it alone was moderately effective for some people: Those who lost weight on their own shed an average of 10 pounds.

While the do-it-yourself dieters were somewhat less satisfied with their initial weight loss than were customers of commercial diet programs, those who did lose weight were a bit more satisfied with their ability to keep the weight off. The changes they made on their own may have been easier to sustain than the more artificial changes imposed by an outside program.

The strategies used by the do-it-yourself group were, by and large, simple and sensible. Those people ate less food, especially fatty foods, snacks, and desserts, and they exercised more—all changes, of course, that benefit health even when they don't produce weight loss.

Hospital-based programs. Of the respondents who used professionally managed programs to lose weight, 6 percent chose programs

offered by local hospitals. Hospital-based programs vary enormously in scope and cost, from free or low-cost nutritional counseling to elaborate, physician-supervised liquid fasts. Overall, people who enrolled in hospital programs lost about as much weight, and kept it off about as well, as people in commercial programs—and they had fewer complaints about the hospital-based programs.

Commercial diet programs. More than 80 percent of the readers who sought help in losing weight chose one of the five largest commercial diet programs. These programs generally attract women who have a moderate weight problem and men who are moderately to seriously overweight. The women in these programs averaged 167 pounds when they started and a body mass index, or BMI, of 28; the men, 217 pounds and a BMI of 31. (A BMI of 25 or less is considered desirable, while most people with a BMI of 30 or more are seriously overweight.)

But diet programs also attracted a significant number of people—about 30 percent of the readers who used them in our survey—who had a BMI of 25 or less. Such people have no clear medical reason to try to lose weight.

These programs all include a low-calorie diet of about 1000 to 1500 calories a day and some kind of counseling to help dieters deal with the temptations presented by eating out or social occasions. All claim to stress exercise as much as diet. But we found that most of them, in prac-

tice, give exercise second billing at best.

Liquid fasts. These are the most drastic weight-loss programs, designed for people with a serious weight problem. Only about 6 percent of the respondents who lost weight with professional help had used liquid fasts. These fasting programs require people to give up solid foods altogether for a time and subsist on flavored liquid formulas that supply between 450 and 800 calories a day. Dieters typically fast for three months, during which time they should receive counseling on how to improve their eating habits. Then they are gradually weaned off the formula and put back on solid foods.

These near-starvation rations produce very fast weight loss but often cause medical complications. The informed-consent form for *Optifast* clients warns that they may experience such "adjustments" as dizziness, sensitivity to cold, slower heart rate, brittle nails, rashes, fatigue, diarrhea or constipation, muscle cramps, and bad breath. Weight loss from very-low-calorie diets is known to cause gallstones, and has been linked to potentially fatal heart-rhythm disturbances—particularly in relatively thin people who try the programs.

Liquid-fast programs are available only through hospitals or doctors' offices and require regular physical checkups and blood tests. They generally cost between $2000 and $3000.

The eight programs we evaluated are essentially based on a single prin-

---

THE KEY PROBLEMS

We asked readers to tell us about the problems they encountered with different weight-loss programs. Here are the key problem areas for the eight programs in our survey; the programs that were more or less likely than the average to cause these difficulties for our readers; and the percent of readers who had that problem with each of those companies.

Did the program have higher costs than you were led to believe? More likely to have higher costs: Jenny Craig (47%), Nutri/System (47%). Less likely: Weight Watchers (7%), HMR (17%).

Was there strong pressure to buy the program's products? More pressure: Jenny Craig (55%), Nutri/System (55%). Less pressure: Weight Watchers (5%).

Was there strong pressure to join or stay in the program? More pressure: Nutri/System (34%), Jenny Craig (31%). Less pressure: Medifast (11%), Weight Watchers (12%).

Was the dieting method artificial and difficult to incorporate into daily life? More artificial: Medifast (40%), Optifast (37%), Nutri/System (31%). Less artificial: Weight Watchers (6%).

Were you always hungry? More hunger: Medifast (22%). Less hunger: Weight Watchers (10%).

ciple: cutting calories. But we found significant differences in their approaches and in our readers' satisfaction with them. Here are the pros and cons of each.

Weight Watchers

Weight Watchers, founded by a self-described Brooklyn housewife in 1963, is the oldest of the weight-loss programs we evaluated. It holds an overwhelming market share. In our survey, it was chosen by 43 percent of those who used professional help to lose weight, far more than the number using any other program. Readers who chose *Weight Watchers* were also significantly more satisfied than those who went to any of its competitors.

"*Weight Watchers* is the only place I ever send anyone," says Janet Polivy, a University of Toronto psychologist who treats people with eating disorders and generally warns clients away from the very idea of dieting. "*Weight Watchers* is the most sensible," she says.

Of all the programs we evaluated, *Weight Watchers* is the only one that relies exclusively on group counseling. Each counselor employed by *Weight Watchers* is a former client who has achieved and maintained his or her "goal weight" on the program. Gaining it back is grounds for dismissal.

Dieters pay an enrollment fee—a CU staffer paid $15 at a local outlet—and are given a diary to record their goal weight and the results of a weekly weigh-in. They are then entitled to attend any weekly *Weight Watchers* session anywhere as long as they pay the weekly meeting fee ($12 at the center we visited, but it varies from place to place). Some groups are held in *Weight Watchers* retail outlets, while others meet in community centers or churches, or at work.

The program costs significantly less than the others we rated: Questionnaire respondents spent an average of $110 for several months' worth of counseling. *Weight Watchers* is also the only diet program that doesn't require customers to buy any company-brand foods or nutritional supplements. (It does, however, shower participants with cents-off coupons for the many types of *Weight Watchers*-brand foods sold in supermarkets.)

The *Weight Watchers* diet is a standard low-calorie regimen, high in carbohydrates and low in fat. According to *Weight Watchers* material, if a dieter is losing more than 1 percent of body weight per week—that usually translates into 1½ to 2 pounds—then he or she will be instructed to eat more to slow down the rate of loss. This practice, unique among the programs we studied, fits with current medical thinking about the hazards of too-rapid weight loss.

Weight Watchers clients in our survey did no better at losing weight than people on other commercial diets. Nevertheless, our *Weight Watchers* respondents said they were more satisfied with their weight loss and with their overall experience than were people who went to any other diet chain. Compared with customers of the typical diet program, *Weight Watchers* customers experienced less sales pressure, had fewer problems with the diet, felt less hungry, and were less often surprised by unexpectedly high costs.

Company-food programs

Nutri/System, chosen by 18 percent of our respondents, and *Jenny Craig,* chosen by 11 percent, each require that dieters buy and consume only company-brand foods (except for a few items such as fresh dairy products and produce). *Jenny Craig* sells both frozen and shelf-stable foods, while *Nutri/System* has shelf-stable selections only. The foods cost about $60 to $70 every week for most participants; the cost drops slightly as you approach your goal weight and start eating some regular food. In addition, readers who used these programs paid higher fees than those who chose *Weight Watchers*—an average of $189 for our *Jenny Craig* respondents and $292 for *Nutri/System.*

The companies assert that their prepackaged meals help dieters learn "portion control" by giving them a sense of how much food they can eat to maintain a given calorie level, and also free them from the need to weigh or measure every morsel they ingest. That rationale aside, the prepackaged foods have a clear benefit for the companies: The annual report for *Jenny Craig Inc.* notes that, in 1992, food sales accounted for 90 percent of revenues from the company's centers.

The mandatory food purchases irritated our readers. More than half complained that the two companies

Moving into maintenance

Name: Saralyn Ingram
Program: Weight Watchers
Experience: Finished losing 17 pounds two months ago.
Comment: "My weight had crept up; Weight Watchers helped me lose it. Now I plan to keep the weight off by walking about half an hour almost every day."

SLIM-FAST AND DYNATRIM

DISAPPOINTING DIET DRINKS

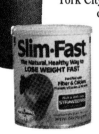

What do L.A. Dodgers manager Tommy Lasorda and former New York City mayor Ed Koch have in common? Both lost a lot of weight on *Slim-Fast,* the nation's most widely used over-the-counter meal-replacement drink. And both took part in a multimillion-dollar advertising campaign that helped build the meal-replacement market into a $1.3-billion business by 1990.

Today, *Slim-Fast* and other low-calorie powdered drink mixes are losing popularity as quickly as they gained it: Sales plunged 44 percent between 1991 and 1992. Why the drop? Probably because consumers nationwide lost about as much weight on these products as respondents to our questionnaire did: not very much.

It wasn't for lack of trying. Meal-replacement diet drinks were the second most popular weight-control strategy among our respondents, after self-help: 24 percent reported using *Slim-Fast, Ultra Slim-Fast,* or (less commonly) *Dyna-Trim.* Most of these people used the drinks (which contain protein, sugars, fiber, vitamins, and minerals) to replace about one meal a day or less—unlike people on liquid fasts, who give up food entirely for a time. Only one-sixth used the diet drinks for more than half their meals.

Men who tried meal replacements lost an average of 4 percent of their starting weight; women, only 3 percent. Moreover, two-fifths of the group lost less than five pounds, and one-fifth actually managed to gain five pounds or more.

Many of our respondents also felt that the low-calorie shakes were a poor substitute for real food. More than one-third said they were "always hungry" while using the drinks. Nearly as many complained that drinking a meal instead of eating one was "artificial," and said that they started to regain weight as soon as they stopped using the products.

applied "strong pressure to buy their products"—by far the highest response on this problem area. Yet when one of our staffers asked to buy sample foods before signing up for the full program, to make sure she liked them well enough to face the prospect of eating them for several months straight, her request was politely but firmly turned down at both programs.

Both *Nutri/System* and *Jenny Craig*

use one-on-one counseling for clients, augmented by group classes in behavior modification. Business is generally conducted in a storefront facility, which also serves as a pickup point for the week's supply of food.

In their literature, both these programs make reference to exercise. But at one *Jenny Craig* outlet, a CU staffer was told that if she wanted the set of walking-program audiotapes, she would have to purchase a special

$94 "Lifestyle Counseling Package."

The two programs' literature seems designed to inspire rather than inform. *Jenny Craig* gives prospective customers a slick brochure that focuses more on the company's new rebate offers than on specifics of the weight-loss program itself. The brochure is illustrated with a number of full-color, full-length photographs of a young woman said to have lost 62 pounds on the program and to have gone from a size 16 to a size 6. The same preoccupation with clothing dominates the *Nutri/System* promotional materials. The company's "Nutri/Size Your Body" advertising campaign has featured slimmed-down, satisfied customers holding up billowing clothing from their fatter days.

Such ads have drawn criticism from many clinicians specializing in weight loss. "Those commercials make me go absolutely ballistic," exclaims David Schlundt, a Vanderbilt University psychologist who treats people with eating disorders. "The majority of people who need to lose weight would be much better off if they dropped to a size 12; their chances of dropping to a size 6 are almost zero. These ads are not selling health benefits, they're playing on a tremendously emotional issue in people's lives."

Certainly, most *Nutri/System* customers who responded to our questionnaire won't be in a size 6 anytime soon. Our average woman who used *Nutri/System* started at 167 pounds and ended up, six months after completing the program, with a net loss of just over 11 pounds.

Other diet plans

The remaining two diet chains of the five in our survey, *Diet Center* and *Physicians Weight Loss Center (PWL)*, were chosen by the smallest number of readers. They provide a mix of elements found in other programs: They focus on diet plans using ordinary foods, as *Weight Watchers* does, but use individual counselors as *Jenny Craig* and *Nutri/System* do. *PWL* also requires dieters to spend about $20 a week for a daily nutritional supplement, while *Diet Center's* plan includes a daily vitamin pill as part of the fee for the program.

Until the late 1980s, *PWL* had by far the lowest-calorie plan of any of the commercial companies, offering a mere 700 calories a day. In 1990, the company increased its daily calorie count to between 900 and 1000—

DEXATRIM AND ACUTRIM

PILLS: STILL NO PANACEA

The perfect diet pill would work in low doses, cause no side effects, have no potential for abuse, and be safe enough to take for a lifetime. Unfortunately, it doesn't exist.

Researchers agree that the diet pills now on the market fall short of the ideal. They include over-the-counter appetite suppressants such as *Acutrim* and *Dexatrim*, which contain phenylpropanolamine (PPA), a stimulant chemically similar to amphetamine; the prescription drug fenfluramine *(Pondimin)*, which acts on the brain chemical serotonin; and the prescription drug phentermine *(Ionamin)*, an amphetamine-type stimulant and appetite suppressant.

Only 6 percent of our questionnaire respondents had tried over-the-counter appetite

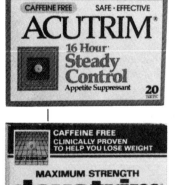

suppressants, and they were generally unhappy with the drugs. Less than 5 percent of those who had tried the pills said they were very satisfied or completely satisfied with how well these medications helped them to lose weight and keep it off. In contrast, half were very or completely *dis*satisfied with the results.

Many people who tried the pills also found the experience itself unpleasant. More than 30 percent said they always felt hungry, even though the drugs are supposed to keep hunger at bay. And just over 20 percent experienced physical side effects such as dizziness or nausea. That's not surprising, since the PPA in *Dexatrim* and *Acutrim* revs up the central nervous system.

Some researchers have argued that better drugs, used as part of a sophisticated weight-

control program, could yield better results. Their hopes have been raised by an ambitious, four-year study conducted at the University of Rochester, which received a great deal of publicity when it was published in 1992. In this study, more than 100 severely overweight adults took varying combinations of fenfluramine and phentermine, or a placebo, and also went through a behavior-modification program designed to improve their diet and exercise habits. The drug treatment group achieved and maintained a significantly greater weight loss than the placebo group.

Close inspection of the study, however, shows that this two-drug regimen is no miracle fat cure. Three years after beginning the study, most participants in all groups—those who were still on the drugs as well as those on placebos—were steadily gaining back the weight they had lost. Those on the drugs were slightly thinner than those on placebos—but even so, the majority were less than 10 percent below their starting weights. Many patients were bothered by the drugs' side effects—dry mouth, nervousness, and sleep disturbances—through the entire course of the study. Finally, people given the real drugs were having an even harder time staying on their diets than people given placebos, even though the drugs are supposed to dampen appetite. These are serious problems, because treatment may have to last indefinitely to be effective; several studies have shown that people who lose weight with the help of drugs almost invariably regain it when the drugs are discontinued.

Many obesity experts still believe that more research should be done on long-term drug treatments for severely overweight people, especially those with life-threatening conditions such as diabetes. But for most people—especially those who are only moderately overweight—the relative ineffectiveness of these drugs, their known side effects, and the unknown hazards of long-term treatment should discourage their use.

still on the low side, but within the range for regular diet programs. Nevertheless, our survey showed that *PWL* did not produce significantly better weight loss or weight maintenance than other programs that allow their clients more food.

Liquid fasts: A last resort

In our survey, people on these programs lost a great deal more weight than customers of regular diet programs—an average of 15 to 20 percent of their starting weight, versus 8 to 12 percent for the diet programs—in about the same amount of time. However, they also regained the weight quickly.

Liquid fasts are generally appropriate only for people with a BMI in the 30s, or people with BMIs in the high 20s who have a serious weight-related risk factor, such as severe high blood pressure or diabetes. Most readers who used liquid fasts fit those criteria: The men weighed on average 250 pounds to start, and the women 203 pounds, with BMIs of 35 and 34 respectively.

But we also found that one-sixth of our respondents who tried liquid fasts said they had a BMI of 25 or less when they started the program: They were not actually overweight at all. For such people, going on a liquid fast could pose a serious risk to health.

Although they produced roughly comparable weight-loss results, the three liquid-fast programs we evaluated—*Health Management Resources (HMR), Medifast,* and *Optifast*—got different marks from our respondents. Clients of *HMR* were the most satisfied with the program overall, and complained less frequently than *Optifast* or *Medifast* clients about unhelpful weight-loss counselors and unexpectedly high costs. *HMR* has now become the market leader among liquid fasts, surpassing *Optifast* in sales. Readers who went to either *HMR* or *Optifast* maintained their weight loss significantly better than *Medifast* customers after six months.

People who tried *Optifast,* the oldest of the liquid-fast programs, lost 45 pounds on average and had gained back 15 pounds six months later. That relapse rate is similar to the study of customers that we were sent by *Optifast,* the only weight-loss company we contacted that had done a careful scientific study of its success rate. (*Optifast* was also the program Oprah Winfrey used when she lost 67 pounds in a highly publicized

effort a few years ago—and then, just as publicly, gained it all back.)

Recommendations

Despite their sales pitches, there is no evidence that commercial weight-loss programs help most people achieve significant, permanent weight loss. If you want or need to lose weight, you would probably do well to try to reduce on your own, or through a free hospital-based program, before spending money on a commercial weight-loss center.

Some people may find they can control their weight better if they have outside support, which is essentially what the commercial programs supply. Any program can produce significant weight loss fairly rapidly. The trick is in keeping it off—and the great majority of dieters don't.

We did find that about one-fourth of our readers who used commercial diet programs were able to keep off most of the weight they'd lost for two years. But we found nothing that gave us a clue to their success; successful maintainers were not significantly different from ordinary dieters in terms of the time they had spent in the weight-loss program, their starting weights, or their sex.

Since no diet program was especially effective, anyone who wants to play the commercial-diet game should choose a program on the basis of cost, comfort, and common sense. By those criteria, *Weight Watchers* was our readers' clear

favorite. It costs less than the others, emphasizes healthful dietary habits, encourages relatively slow weight loss, and generally appears to provide the most satisfying, supportive experience. In contrast, *Nutri/System* and *Jenny Craig* cost more, are more likely to use high-pressure sales tactics, and were not as satisfying to clients overall.

No one should go on a liquid-fast program without a compelling medical reason to do so. Among the liquid-fast programs, *Health Management Resources* seems the best, in terms of our readers' satisfaction.

None of the diet programs we investigated give top priority to increasing physical activity, a change that researchers now unanimously agree is critical to lasting weight loss. If you use one of these programs, you should be prepared to find a way to exercise on your own.

Most important, given the strong likelihood that any weight lost on a reducing diet will be gained back promptly, we recommend that anyone contemplating a diet think seriously about whether losing weight is necessary or desirable in the first place. As our survey and others have shown, many people diet even though they are not overweight. For reasons the previous report makes clear, the majority of dieters would probably do better to forget about cutting calories, focus on exercising and eating a healthful diet, and let the pounds fall where they may.

A rare success

Name: Carol Sherwin
Program: Diet Center
Experience: Lost 40 pounds seven years ago; has kept it all off.
Comment: "It's still a very difficult struggle. One thing I learned on the program was to think about what I was eating all the time, and I still do that—I think about every single bite."

RATINGS Weight-loss programs

Diet programs and liquid-fast programs are listed separately. For each type, individual programs are listed in order of readers' overall satisfaction, based on responses to CU's 1992 Annual Questionnaire.

Results reflect our readers' experiences with these programs from January, 1989 through spring 1992, and may not be representative of the experiences of the population at large.

	Satisfaction with program overall [1]						Satisfaction with weight loss	Satisfaction with maintenance [2]	Percent of weight lost [3]	
	0%	20%	40%	60%	80%	100%			End of program	6 mos. after end
Diet programs										
Weight Watchers							74%	54%	8%	5%
Jenny Craig							65	35	11	6
Physicians' Weight Loss							65	37	12	7
Diet Center							68	38	10	6
Nutri/System							63	34	11	7
Liquid-fast programs										
Health Management Resources							82	43	20	15
Optifast							73	24	20	12
Medifast							65	23	15	8

[1] *All satisfaction ratings give the percent of respondents saying they were either "completely," "very," or "fairly well" satisfied, the top three levels of a 6-point scale that included three levels of dissatisfaction as well. Differences of about 5 percentage points in this and other satisfaction measures can be considered meaningful.*

[2] *Based on readers who had lost 3 lbs. or more and who had been out of the program for 6 mos. or longer.*

[3] *The median percent of starting weight that readers reported they had lost at the time they ended the program, and the net loss 6 mos. after they ended the program. Differences of 4 percentage points are meaningful.*

Causes of Obesity in Infants

Susan B. Roberts PhD • Scientist II • USDA Human Nutrition Research Center on Aging • Tufts University • Boston

Overweight adults have well-established risks for early death from cardiovascular and cerebrovascular disease, diabetes, and colon cancer, as well as increased risks of orthopedic disorders and psychological dysfunction. However, such risks have not been established for obese and overweight infants.

Instead, the principal hazard of obesity in infancy is remaining obese, and therefore being susceptible to the disorders that afflict obese adults. This is an important concern, because many obese adults were overweight as infants. Furthermore, it is suspected that obesity which develops early in life may be more difficult to treat than obesity developing later on.

For these reasons, prevention and even treatment of obesity in infants are desirable goals—but are they safe and feasible?

Obesity in infancy results from energy intake exceeding both energy expenditure as well as the energy required for normal growth. This energy imbalance can theoretically result from excessive energy intake or from abnormally low energy expenditure, or indeed a combination of these two factors.

It is often assumed that excessive energy intake, promoted by early weaning and the use of artificial formulas, is the cause of infant obesity. The scientific basis for this belief originated with the "fat cell hypothesis" of obesity which suggested, on the basis of studies of laboratory rodents, that overeating early in life leads to an increased number of fat cells in the body and hence to an increased total body fat content (*J Clin Invest* 47:2091, 1968).

Recent studies, however, have not supported the early research and have instead indicated that susceptible infants can become overweight while consuming no more energy than normal weight infants (*N Engl J Med* 318: 461, 1988). In these cases, reduced energy expenditure for physical activity may be an important cause of the abnormal fat deposition.

In light of these new findings, what, if anything, should be done to prevent and treat obesity developing in infancy when no endocrinopathy is apparent? It can be impossible for the physician to determine with certainty the contributions of overeating and reduced physical activity to the development of obesity in a patient; accurate techniques for this purpose (*Can J Physiol Pharm* 67:1190, 1989) are expensive and not widely available, and the alternatives (records of food intake and activity made by parents) may well be unreliable.

In the absence of means to determine the exact cause of excess weight gain in an individual infant, it is necessary to consider the potential risks of the available options for prevention and treatment.

Dietary restriction is the commonly used method. The risks are not well understood but may well be comparable to those associated with weight loss in adults and therefore could include possible micronutrient deficiencies as well as reduced spontaneous physical activity, lowered body temperature, and reduced immunity. Even a small chance of these complications occurring in infancy is unacceptable; and, for this reason, significant dietary restriction should not be a preferred from of treatment for obesity.

However, obesity control through long-term prevention of overeating may be a more acceptable form of dietary management. These suggestions are consistent with the American Academy of Pediatrics recommendation that low-calorie diets should not be used during the first year of life (*Pediatrics* 72:253, 1983).

Increasing physical activity is another option to prevent and treat obesity. However, it is recognized that infant exercise programs can be dangerous; and so they may also carry unacceptable risks. Physical activity can theoretically be increased in a safe and acceptable manner by increased parent-child interactions. The value and success rate of this method is uncertain because it has not been tested experimentally.

It would appear that there are currently few methods for the prevention and treatment of obesity in infants that are completely free from risk, although new methods may become available with further research.

When deciding whether to treat obesity in an infant, it is also necessary to take into consideration the fact that only about one in nine obese infants are reported to remain obese. Thus, in only about 10% of cases will the prevention or treatment of obesity in infancy result in stabilization or loss of fat mass that would not occur naturally during childhood. In other words, many more infants become obese during the first year of life than would benefit from the possible advantages of routine prevention or treatment.

Suggested reading

Charney E et al: Childhood antecedents of adult obesity. *N Engl J Med* 295:6, 1976

Gortmaker SL et al: Increasing pediatric obesity in the United States. *Am J Dis Child* 141:535, 1987

Roberts SB: Early diet and obesity, in *Nutrition in the Second Six Months,* Raven Press, New York (in press)

Schurch B, Scrimshaw NS: Chronic energy deficiency: consequences and related issues. Nestle Foundation, Lausanne, Switzerland

... An Editorial View

Dr. Roberts' article provides a synopsis of more recent developments, including important observations of her own, regarding the etiology of obesity in infancy. As in all age groups, evidence for safe and prolonged reversal of the obese state in children is minimal. However, there is evidence that it may be possible to identify many infants at greater risk of remaining obese children and adults. These appear to be those infants with one or two obese parents and who gain weight very rapidly in infancy.

The editorial board questions whether, in such infants, "prevention of overeating" may need to begin earlier in life than suggested by Dr. Roberts. The results of at least one study have indicated that such intervention may be effective (*Pediatrics* 61:360, 1978). However, the editorial board agrees that, for most chubby babies, body weight tends to return to normal range by school age.

Food Safety

In 1906, with the passage of the first Food and Drug Act,
the federal government began to assume some responsibility for food safety. Increased governmental involvement has been an inevitable trend ever since. With the
1950s came a fear that chemicals in the food supply might
be carcinogenic. Congress responded by requiring increased testing of additives. The Delaney Clause prevented the use of any additive found to induce cancer in
man or experimental animals. There were stricter regulations covering the testing of new additives. The GRAS
(Generally Recognized as Safe) list of additives identified
those believed by scientists to be safe for human consumption. This list is periodically revised, and testing and
retesting of some additives continue. The FDA governs all
of these procedures, and books of regulations cover all
aspects of food production and service.

The concept in the quote at the top of this page is not
new. A sixteenth-century physician, Parcelsus, said "All
things are poison. Nothing is without poison. Solely the
dose determines that a thing is not poison." Thus, it is
appropriate for critics to question the continued usefulness of the Delaney Clause. When this law was passed,
they argue, only about 50 carcinogens were known. Today
thousands are known, and advances in analytical methods enable the detection of amounts with no biological or
toxicological significance, causing products to be banned
needlessly. Some prominent scientific groups believe that
the FDA should be allowed to not "concern itself with
trifles." This is known as a "de minimis" policy.

But today's consumers frequently fail to assess risk and
benefit rationally. With little knowledge to draw upon, they
do not understand that even an essential nutrient can be
both life-giving and life-threatening. Sodium, for example,
is absolutely necessary, but if put into an infant's formula
instead of sugar, it can (and has) resulted in death. Likewise, explorers have become very ill from eating a small
portion of polar bear liver due to its excessive vitamin A
content.

Given the complexity of biological interactions, the
uniqueness of each human organism, and the multitude
of chemicals potentially interacting, few knowledgeable
people would contend that the absolute safety of anything

can be assured. Yet activist groups demand just that and
have become experts at escalating a minor or nonexistent
issue into a major catastrophe. It has been argued that if it
takes television programs like "60 Minutes" or a partisan
political group such as the National Resources Defense
Council (NRDC) to create a public issue, then it probably
is not a safety issue at all. The Alar-treated apple scare,
described in the article "Scientists Urge Skepticism of
Reports About an Unsafe Food Supply," is a good example. Because public reaction to food safety issues has
become so strong and misguided, the first five articles in
this unit are devoted to putting perspective into threats to
food safety. Here you will find discussions of pesticides,
gene splicing, artificial sweeteners, and irradiation.

Food irradiation (see article 46), is partially a food
safety issue and certainly a political issue, but not the
health threat loudly proclaimed by the activist group Food
and Water, Inc. While irradiation does not produce radioactive food, it does prolong the shelf life of fresh produce
and destroys bacteria that cause food-borne diseases.
The first commercial food irradiation plant is currently
operating in Florida, and a market test in Chicago proved
that irradiated strawberries, with their longer shelf life, can
outsell nonirradiated berries 20 to 1. Meanwhile, the
world's largest spice company does not irradiate only
because of negative public reaction.

The debate over gene-altered food has continued for
more than a decade, and it remains highly controversial.
Among other benefits, proponents point to longer shelf
life, crops resistant to drought or cold, and lower-starch
potatoes that will absorb less fat when fried. Critics say
that there are safety risks, that even greater problems will
arise if bugs become immune to crops' new insect-resis-
tant qualities, and that big companies will exploit the
opportunities with little regard for negative effects.

Clearly, one legitimate health and safety concern is food
spoilage. Preserving food safely for later consumption is
absolutely necessary in today's society. Canning, discussed in "The Canning Process: Old Preservation Technique Goes Modern," was an invention in response to
Napoleon's demand for better methods of preserving food
for his troops. Now, a century and a half later, this process
is used for more than 1,500 food products. New canning
methods permit packaging in paperboard and plastic as
well as metal and glass.

Food-borne illnesses continue to be a major threat to
health. Total costs of those illnesses consume nearly $10

billion annually, and the estimated number of yearly cases varies from 6 to 100 million. The late 1992 outbreak of food poisoning in Washington State is an extreme example: hundreds became ill, and there was at least one fatality. In that case, the culprit was rare hamburger. Many people are fond of blaming the packing industry and food inspection procedures for the presence of illness-producing organisms, but the outbreak could easily have been prevented with proper food handling procedures—something we can all control.

Furthermore, most of us assume that food-borne illness is caused by poorly handled food at restaurants. It is revealing to discover, however, that each of us is his or her own worst enemy. Properly handled food in home kitchens would reduce the incidence of disease dramatically. This always includes conformance with rules governing bacterial growth, time, and temperature. New information also presents a forceful case for something very simple: using wooden—not plastic—cutting boards, as bacteria apparently die quickly on the wooden boards but not on plastic ones. One very common bacterial cause of food-borne illness is salmonella, and we are frequently warned about "serving up salmonella for dinner" with either the chicken or the egg, as article 50 indicates. Other food-borne illnesses are discussed in article 48.

While everyone would agree that it is appropriate to raise questions about the safety of our food supply, there is sometimes disagreement on the extent of the problem and on how to solve it. As consumers, we must accept personal responsibility for safe food handling. We must also continue to expect our regulatory agencies to do their best. Problems arising over the safety of food supplies can be documented throughout history. Clearly, solutions are not easy.

Looking Ahead: Challenge Questions

If you were to consume only those foods for which complete safety could be proved, what would you eat?

How can risk versus benefit be reasonably assessed in making decisions about the safety of an additive or process?

How would you rank order three issues of food safety that you think are the most important? Why?

What measures do you believe would be effective in counteracting misinformation about food safety?

Observe yourself when you handle food. In what ways might you be the vector of food-borne illness?

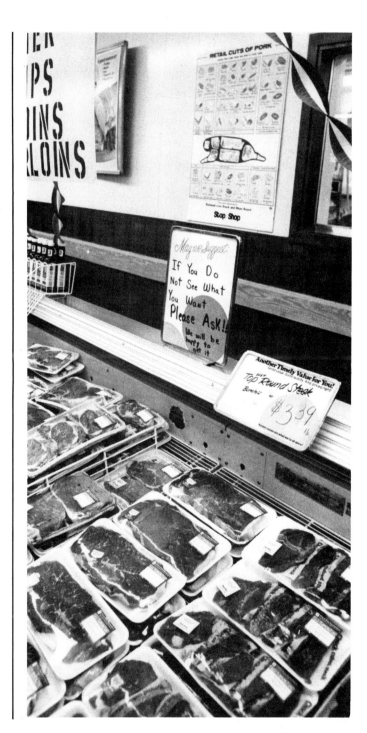

Scientists Urge Skepticism Of Reports About an Unsafe Food Supply

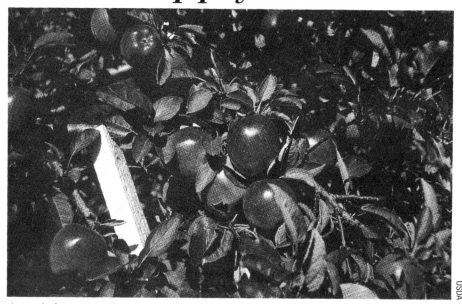

A panel of experts gathered to assure the public that the American food supply is safe.

USDA

Laurie Hayes

In early 1989, hysterical moms poured thousands of gallons of apple juice down the drain in response to reports by a special interest group claiming that Alar-treated apples posed a significant risk to their children. On the three year anniversary of the Alar-scare, a panel of scientists held a press conference to declare that apples never posed a public health risk and called upon regulatory authorities, the media and consumers to be more discerning the next time they hear claims that America's food supply is unsafe.

On Feb. 26, 1989, the television program "60 Minutes," in collaboration with the Natural Resources Defense Council, released a non-peer reviewed study alleging that Alar, a chemical growth regulator used for years by apple farmers, posed an "intolerable" risk of cancer, especially to children. Panic ensued throughout the U.S. as consumers stopped buying apples. Apple farmers experienced economic chaos as their harvest plummeted in value, losing more than $100 million in the following months.

"I think it's important to remember the Alar scare because it was such a disaster for the American people," stresses former Surgeon General of the U.S. Dr. C. Everett Koop, principal speaker of the panel. "On faulty evidence, exaggerated evidence, the apple industry was destroyed for a year. Mothers and children were frightened out of their wits."

In the aftermath of the scare, apples were tossed out and removed from the marketplace and housewives threw out countless unopened jars of applesauce. "And then there was that intrepid, courageous New York State trooper who stopped a school bus and went and extracted an apple from the lunch bag of one of the students in the cab," Koop recalls.

"A story which started as somebody's whim and pet peeve became a national scandal," he says, "and what we are trying to do is remind people that you have got to have a scientific background before you have headlines."

The panel, which also included Dr. Elizabeth Whelan, president of the American Council on Science and Health, Dr.

Alan Moghissi, former staffer at the Environmental Protection Agency, Dr. Joseph Rosen, professor of Food Science at Rutgers University, Dr. M. Ralph Reed, senior medical advisor at the American Medical Association and Herbert Slenker, an Ohio apple farmer, joined the World Health Organization and the British government in attesting that Alar does not pose a public health hazard.

The prestigious science publications *Science* and *Issues in Science and Technology* have respectively called the claims against Alar "dubious" and "based on arguable math." Three years after the scare, the scientific consensus is that Alar never posed a risk of cancer to adults or children.

"At the time of the 'great Alar scare,' I attempted to put things in perspective, but it seemed to me that the public only wanted to hear from the alarmists, the movie stars or T.V. personalities," Koop notes.

"It's interesting that Surgeon General's warnings are almost always 'Don't do something,'" Koop muses. "When the Alar scare came along I was faced with the opportunity of saying, 'Do something, eat an apple.'

"But at that time, the emotional content of the press was so great that my warning appeared on the seventeenth page of the *Washington Post*."

Indeed, Koop adds, there are signs seen today in some grocery stores certifying that their apples have not been treated with Alar.

"As a pediatric surgeon, I care deeply about the health of children, and if Alar ever posed a health hazard, I would have said so then and would say so now," he adds.

ACSH sponsored the press conference to demonstrate that a much larger problem still exists, according to Whelan. "The Alar scare is but one sorry example of what can happen when politics and hysteria prevail over science in determining alleged human cancer risks. "America's food supply is the safest and most cost-

By Laurie Hayes. From *ChemEcology,* Vol. 21, No. 4, April 1992, pp. 4-5. *ChemEcology* is a publication of the Chemicals Manufacturers Association. Reprinted by permission.

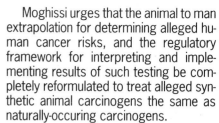

effective to produce in the world," she says. "Withdrawing from the market useful, safe products of modern technology, such as Alar, will discourage researchers from bringing similarly useful products to the market because there will be little incentive to invest in a technology that can be compromised by irrational or unscientific regulatory decisions in the future."

ACSH is not calling for the return of Alar to the market, Whelan emphasizes. "What is at stake here goes way beyond Alar in apples," she says. "The ultimate resolution of the issue we are addressing will determine whether or not the United States will continue to have the safest, most abundant and enviable food supply in the world or whether we will in the future face major crop losses, deteriorated quality of food and higher prices because of fear and ignorance."

Apple grower Slenker stresses the importance of the continued availability of new and improved pesticides to our nation's crops. "Insects and disease have the ability to adapt to their environment no matter how hostile it may be," he says. "We need new pesticides coming out all of the time to keep ahead of that ability to adapt.

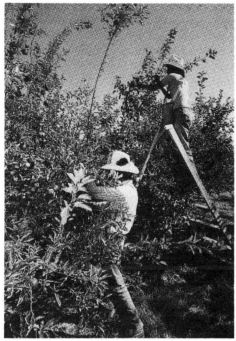

Apple farmers lost $100 million in the months after the scare.

"But we are not getting them," Slenker warns. "And the failure to control any one insect or disease can cause the loss of an entire crop." As evidence of this, Slenker cites the recent devastation caused by the outbreak of white flies that became resistant to pesticides in California.

Koop and Whelan agree that yet another hazard of the scare was its effect of drawing attention away from the known effects of human cancer such as cigarette smoking and overexposure to sunlight. "By focusing on a strawman, (the American public) feels that they are doing something to improve their health, and in doing so they actually neglect the very things that they could be doing to improve

their health," Koop notes. "They could do this more legitimately, more readily and with greater effect if they worried about not smoking, not drinking, getting exercise and eating a balanced diet."

Despite this, reports continue to surface about dangers in our nation's food and consumers are increasingly confused about what to believe.

"Some so-called consumer advocates continue to tell the public that cancer causing pesticides are present in our food supply and that they and their children are at extreme risk," Koop says. "And I want to say that this is simply not true. We have a number of serious health crises in America today, but food safety is not one of them.

"Some pesticides," Koop continues, "when given to some laboratory animals in extremely high doses cause tumors. Even if residues of such pesticides are found on some foods, which they are, it is at such minuscule levels as to pose no risk to human health. So the conclusion that I have come to is that there is no scientific evidence that residues from the lawful, proper application of pesticides results in illness or in death."

"The Alar controversy is a classic example of poor science, poorly applied societal decision, resulting in a poor final decision," concurs former EPA official Moghissi.

Moghissi is not proud of EPA's response to the Alar scare. "I plead guilty," he says. "I'm proud of a number of things that EPA has done and less proud of some other things and Alar and risk assessment is one of those that I am less proud of."

The time has come for this country to insist upon truth in risk assessment, according to Moghissi. "Risk assessment is not supposed to be conservative, liberal, Republican, Democratic, or whatever party ideology may be around," he stresses. "Risk assessment is supposed to be truthful."

Moghissi urges that the animal to man extrapolation for determining alleged human cancer risks, and the regulatory framework for interpreting and implementing results of such testing be completely reformulated to treat alleged synthetic animal carcinogens the same as naturally-occuring carcinogens.

"There is a myth that all manmade chemicals are the ones that cause cancer and natural chemicals do no," he says. "That is nonsense. It is in fact highly likely that there are more natural carcinogens than manmade carcinogens, if for no other reason than because there are a lot more natural chemicals than there are manmade chemicals.

"Nature is not benign," Moghissi continues, "but instead of banning peanuts and corn, which contain trace amounts of the natural human carcinogen aflatoxin, we set tolerance levels for 'safe consumption.'

"The human body doesn't know the difference between natural and synthetic carcinogens," he adds. "Instead of banning a synthetic chemical outright because it contains a trace amount of an alleged human carcinogen, we likewise need to set safe tolerance levels. Current law doesn't allow for this methodology."

Moghissi and the rest of the panel therefore asked that the media be skeptical of future reports of dangers with our nation's food supply and urged them to seek out sound science to confirm or disprove such reports.

There are two different kinds of groups who are concerned about human health and the environment, Moghissi says. "Those of us who rely on science as the basis for decision making and those who rely on ideology rather than science. It's imperative that you folks in the media insist upon outstanding science and nothing less than that as the basis for decision-making in environmental protection."

Without this reliance on sound science, Koop stresses, the media and the public is bound to be duped again.

"False alarms about alleged cancer-causing effects of produce could very seriously adversely effect the availability of safe, abundant and affordable food supplies in this country," he reiterates. "And we really cannot afford any more baseless scares about the food supply. We owe it to ourselves and the health and economy of the country to take a hard, critical and very scientific look at the next charge that is presented to us about the safety of the American food supply."

Hot Potato

Will safety questions curb public appetite for gene-spliced food?

While some companies were focusing on the enormous potential of gene splicing to produce new drugs from modified cells, other entrepreneurs saw in biotechnology the promise of a second "Green Revolution." A group of small start-ups, agricultural chemical giants, seed producers and food processors devoted their efforts to developing plants with new genetic traits of value to consumers and farmers, such as better nutrition and taste, longer shelf life and resistance to diseases and pesticides.

Nearly a decade after the first drug produced by biotechnology received marketing approval from the Food and Drug Administration, genetically engineered foods still await their debut. Agricultural biotechnology firms are finding that the same science that lifts hopes in the clinic raises fears around the kitchen table. Top New York City chefs are loudly threatening to boycott what one wag has dubbed "Frankenfood," and groups critical of biotechnology, such as Jeremy Rifkin's Foundation on Economic Trends, promise legal challenges to the FDA.

Apprehensions about the safety of genetically engineered foods began flaring like a grease fire in a deep fryer when the FDA announced in late May that plants modified by genetic engineering will in most cases be treated just like any ordinary garden variety. New plants, whether they are produced through techniques of biotechnology or conventional breeding, do not require any special review to gain market approval, the agency decreed. The FDA also decided that genetically engineered foods need not be labeled as such simply because they are produced by that process. Changes that result in products significantly different from what consumers expect—for instance, high-fiber potatoes or oranges low in vitamin C—will warrant some kind of informational labeling, the FDA says.

Critics charge that the public has the right to know what it is buying. They point out that the FDA currently leaves the responsibility for food safety to producers, and they question the wisdom of extending that trust to purveyors of unproved technology. "The FDA is counting on companies' coming to them; otherwise, they're saying you don't have to talk to us," declares Rebecca J. Goldburg, senior scientist at the Environmental Defense Fund (EDF).

The New York-based environmental group has proposed its own ideas for safety and labeling rules under the title *A Mutable Feast: Assuring Food Safety in the Era of Genetic Engineering.* "While I don't think most genes will be hazardous, I do think we have to look for exceptions, not the rule," Goldburg says. The EDF is particularly concerned about plants engineered to contain pesticides; it also fears that the potential for allergy problems will rise as genes are transferred among organisms. Rifkin plans to emphasize allergenicity in his Pure Food campaign as well.

For their part, companies say the technology to insert new genes permits them to do what plant breeders have been doing for thousands of years—only more rapidly and with greater specificity. "Single-gene modifications are actually less likely to cause unexpected negative traits than is traditional breeding because far less genetic material is exchanged," asserts Vic C. Knauf, vice president for research at Calgene in Davis, Calif.

The first genetically engineered vegetable is slated to appear at the produce counter in mid-1993 or early 1994. The Flavor Saver tomato engineered by Calgene contains "antisense" RNA sequences to block production of an enzyme that hastens rotting. Other food crops that various companies are currently field-testing include squash, cantaloupe, cucumbers, potatoes, corn and such oilseeds as cotton and canola [*see box*].

Beyond the first wave of bioengineered plants is a "more complex and subtle second generation" that will not approach market for another five to 10 years, says John C. Sorenson, executive director of vegetable research for Asgrow Seed Company in Kalamazoo, Mich. "We're now moving to understand the metabolic basis of plant disease and to interfere with that process," he notes. In addition, some laboratories—for instance, the U.S. Department of Agriculture's Agricultural Research Service in Lubbock, Tex.—are experimenting with "thermostat" genes believed to determine the narrow ranges of temperature at which plants grow best. Transfer of these traits and others, including resistance to drought, salt and even

Major Developers of Genetically Engineered Foods

Asgrow Seed Company, Kalamazoo, Mich. Field-testing yellow squash, cucumbers and cantaloupes genetically vaccinated against four common plant viruses. Also developing genes for resistance to fungus and bacteria to protect these and other fresh-market vegetables, including lettuce and carrots.

Calgene, Davis, Calif. Flavor Saver tomato with "antisense" RNA that allows vine ripening and longer shelf life will debut commercially, possibly in 1993. Testing canola (rapeseed) engineered to produce laurates and stearates found in tropical oils, for food processing and soap manufacture. Has also modified canola to produce a highly hydrogenated oil for margarine.

DNA Plant Technologies, Cinnaminson, N.J. Field-testing tomatoes that produce the enzyme chitinase, which repels fungi responsible for post-harvest rot, and tomatoes with an enzyme that extends vine ripening. Developing tomatoes with "antifreeze" genes from winter flounder. Also working with Du Pont on a genetically engineered canola that produces a high-temperature frying oil that is low in saturated fat.

Monsanto, St. Louis, Mo. By incorporating genes from soil bacteria, the company is developing a high-solids, low-moisture potato that will absorb less fat during deep frying and a tomato with delayed ripening. Also developing potatoes and tomatoes engineered to resist viral disease as well as potatoes protected against insects. Testing herbicide-resistant cottonseed for oil.

Pioneer Hi-Bred, Des Moines, Iowa Testing sunflowers and canola with altered amino acid profiles to make oils that are more nutritious and lower in saturated fat. Also developing high-methionine soybeans for livestock feed, corn resistant to insects and disease, and alfalfa resistant to alfalfa mosaic virus.

heavy metals, could help crops grow on land that is currently not arable.

Now that scientists are beginning to reap the benefits of agricultural biotechnology, companies and regulators alike are eager to soothe public concerns. "It isn't that we're not asserting authority and giving everything away," argues Eric L. Flamm, a microbiologist in the FDA's Office of Biotechnology. "It just happens that most of the modifications we know of are trivial from a public health point of view." Although regulators insist genetically engineered plants are not inherently dangerous, neither are the foods inevitably safe, they concede. The same legal provisions allowing the FDA to prevent sales of contaminated shellfish could also be used to yank a genetically engineered product, Flamm says. "Everybody knows—one phone call and it's off the market," he adds.

To fend off critics, the FDA has already issued guidelines on potential problem areas for genetically engineered crops. Companies should first consider the basic characteristics of a new substance, the agency advises. Something substantially similar to the proteins, fats and carbohydrates already in the diet would generally be considered safe. But in some cases—for instance, when a protein's function is unknown or unusual—that substance might be subject to regulation as a food additive. Two sweeteners being considered for development in plants, thaumatin and monellin, are likely to incur such scrutiny, Flamm says. Unlike most sweet substances, which are carbohydrates, these are proteins.

In addition, Flamm warns that companies should be aware of, and look for, natural toxins likely to be found in both the parent plant and the organism donating genetic material. For example, plant breeders routinely monitor new varieties of squash, celery and potatoes, which are notorious for producing toxic metabolites.

The FDA also wants companies to ensure that engineered plants have the same range of nutrients as do conventional varieties. The agency says it will come down hardest on potential allergens. "Our concept is if you're moving a gene from an allergen, you are moving the allergen," Flamm declares. Plants modified with DNA from wheat, nuts, legumes, milk, eggs and shellfish will require labeling unless companies can conclusively prove the new food inherits no allergenicity, he says.

Some developers of genetically engineered plants do not object to labeling requirements. Calgene, for one, plans to highlight the fact so consumers know why Flavor Saver will cost three to four times the going rate for a store-bought tomato. But labeling agricultural commodities, such as grains, would present problems, says Edward W. Raleigh, Du Pont's manager of biotechnology regulatory affairs. "It's one thing to label an identity-preserved product and quite another to label something that is processed industrially, like corn," he notes. There are so many truckloads, grain elevators and vats between the farm and the consumer that tracking a shipment of gene-spliced corn all the way to a tortilla chip or bottle of oil would be almost impossible.

Moreover, it is still unclear precisely what kind of information consumers want from labeling of genetically engineered food, says Alan Goldhammer, director of technical affairs for the Industrial Biotechnology Association in Washington, D.C. Do they want to know if a gene put into a tomato comes from a soybean? Do they want to know that an enzyme called polygalacturonase is being blocked with antisense RNA? "There is now a way of assuring safety of genetically engineered plants," Goldhammer declares. "It is easy to communicate on a scientific level; our challenge now is to communicate to the society at large," he says.

Even the Agricultural Biotechnology Research Advisory Committee, which reviews field-trial requests submitted to the USDA, could use some tutoring, observes Alvin Young, director of the USDA's Office of Agricultural Biotechnology. "From a scientist's point of view, a gene is just a functional unit that causes certain reactions," Young says. He acknowledges that there are deeper issues to be addressed. "We need some really good thinkers" to assist regulators in their responses to societal concerns about agricultural biotechnology, he emphasizes.

To get the ball rolling, Young has asked W. Steven Burke of the North Carolina Biotechnology Center in Research Triangle Park to prepare a set of draft guidelines. Young intends to use the document, when it is submitted next March, to open up the first major discussion on ethics and personal, cultural and community beliefs surrounding genetically engineered food. If education makes consumers more comfortable with the idea of moving genes, then public awareness programs may well ease acceptance of agricultural biotechnology. Yet logic is rarely a match for instinct, especially when it comes to food. —*Deborah Erickson*

Is the artificially sweetened stuff the right stuff?

Americans have developed an artificially sweet tooth. In addition to eating, at last count, some 1,500 artificially sweetened foods—everything from chewing gum to pudding to yogurt to the 5.4 billion gallons of diet soda pop we guzzle annually—we're continually adding new kinds of sugar substitutes to our diets. Just this month supermarkets have begun selling the newest form of artificially sweet stuff: NutraSweet Spoonful, an aspartame-carbohydrate blend that has the same sweetening power as sugar and measures out the same way by the spoonful but has only two calories per teaspoon as opposed to sugar's 16. As much as Americans' taste for artificial sweeteners has intensified, however, some nagging questions about them remain: Do they actually help people keep weight down? Can any, like saccharin, cause cancer? Does aspartame bring about headaches? If you are one of the 100 million consumers who use artificial sweeteners, what follows will provide some much needed clarification.

A lightweight in the 'losing' battle?

The controversy began six years ago in England, where a group of researchers found that aspartame, marketed under the trade name Nutra-Sweet, appears to stimulate appetite and, presumably, the eating of more calories in the long run than if a person simply consumed sugar. When the researchers asked a group of 95 people to drink plain water, aspartame-sweetened water, and sugared water, they said that overall they felt hungriest after drinking the artificially sweetened beverage.

The study received widespread media attention and stirred a good deal of concern among the artificial-sweetener-using public. However, its results were questionable at best, since the researchers did not go on to measure whether the increase in appetite did actually translate into an increase in eating. The two do not necessarily go hand in hand.

In the years that followed, more than a dozen studies examining the effect of aspartame on appetite—and eating—were conducted. And after reviewing every one of them, the director of the Laboratory of the Study of Human Ingestive Behavior at Johns Hopkins University, Barbara Rolls, PhD, concluded that consuming aspartame-sweetened foods and drinks is not associated with any increase in the amount of food eaten afterward.

There is also scant evidence that appetite and eating habits will be altered by saccharin, the artificial sweetener sold as Sweet 'N Low. Thus, it appears that calorie-conscious consumers who use the two popular sweeteners needn't worry that they are undoing their efforts to save calories by altering their appetites.

Whether people undercut their efforts by allowing themselves more calorie-eating leeway than artificial sweeteners actually provide, however, is another matter. That is, although reaching for, say, a diet soda pop instead of a sugar-sweetened beverage clearly saves calories, drinking diet soda pop to justify eating a piece of chocolate cake or a hot fudge sundae won't do the trick. It's when calorie watchers *replace* sugary foods with artifi-

---

How (artificially) sweet it is

Sweetener *(trade name)*	Sweetness compared with sugar	Uses
Aspartame (NutraSweet)	180 times sweeter	Can be used to sweeten cold foods and beverages; cannot be used during cooking or baking at high temperatures because heating causes it to break down. It can, however, be added to cooked products after heating.
Acesulfame K (Sunette)	200 times sweeter	Can withstand high temperatures and therefore be used in cooking and baking as well as in cold foods and beverages.
Saccharin	300 times sweeter	Can withstand high temperatures and be used in cooking and baking along with being added to cold items.

From *Tufts University Diet & Nutrition Letter,* Vol. 10, No. 7, September 1992, pp. 4-6. *Tufts University Diet & Nutrition Letter,* 53 Park Place, New York, NY 10001.

cially sweetened items that the savings add up, not when they *add* them to a diet on top of fatty, sugary, high-calorie dishes.

A cancer connection?

For many artificial sweetener users, the issue is not whether sugar substitutes increase appetite and eating but whether they contribute to cancer and/or other ills. Small wonder, then, that when this past spring scientists at the University of

Nebraska released research results suggesting that saccharin causes cancer not in people but only in rats, their news made national headlines. To the scientific community, however, the conclusion reached by the Nebraska scientists was just one more addition to a large body of accumulated evidence that already indicates saccharin is safe. It's true that in 1977 Canada's Health Protection Branch, akin to the U.S. Food and Drug Administration, released a major study indicating that saccharin causes bladder cancer in rats—a finding that prompted the FDA to propose a ban on the sweetener. But a person would have to drink

---

When the FDA proposed a ban on saccharin in 1977, consumers were so upset (saccharin was the only "calorie saver" on the market at the time) that they sent tens of thousands of letters to the FDA protesting it. To stifle the clamor, Congress postponed the saccharin "prohibition" until more research could be completed—a delay that has been extended repeatedly ever since.

---

850 cans of diet soda pop daily in order to take in the amount of saccharin consumed by the rats in the Canadian study. Moreover, since the announcement of the Canadian report, studies in both animals and humans have failed to show a definite connection between saccharin use and the risk of suffering bladder cancer. In fact, six separate investigations involving more than 5,000 people with bladder cancer conducted during the 1970s and 80s did not find any association between artificial sweetener consumption and that disease. The same goes for the largest study to date, carried out by the National Cancer Institute. Saccharin did not raise the risk of cancer overall among some 9,000 men and women the Institute observed.

The American Medical Association's Council on Scientific Affairs goes so far as to say that evidence indicates that saccharin use "is not associated with an increased risk of bladder cancer." The National Academy of Sciences echoes that position in its *Diet and Health* report. The use of food additives such as saccharin, it says, "does not appear to have contributed to the overall risk of cancer in humans." The only people who might

want to consider limiting the amount of saccharin in their diets are mothers-to-be. While the sweetener has never been proved to pose a hazard to pregnant women and their unborn children, that it might cause them harm has not been ruled out.

A second artificial sweetener that has come under fire as a possible cancer promoter is acesulfame K, marketed as Sunette in a sugar substitute called Sweet One and found in foods such as puddings and gum. Soon after the substance was approved for use in 1988, critics charged that some evidence suggested it might cause tumors in rats. But when the FDA reviewed the studies conducted on the sweetener, it found that over time, rats who ate acesulfame K ended up with no higher incidence of tumors than would be expected to occur naturally during their lifetimes.

Other health concerns

One artificial sweetener that is not typically accused of causing cancer is aspartame. But it most certainly has been blamed for a number of other ills. Since its introduction in 1981, the government has received thousands of complaints accusing it of causing everything from headaches to nausea to mood swings to anxiety. Still, years of careful scientific study conducted both before and after the sweetener's entering the market have failed to confirm that it can bring about adverse health effects. That's why the Centers for Disease Control (the government agency charged with monitoring public health), the American Medical Association's Council on Scientific Affairs, and the Food and Drug Administration have given aspartame, one of the most studied food additives, a clean bill of health.

In December, the NutraSweet Company's patent on aspartame will expire, which means other companies will be able to manufacture the sweetener and put it on the market for the first time since its introduction in 1981. Thus, you may soon be seeing aspartame on products labeled with trade names other than NutraSweet.

Granted, the FDA has set forth an "acceptable daily intake" of 50 milligrams of aspartame per kilogram of body weight. To exceed the limit, however, a 120-pound (55 kilogram) woman would have to take in 2,750 milligrams of aspartame— the amount in 15 cans of aspartame-sweetened soda pop, 14 cups of gelatin, 22 cups of yogurt, or 55 six-ounce servings of aspartame-containing hot cocoa, as the following list illustrates. A 175-pound (80 kilogram) man would have to consume some 4,000 milligrams of the sweetener—the amount in 22 cans of soda pop or 32 cups of yogurt—to go over the limit.

	Milligrams of aspartame
Equal sweetener, 1 packet	35
Soda pop, 1 12-oz can	180
Beverage made with powdered drink mix, 1 cup	120
Gelatin, 1 cup	190
Pudding, 1 cup	50
Yogurt, 1 cup	124
Hot cocoa, 1 cup	50
Cereal, 1 cup	55
Instant tea, 1 cup	80
Wine cooler, 12 ounces	89

Only one small group of people must be certain to stay away from aspartame: those born with a rare metabolic disorder called phenylketonuria, or PKU. The estimated one person in every 12,000 to 15,000 who has it is unable to properly metabolize an essential amino acid in the aspartame called phenylalanine. Once a child consumes it, it builds up in the body and can ultimately cause such severe problems as mental retardation. To help people with PKU avoid the substance, labels on cans of soda pop and other aspartame-sweetened foods must carry the warning "Phenylketonurics: Contains Phenylalanine."

The future's looking sweeter than ever

While aspartame, acesulfame K, and saccharin are the only artificial sweeteners available in the U.S. today, a number of others have been developed by manufacturers trying to get a piece of the $1.3 billion a year artificial sweetener "pie." Among them:

Alitame: Made from amino acids, the building blocks of protein, this product is 2,000 times sweeter than sugar. The manufacturer of alitame, Pfizer, Inc., filed a petition for approval with the FDA six years ago. Approval is still pending, but if it comes to pass, the sweetener could potentially be used in almost all types of food to which sweeteners are added—from baked goods to hot and cold beverages to candies to drugs.

Stevioside: Currently used in 10 countries, including Japan, Paraguay, and Brazil, stevioside is extracted from the leaves of the stevia, a South American shrub now grown in other subtropical regions such as Asia and parts of California. The substance is 300 times sweeter than sugar, but it

significantly alters the taste of foods and beverages and can leave a strong aftertaste.

Sucralose: Six hundred times sweeter than sugar, sucralose is a derivative of table sugar, or sucrose, that has been tested extensively for safety. Currently the FDA is considering a petition for use of sucralose in 15 foods and beverages such as fruit spreads, milk products, and salad dressings, as are officials in Canada, Australia, and the European Community.

A sweetener's standing goes sour

In 1937 a scientist at the University of Illinois by the name of Michael Sveda happened to lay a lit cigarette on a pile of crystal-like powder he was experimenting with. When he picked up the cigarette and inhaled, he noticed that a bit of the powder that lingered on it tasted sweet. What Sveda had discovered, albeit accidentally, was the sweetener cyclamate, an acid derivative 30 times sweeter than sugar.

Cyclamate entered the marketplace in the early 1950s and reigned as the champion sweetener throughout the 60s. In 1970, however, the Food and Drug Administration banned it after learning it causes bladder tumors in laboratory animals. Three years after the ban was put into place, cyclamate's manufacturer, Abbott Laboratories of North Chicago, asked the FDA to allow the substance to be placed back on the market. But after reviewing the research Abbott Laboratories used to support that request, the FDA told the company that it had not indicated "to a reasonable certainty" that cyclamate was safe for human consumption.

In 1982, armed with more data regarding the safety of cyclamate, Abbott again petitioned the FDA to allow its sale. The FDA called on its Cancer Assessment Committee to review the data, a process that took two years. This time around, the committee concluded that the evidence on cyclamate indicated it *is* safe. Yet in a separate review by the National Academy of Sciences a year later, it was found that while cyclamate did not appear to be carcinogenic in and of itself, some evidence, albeit tenuous, suggested that it may promote the growth of tumors when it hooks up with other carcinogens. To this day Abbott Laboratories continues to campaign for allowing the sweetener back into the marketplace.

ASPARTAME

Aspartame, discovered in 1965, was introduced in the U.S. in 1981. It is best known to the public by the trade names NutraSweet® and Equal®.

The aspartame molecule consists of two amino acids linked together: aspartic acid and the methyl ester of phenylalanine. The two amino acids in aspartame occur naturally in foods as protein components. Methanol is formed during the digestion of aspartame. Methanol also occurs naturally in some foods and is produced by the digestion of other food constituents. Aspartame itself does not occur naturally.

Aspartame provides four calories per gram—as many calories as protein or sugar. It is roughly 180 times sweeter than sugar, however, so only very small amounts which provide

Aspartic Acid | Phenylalanine | Methanol

very few calories are necessary to sweeten a food or beverage.

Aspartame is used in a wide variety of foods and beverages and as a table-top sweetener. Aspartame is unstable if subjected to prolonged heating, so it is not suitable for use in cooking or baking. It also breaks down

in liquids during prolonged storage. However, control of the distribution system has allowed aspartame to be used successfully in liquid products including carbonated beverages.

Foods and beverages that contain aspartame must carry a label statement indicating that the product contains phenylalanine. This statement is for the benefit of the small number of individuals (those with the hereditary disease phenylketonuria) who must strictly limit their intake of this amino acid from all food sources. Normal, healthy individuals do not need to restrict their intake of foods containing phenylalanine, because their bodies produce ample amounts of the enzyme that breaks down this substance.

Aspartame-sweetened products that might be used in recipes carry a second required label notice stating that the product should not be used in cooking or baking. This is not a health warning; its purpose is simply to inform people that aspartame may not work as a sweetener under those conditions.

Regulatory History: U.S.

Aspartame was originally approved by the FDA in 1974. In 1975, before the sweetener had appeared on the market, its clearance was temporarily postponed until two objections raised by parties who questioned its safety could be resolved. Later, questions arose concerning the authen-

ticity of some of the scientific studies supporting aspartame's safety.

After extensive investigations, all of these issues were resolved, and aspartame was approved for use in dry foods in 1981. In 1982, the manufacturer submitted a second petition to FDA, requesting approval for use in carbonated beverages; this approval was granted in 1983. Subsequently, FDA has approved the use of aspartame in many additional product categories, including multivitamins, frozen desserts, fruit drinks and yogurt.

On several occasions, petitions have been filed with FDA requesting that the agency ban aspartame or refuse to approve additional uses. FDA has denied each of these requests, stating that the safety issues raised by the petitioners have already been resolved and that no new, valid data supporting the petitioners' objections have been presented.[1] Both federal courts and the General Accounting Office have reviewed the process by which FDA approved aspartame and have concluded that the agency followed appropriate procedures.

Regulatory Status: Canada

Canadian authorities approved aspartame for use in table-top sweeteners and a wide variety of foods, including carbonated beverages, in 1981.

Reprinted from *Low-Calorie Sweeteners*, March 1993, pp. 5-13, 24-26. *Low-Calorie Sweeteners*, a publication of the American Council on Science and Health, New York, NY.

Safety

Aspartame is one of the most thoroughly tested substances in the U.S. food supply. A comprehensive set of safety studies was completed before its approval, and many additional investigations have been conducted since the sweetener went on the market.[2] Many authorities, including the Joint Expert Committee on Food Additives of the FAO/WHO, the European Community and the American Medical Association,[3] have evaluated the scientific evidence on aspartame and concluded that it is a safe food additive. It is particularly worthy of note that there is a large body of data on aspartame's safety in human subjects, as well as in experimental animals.

Levels of Consumption
No food substance can be classified unequivocally as safe or unsafe. Instead, safety depends on the amount of the substance present in the diet. Natural food constituents, including such familiar substances as vitamin A, iron, salt and even water, are unsafe in excessive amounts. The same is true of aspartame and other food additives.

FDA has set the maximum acceptable daily intake (ADI) of aspartame at 50 milligrams per kilogram of body weight per day (mg/kg/day). The ADI is an estimate of the amount of a food additive that can be consumed daily for a lifetime without adverse effects. It is not an absolute limit that must never be exceeded on any one day. A person may occasionally consume amounts of a food additive in excess of the ADI without harm.

Prior to aspartame's approval, experts made several estimates of the amount of the sweetener that people would consume. Although these projections deliberately exaggerated typical consumption patterns in order to account for heavy users of the product, they indicated that intakes would be well below the ADI.

For instance, it was projected that if aspartame replaced all of the sucrose (table sugar) in the U.S. diet, average consumption would be approximately 8.3 mg/kg/day. If it replaced all of the carbohydrates (sugars plus starches), average consumption would be about 25 mg/kg/day. Another type of estimate indicated that the 99th percentile of aspartame consumption (the level exceeded by only one out of 100 people) would be 34 mg/kg/day.

As a condition of aspartame's approval, FDA has required its manufacturer to monitor the actual use levels of the product.[4] This surveillance has shown that consumption levels are well below the ADI of 50 mg/kg/day. In surveys conducted between 1984 and 1989, the 90th percentile of aspartame consumption among aspartame users ranged from 1.6 to 2.3 mg/kg/day. The 90th percentile (the level exceeded by only one out of ten people) is the level FDA considers most meaningful in evaluating the exposure of a high level consumer of a product. The 99th percentile in two recent surveys was 5.8 and 6.5 mg/kg/day.[5]

Similar findings have been reported in other countries. For instance, a 1987 Canadian survey showed that 90th and 95th percentile intakes for the total population were 3.8 and 5.2 mg/kg/day, respectively.[6]

It has been speculated that children, because of their lower body weights, might consume excessive amounts of aspartame. It has also been suggested that diabetics and dieters, many of whom make an effort to seek out products made with low-calorie sweeteners, might exceed the aspartame ADI. However, ongoing surveillance indicates that all of these special population groups are consuming amounts of aspartame well within acceptable limits.

Recent U.S. surveys showed that the 99th percentile of aspartame consumption by children in all age groups ranged from 3.0 to 8.3 mg/kg/day.[5] In Canada, 95th percentile consumption levels for various age groups of aspartame-using children ranged from 5.7 to 12.3 mg/kg/day.[6] The 99th percentile of aspartame

consumption among U.S. diabetics in two recent surveys was 8.0 and 8.3 mg/kg/day; among individuals on active weight-loss programs it was 5.6 and 7.3 mg/kg/day.[5] In Canada, 95th percentile consumption levels for both diabetics and dieters were less than 15 mg/kg/day.[6]

Breakdown of Aspartame in the Body
In the safety testing of a new food additive, researchers investigate a wide variety of possible health effects. To focus on those areas of greatest importance, however, it is necessary to know what happens to the additive in the body after it is consumed.

Aspartame, which resembles a tiny piece of protein, is digested like a protein fragment. The body breaks it down into its components: phenylalanine, aspartic acid and methanol. These components are handled just as if they had been derived from other dietary sources.

All three components are present in many foods and are safe as consumed in normal diets. All three can be harmful if present in extremely large amounts in the body; the same is true of all normal food components. Much of the safety testing of aspartame focused on studies designed to determine whether consumption of normal or even unusually high levels of aspartame would lead to increases in the amounts of these substances in the body to levels that might be associated with adverse effects.

The Components of Aspartame
In pre-approval studies, aspartame was administered to human volunteers in doses of up to 200 mg/kg at a single sitting. Even at this high dose, blood levels of aspartame's three components remained well below levels that are considered unsafe.[7]

More recently, volunteers received 75/mg/kg of aspartame daily for 24 weeks. This does is one-and-a half times the ADI and approximately 30 times the 90th percentile aspartame consumption level. All of aspartame's three components were metabolized normally; toxic levels of these substances did not accumulate in the blood, and the volunteers did not experience any adverse effects.[9]

Many foods have higher levels of phenylalanine, aspartic acid or methanol than those found in aspartame-sweetened products. For example, a glass of skim milk has approximately 13 times more aspartic acid and six times more phenylalanine than the same size serving of an aspartame-sweetened beverage.[2] Four to five times more methanol is produced during digestion of tomato juice than from the same amount of an aspartame-sweetened beverage.[2]

The use of aspartame causes only a small increase in the total intake of its components. It has been calculated that a 90th-percentile consumer of aspartame-sweetened products would increase his or her daily consumption of phenylalanine and aspartic acid by one to two percent.[5] Such changes are well within the range of variation caused by day-to-day differences in protein intake and are clearly not harmful.

Breakdown Products
When aspartame is stored for prolonged periods of time or exposed to high temperatures, it may break down. The breakdown products include the components discussed above as well as the diketopiperazine (DKP) derivative of aspartame. This derivative has been subjected to safety tests in animals similar to those conducted for aspartame itself. No problems were found.[10]

Trace amounts of beta-aspartame, a molecule that is the mirror image of aspartame, may also be present in aspartame-sweetened products subjected to prolonged storage. Safety tests on beta-aspartame have been conducted, and no problems have been discovered.

Cancer Studies
As with all new food additives, aspartame was evaluated through ani-

mal tests to determine whether it had the potential to cause cancer. During the process of evaluating aspartame's safety before its approval, two of these animal cancer tests became controversial.[11]

One group of scientists, from an independent review panel commissioned to assess these studies, contended that the studies had unusual features that made them impossible to evaluate. The scientists also stated that the data did not exclude the possibility that aspartame might be linked to an increased risk of brain tumors in rats.[12] These scientists recommended that the studies be repeated. A second group of scientists, from the FDA's Bureau of Foods, argued that the data could be evaluated and that appropriate analysis showed no evidence of an association between aspartame and brain tumors in rats.[13]

The FDA Commissioner agreed with the Bureau of Foods and decided that additional studies on this subject were not necessary.[4] A later study on a different strain of rat also supported the conclusion that aspartame does not cause brain tumors.[14]

Special Population Groups

Concerns have been expressed that while aspartame is safe for most people, it might be unsafe for certain population groups such as children, diabetics, people on weight-reduction diets, lactating women or people who carry the gene for phenylketonuria. However, aspartame has been tested and found to be safe in all of these population groups.[2]

Low-calorie sweeteners are not intended for use by very young children, since this age group has no need to restrict caloric intake. However, normal quantities of aspartame are not toxic to young children. A series of studies in one-year-olds showed that they metabolize aspartame's components as effectively as adults do.[15] Aspartame has also been

shown to be safe for older children and adolescents.[16]

The safety of aspartame in phenylketonuria (PKU) carriers has been investigated extensively. (PKU carriers inherited the gene for PKU from only one parent. Those who inherited the gene from both parents actually have the disease.) PKU carriers are essentially normal, with no symptoms of the disease, and they do not require special diets. However, they do have a diminished ability to metabolize phenylalanine. Both short- and long-term tests in PKU carriers have shown that they do not develop harmful blood phenylalanine levels after consumption of normal or even unusually high doses of aspartame (as much as twice the ADI).[17]

Charges have been made that aspartame is dangerous to pregnant women because its consumption might lead to dangerously high blood phenylalanine concentrations in the fetus. The scientific evidence does not support these charges. Normal consumption of aspartame is safe for normal pregnant women.[2] Harmful amounts of the component amino acids do not accumulate in the fetus.[18] Studies in experimental animals indicate that there is a large margin of safety for aspartame consumption in pregnancy; fetal abnormalities did not result even when animals were fed aspartame at doses far greater than those consumed by humans.[19]

A few women have abnormalities of phenylalanine metabolism in which consumption of a normal diet leads to blood phenylalanine levels high enough to damage a fetus. Unfortunately, this condition may not be diagnosed, since the women themselves show no symptoms, and therefore the mothers may not be placed on the special diet needed to protect the fetus. Since aspartame supplies only a small proportion of dietary phenylalanine, its use does not add significantly to the hazards faced by expectant mothers with undiagnosed abnormalities of phenylalanine metabolism.

Behavioral Effects

Aspartame has been alleged to have adverse effects on mood or behavior because it can change brain chemistry. Scientific evidence does not support this claim.

Recent scientific research indicates that normal consumption of ordinary dietary components may influence mood and behavior. Animal studies suggest that brain chemicals called neurotransmitters may play a role in these effects. The changes in neurotransmitter levels produced in this way are normal physiological variations; they do not constitute a health hazard.

Since the amino acid phenylalanine is one of the many food components that can affect neurotransmitter levels, it has been speculated that aspartame might influence behavior. However, since the amount of aspartame that people consume is small, dramatic (or even readily detectable) effects are highly unlikely.

A number of studies in human subjects have examined the psychological and behavioral effects of consuming aspartame. Aspartame was not found to affect mood, cognition or behavior in any of these studies.[2]

Animal research confirms that aspartame does not have significant effects on behavior. For example, infant macaque monkeys were fed aspartame for long periods of time in doses far beyond those that would ever be consumed by humans. Standard tests of primate behavior showed no differences between these monkeys and otherwise similar monkeys that had not consumed aspartame.[10] A lack of behavioral effects has also been demonstrated in rodents.[2]

Possible Adverse Reactions

Both the FDA and the Centers for Disease Control (CDC) have investigated reports from consumers who believe that they have experienced adverse reactions as a result of consuming aspartame.[20] Reports of possible adverse reactions have also appeared in medical journals.

Such reports are to be expected. When an individual develops a health problem, it is natural for him or her to try to figure out the cause. Aspartame is an obvious candidate. Indeed, it may be the most conspicuous new ingredient ever introduced into the American food supply. However, the mere fact that a person consumed aspartame and later experienced an unpleasant symptom does not establish a cause-and-effect relationship.

Most of the alleged adverse reactions to aspartame have involved mild symptoms common in the general population, such as headaches, skin rashes, mood changes or menstrual irregularities. Claims that aspartame can cause serious problems, such as impaired vision or epileptic seizures, have not be substantiated.

Allegations about visual impairment were apparently prompted by concern over aspartame's methanol content. Large doses of methanol, when converted to formic acid in the body, can indeed affect vision. However, the doses of aspartame consumed by humans do not increase blood methanol concentration to toxic levels and do not produce a detectable increase in blood formic acid levels.[8]

FDA's evaluation of reported cases of eye damage allegedly linked to aspartame found no evidence of a cause-and-effect relationship.[21] In many instances, the vision problems were attributed to other factors, such as diabetes or the use of medications.[21]

No cases of epileptic seizures in humans attributable to the consumption of aspartame have been documented.[2] The idea that aspartame might cause seizures is apparently based on a misinterpretation of experiments in which extraordinary doses of aspartame or phenylalanine may have potentiated the induction of seizures by seizure-producing drugs or other agents in susceptible strains of rats.[22] These effects were seen in only a few of the many animal models of epilepsy, did not occur when aspartame alone was administered and are not seen at aspartame

doses typical of human exposure.[23] The consumption of aspartame is considered safe for persons with seizure disorders.[23]

In 1992, FDA researchers published a detailed report on 251 seizure cases allegedly linked to aspartame that had been reported to their agency during the years 1986–90. They found no meaningful association between these seizures and the consumption of the sweetener and concluded, "The fact that some people have a seizure shortly after consuming the food additive does not indicate a causal relationship. . . . The analyses presented here do not indicate any unusual or significant association that would warrant clinical studies at this time."[24]

The CDC concluded in 1984 that the available data "do not provide evidence for the existence of serious, widespread, adverse health consequences attendant to the use of aspartame."[25] That conclusion remains valid today, after eight more years of extensive use and continued monitoring of the sweetener.

As with any drug, food component or other substance, it is possible that there may be rare adverse reactions in some individuals that truly are linked to aspartame. To date, however, evidence for their existence is limited. In fact, two groups of scientists who attempted to study aspartame allergy found it difficult to locate people who believed themselves allergic to aspartame despite extensive recruitment efforts. Of the small number of subjects who did participate in the investigations, none proved to have a true sensitivity to the sweetener.[26,27]

In a few instances, individuals have reported that they consistently developed particular symptoms (mostly rashes or skin eruptions) after consuming aspartame, and the physician treating the patient found that the symptoms were reproducible.[28] "Reproducible" means that the symptoms consistently appeared after aspartame was consumed and disappeared when aspartame was excluded from the patient's diet.

Whether these cases represent isolated instances of aspartame sensitivity is unclear, since investigations in single patients do not have the same scientific significance as well-controlled studies involving larger numbers of subjects.

One such well-controlled study has provided no evidence for the existence of adverse reactions to aspartame. In this clinical trial, 108 volunteers received 75 mg/kg (one and a half times the ADI) of aspartame or an inactive placebo daily for 24 weeks.[9] The study was conducted under "double-blind" conditions, meaning that neither the volunteers nor the researchers knew who was receiving aspartame and who was receiving a placebo until after the end of the experiment. No differences were found between the aspartame and placebo groups in the number or types of physical symptoms experienced during the study.

The possibility that aspartame might act as a dietary trigger of headache in patients prone to migraine or other types of recurrent headaches has been investigated. Two controlled scientific studies of this subject have been reported. In one, patients receiving aspartame experienced more headaches than those receiving an inactive placebo.[29] In the other, no difference was found in the effects of aspartame and placebo.[30] Other researchers have argued that each of these studies had important methodological limitations.[31,32] One authority has suggested that physicians should alert patients with recurrent headaches to the possibility that aspartame might increase the frequency of their attacks. He emphasizes, however, that an outright prohibition of aspartame consumption by headache patients is not needed.[33] Others contend that current evidence does not warrant even such mild cautionary advice to patients.[31]

Conclusion

The low-calorie sweetener aspartame has been used in the U.S. and many other countries for a decade. Extensive scientific evidence, including an unusually large number of studies in human subjects, is now approved for a wide variety of uses, levels of consumption remain well within safe limits.

Notes

1. For the most recent action of this type, see U.S. FDA. Aspartame: denial of request for hearing on final rules. *Federal Register* 57(20:3698–3701, Jan 30, 1992.

2. Aspartame safety studies conducted through 1989 were reviewed in Butchko, HH and FN Kotsonis. Aspartame: review of recent research. *Comments on Toxicology* 3: 253–278, 1989. Newer studies and those of particular interest are cited specifically below.

3. Council on Scientific Affairs, AMA. Aspartame, review of safety issues. *Journal of the American Medical Association* 254: 400–402, 1985.

4. U.S. FDA. Aspartame: commissioner's final decision. *Federal Register* 46(142):38284–38308, July 24, 1981.

5. Butchko, HH and FN Kotsonis. Acceptable daily intake vs. actual intake: the aspartame example. *Journal of the American College of Nutrition* 10:258–266, 1991.

6. Heybach, JP and C Ross. Aspartame consumption in a representative sample of Canadians. *Journal of the Canadian Dietetic Association* 50:166–170, 1989.

7. Stegink, LD, LJ Filer, Jr., and GL Baker. Plasma and erythrocyte concentrations of free amino acids in adult humans administered abuse doses of aspartame. *Journal of Toxicology and Environmental Health* 7: 291–305, 1981.

8. Stegink, LD, *et al.* Blood methanol concentrations in normal adult subjects administered abuse doses of aspartame. *Journal of Toxicology and Environmental Health* 7: 281–290, 1981.

9. Leon, AS, *et al.* Safety of long-term large doses of aspartame. *Archives of Internal Medicine* 149:2318–2324, 1989.

10. U.S. FDA. Food additives permitted for direct addition to food for human consumption; aspartame: final rule. *Federal Register* 48(132):31376–31382, July 8, 1983.

11. Interpretation of the disputed studies is discussed in detail in two reports: Koestner, A. Aspartame and brain tumors: pathology issues. Pp. 447–457; and Cornell, RG, RA Wolfe, and PG Sanders. Aspartame and brain tumors: statistical issues. Pp. 459–479. Both in *Aspartame. Physiology and Biochemistry* (LD Stegink and LJ Filer Jr, eds), Marcel Dekker, Inc., New York, 1984.

12. Aspartame: decision of the public board of inquiry, Department of Health and Human Service, FDA. Docket No. 75F–0355. September 30, 1980.

13. Bureau of Foods' exceptions to the decision of the public board of inquiry, Department of Health and Human Services, FDA. Docket No. 75F-0335. December 19, 1980.

14. Ishii, H. Incidence of brain tumors in rats fed aspartame. *Toxicology Letters* 7: 433–437, 1981.

15. Filer, LJ Jr, GL Baker, and LD Stegink. Aspartame ingestion by human infants. In *Aspartame. Physiology and Biochemistry* (LD Stegink and LJ Filer Jr, eds), Marcel Dekker, Inc., New York, 1984. Pp. 579–591.

16. Frey, GH. Use of aspartame by apparently healthy children and adolescents. *Journal of Toxicology and Environmental Health* 2:401–415, 1976.

17. Stegink, LD, *et al.* Repeated ingestion of aspartame-sweetened beverages: further observations in individuals heterozygous for phenylketonuria. *Metabolism* 39:1076–1081, 1990; Stegink, LD, *et al.* Effect of an abuse dose of aspartame upon plasma and erythrocyte levels of amino acids in phenylketonuric heterozygous and normal adults. *Journal of Nutrition* 110:2216–2224, 1980; Stegink, LD, *et al.* Plasma phenylalanine levels of phenylketonuric heterozygous and normal adults administered aspartame at 34 mg/kg body weight. *Toxicology* 20:81–90, 1981; Koch, R, *et al.* Use of aspartame in phenylketonuric heterozygous adults. *Journal of Toxicology and Environmental Health* 2:453–457, 1976.

18. Pitkin, RM. Aspartame ingestion during pregnancy. In *Aspartame. Physiology and Biochemistry* (LD Stegink and LJ Filer Jr, eds), Marcel Dekker, Inc., New York, 1984. Pp. 555–563.

19. Molinary, SV. Preclinical studies of aspartame in nonprimate animals. In *Aspartame. Physiology and Biochemistry* (LD Stegink and LJ Filer Jr, eds), Marcel Dekker, Inc., New York, 1984. Pp. 289–306.

20. Bradstock, MK, *et al.* Evaluation of reactions to food additives: the aspartame experience. *American Journal of Clinical Nutrition* 43:464–469, 1986; Tollefson, L. Quarterly report on adverse reactions associated with aspartame consumption. FDA Memorandum, July 1, 1991.

21. Copestake, P. Aspartame—a bit of a headache? *Food and Chemical Toxicology* 26:571, 1988.

22. Guiso, G, *et al.* Effect of aspartame on seizures in various models of experimental epilepsy. *Toxicology and Applied Pharmacology* 96:485–493, 1988; Diomede, L, *et al.* Interspecies and interstrain studies on the increased susceptibility to metrazol-induced convulsions in animals given aspartame. *Food and Chemical Toxicology* 29:101–106, 1991.

23. Fisher, RS. Aspartame, neurotoxicity, and seizures: a review. *Journal of Epilepsy* 2:55–64, 1989.

24. Tollefson, L and RJ Barnard. An analysis of FDA passive surveillance reports of

seizures associated with consumption of aspartame. *Journal of the American Dietetic Association* 92:598–601, 1992.

25. Centers for Disease Control. Evaluation of consumer complaints related to aspartame use. *Morbidity and Mortality Weekly Report* 33:605–607, 1984.

26. Garriga, MM, C Berkebile, and DD Metcalfe. A combined single-blind, double-blind, placebo-controlled study to determine the reproducibility of hypersensitivity reactions to aspartame. *Journal of Allergy and Clinical Immunology,* 87: 821–827, 1991.

27. Geha, R, *et al.* Aspartame is no more likely than placebo to cause allergic reactions [abstract]. *Journal of Allergy and Clinical Immunology* 89: 184, 1992.

28. Novick, NL. Aspartame-induced granulomatous panniculitis. *Annals of Internal Medicine* 102:206–207, 1985; McCauliffe, DP and K Poitras. Aspartame-induced lobular panniculitis. *Journal of the American Academy of Dermatology* 24:298–300, 1991; Kulczycki, A Jr. Aspartame-induced urticaria. *Annals of Internal Medicine* 104:207–208, 1986; Johns, DR. Migraine provoked by aspartame. *New England Journal of Medicine* 315:456, 1986.

29. Koehler, SM and A Glaros. The effect of aspartame on migraine headache, *Headache* 28:10–13, 1988.

30. Schiffman, SS, *et al.* Aspartame and susceptibility to headache. *New England Journal of Medicine* 317:1181–1185, 1987.

31. Schiffman, SS. Aspartame and headache [letter]. *Headache* 28:370, 1988.

32. Amery, WK. More on aspartame and headache [letter]. *Headache* 28:624, 1988; Various authors. Aspartame and headache [correspondence]. *New England Journal of Medicine* 318:1200–1202, 1988.

33. Edmeads, J. Aspartame and headache [editorial]. *Headache* 28:64–64, 1988.

Good Food You Can't Get

Decades of research have perfected a wonderful way to keep meat, seafood and produce fresher and safer—yet it's not being widely used. Why?

Larry Katzenstein

When more than 500 people got sick and three children died after eating tainted hamburger meat at a fast-food chain earlier this year in the Pacific Northwest, alarms rang nationwide. Public-health officials and meat-industry executives called for new measures to protect the public from such bacteria-induced illnesses. Soon Agriculture Secretary Mike Espy was outlining a plan of action before Congress. Among his suggestions: a wider use of irradiation to destroy harmful bacteria in raw meat. "Irradiating meat may have very important benefits," Espy has said.

In addition to destroying bacteria that cause illnesses, irradiation kills insect pests on produce, eliminating the need for chemical fumigation after harvest. It can also extend the shelf life of food.

Irradiation was first studied in the United States and Europe at the turn of the century. Today it is common overseas. Scores of foods, from apples to frogs' legs, are routinely irradiated in dozens of countries, including Great Britain, France, the Netherlands, Israel and South Africa. But not in the United States—thanks in part to Food & Water, Inc., a consumer group based in Marshfield, Vt., that is leading a nationwide campaign to keep food irradiation from winning public acceptance.

The campaign plays on two of our deepest concerns: anxiety over food safety and mistrust of anything involving radiation. In 1991, for example, Floridians heard this Food & Water radio spot: "Supermarkets have started selling radiation-exposed foods: spices, processed foods, and soon, meats and fruits and vegetables. New studies show that ingesting radiation-exposed foods causes genetic damage, which can lead to cancer and birth defects . . . ."

Such scare tactics have paid off. So far, despite Food and Drug Administration (FDA) approval, just one irradiation plant devoted mainly to food has opened in the United States, near Tampa, Fla. And aside from scattered sales of irradiated produce and spices, Food & Water has fulfilled its pledge: "We *will* stop radiation-exposed food. We will!" But Food & Water's triumph may be a defeat for the American consumer.

What's in a Name? Since it makes food safer by killing potentially harmful microbes, irradiation has been likened to pasteurization. Milk was first pasteurized in the United States a century ago, but health fears delayed widespread use for decades. Many of the arguments voiced against pasteurization are now used against food irradiation. Opponents claim irradiation destroys nutrients, makes spoiled food appear fresh, forms dangerous chemicals and meddles with nature. Such claims have helped persuade New York State to approve a moratorium on the sale of irradiated food and Maine to ban it, except for spices used as ingredients.

The biggest problem with food irradiation is its name. The very word *radiation* is emotionally charged. Add *food* and many people envision poultry and produce that glow in the dark.

In reality, food irradiation doesn't make food radioactive. The process is akin to sending your luggage through an airport scanner. Your suitcases are irradiated, but they don't become radioactive—a point even Food & Water acknowledges.

The procedure is relatively simple. Food travels on a conveyor through a chamber where dozens of "pencils," usually made from cobalt-60 and sealed in stainless-steel tubes, irradiate the food with gamma rays. Because any increase in the food's temperature is negligible, changes in taste, texture and aroma are minimized.

Irradiation can reduce some nutrients, particularly vitamins. But these losses, experts point out, are often less than those resulting from other food-processing techniques, such as cooking, canning or freezing. And for the many Americans who eat poultry—on average we each consume about 87 pounds a year—food irradiation can be nothing short of a blessing.

Poultry is frequently contaminated with salmonella and campylobacter—the two bacteria that cause most food poisonings. The federal Centers for Disease Control and Prevention estimate that more than 20 million illnesses occur each year, causing some 9000 deaths.

Poultry causes more than one million of those illnesses. Thorough cooking kills the organisms, but illness can occur if the meat isn't well cooked or if drippings contaminate hands, a chopping board or utensils. That's where irradiation comes in. Tests by the U.S. Department of

Reprinted with permission from *Reader's Digest*, July 1993, pp. 43-47. Originally appeared in *American Health*, December 1992, p. 60, "Food Irradiation."

Agriculture have shown that irradiation at the dose range prescribed by the FDA kills from 99.5 to 99.99 percent of salmonella in poultry. A few of the bacteria can survive the process, so irradiated chicken (like ordinary chicken) must stay refrigerated and be properly cooked. But since irradiation also kills harmless bacteria that make chicken spoil faster, the bird keeps at least a few days longer in the fridge than a nonirradiated chicken.

Despite such benefits, Food & Water called the FDA's 1990 approval of poultry irradiation "nothing short of a criminal act." It claims it has persuaded 13 major poultry companies to declare they won't irradiate. And its publicity helped bring it $315,000 last year in dues and donations.

False Scenario. Food & Water was founded in 1986 by Dr. Walter Burnstein, a Denville, N.J., osteopath and anti-nuclear activist who asserted that food irradiation was being foisted on the public as a way to get rid of nuclear waste. Cesium-137, which is formed as a waste product when nuclear weapons are made and nuclear power is generated, can be used in irradiation. The group has contended, without documentation, that the government wanted "up to 1000" irradiators built to create a demand for cesium.

Such a nuclear-conspiracy theory "may have been somewhat plausible several years ago," says George Giddings, a food-irradiation consultant, "but today it's absurd. Cesium is now recognized as unsuitable for use in industrial irradiation." Nevertheless, by selling T-shirts stating "The Department of Energy has a solution to the problem of radioactive waste. You are going to eat it," Food & Water still promotes this nuclear scenario.

Despite the scare tactics, proponents of irradiation foresee its more widespread use on several types of foods.

Meat. Food-borne illness isn't limited to poultry. Beef, pork and other red meats account for many cases, including those caused by the tainted hamburgers. Scores of studies show that irradiation can minimize this risk.

Seafood. Tests dating back four decades have found that irradiation kills the bacteria and parasites that infect fish and shellfish, and delays spoilage. Irradiation could provide

the nation's heartland with seafood as fresh-tasting as that on both coasts.

Imported Fruit. Before fruit can enter the United States, it must be certified free of insect pests. In 1984 ethylene dibromide, the fumigant used to treat many fruits, was banned from use on all produce sold in the United States because of concern over cancer-causing residues. Irradiation kills pests without leaving residues, and its use could allow many types of foreign fruit to gain entry. Irradiation could also replace methyl bromide, one of the world's most widely used postharvest fumigants, which some experts say will be phased out by the year 2000.

Spices. Each year Americans consume 850 million pounds of spices, which are often infested with insects and microbes. Unlike the chemical fumigant sometimes used on them, irradiation has proved effective in decontaminating spices without affecting flavor, color or aroma. Yet, less than one percent of the nation's spices are now irradiated, versus the 20 to 30 percent that are treated chemically.

Produce. Currently only a few fruits and vegetables are irradiated. The process can turn some foods—including melons, cucumbers and lettuce—mushy. But many others are good candidates, including apples, pears, onions, mushrooms and tomatoes. Irradiated strawberries last in the refrigerator at least a week longer than untreated ones.

Food irradiation could have its greatest impact in feeding starving people in developing countries, where ten percent of grains and up to half of other crops are lost to rot or insects. But most developing nations have resisted food irradiation, partly because Americans seem opposed. "Developing nations look to the United States for guidance," says Dr. Fritz Käferstein, chief of the food-safety unit of the Geneva-based World Health Organization, which strongly endorses food irradiation. "If the United States won't accept irradiation, it will be extremely difficult for these countries to adopt it. The loss of this technology is resulting in the needless suffering and death of thousands, perhaps millions, of people."

IF IRRADIATED FOOD doesn't become

radioactive, what then is the problem? Critics such as Food & Water claim that irradiation creates chemical residues—including benzene and formaldehyde—that can cause cancer and birth defects. But the FDA and scientists who've researched food irradiation have concluded that the total amount of these chemicals in an irradiated food is extremely low. Indeed, higher amounts occur naturally in many foods. An egg, for example, has more than 100 times as much benzene as an irradiated steak, and formaldehyde levels in apples are much higher than irradiation could ever produce in food.

More ominously, opponents claim that irradiation spawns unique radiolytic products (URPs) that could cause serious health effects. "Irradiation opponents invariably bring these up," says Giddings. "However, URPs are entirely hypothetical, and many years of studying irradiated foods have yet to uncover any."

The search for some hazard in irradiated food has been going on for more than 40 years. That effort, advocates say, has made irradiation the most thoroughly researched of all food-processing techniques.

Numerous short-term safety studies that tested irradiated foods—from chicken and fish to mangoes and onions—on lab animals or cell cultures produced no mutations. Nor were any hazardous chemicals identified in irradiated food. The most comprehensive of the many long-term studies involved numerous generations of mice, rabbits and dogs that were fed poultry completely sterilized by irradiation at about 20 times the standard dose. The outcome: a lifetime diet of irradiated chicken didn't cause cancer, affect nutrition or reproduction, or otherwise harm the animals in any way.

Nevertheless, when Florida's food irradiation plant opened last year, Food & Water's protests and pickets deterred all but one store in that state from carrying irradiated produce. And companies previously considering irradiation beat a hasty retreat after Food & Water and other groups threatened to rally stockholders and consumers against them.

With about 3500 members, Food & Water has successfully created the impression that most Americans oppose irradiated food. But the perception appears to be false. "The activists are simply wrong in claiming the public opposes it," says Christine Bruhn, a food-marketing specialist at the University of California at Davis.

Surveys by Bruhn and others find that most Americans would not reject irradiated products when given information about their benefits.

Proof that consumers will buy irradiated food comes from Carrot Top, a large grocery and produce store in the Chicago suburb of Glenview. Last year owner James Corrigan gave customers a choice between irradiated and nonirradiated strawberries, both $1.29 a pint and picked from the same field at the same time. In one weekend, Corrigan sold 172 cases of irradiated strawberries, versus only six of the nonirradiated ones. His irradiated oranges and grapefruit sold equally well.

"At first I thought it was just the novelty of it," Corrigan says. But continued strong sales have convinced him that "customers overwhelmingly prefer irradiated produce" when given the choice.

Food & Water and other opponents of irradiation ignore the obvious benefits and focus instead on unsubstantiated risks, public-health experts contend. "They've lost sight of what the public interest is," says Dr. Allan Forbes, former director of the FDA Office of Nutrition and Food Sciences. "Food irradiation is safe beyond the slightest question. It's a sad commentary, but it's clear to me that these groups make their living by creating fear about issues like this."

The Canning Process

Old Preservation Technique Goes Modern

Dale Blumenthal

*Dale Blumenthal is a staff writer for
FDA Consumer.*

The steamboat Bertrand was heavily
laden with provisions when it set out on
the Missouri River in 1865, destined for
the gold mining camps in Fort Benton,
Mont. The boat snagged and swamped
under the weight, sinking to the bottom
of the river. It was found a century
later, under 30 feet of silt a little north
of Omaha, Neb.

Among the canned food items re-
trieved from the Bertrand in 1968 were
brandied peaches, oysters, plum tomatoes, honey, and mixed vegetables. In
1974, chemists at the National Food
Processors Association (NFPA) analyzed
the products for bacterial contamination
and nutrient value. Although the food
had lost its fresh smell and appearance,
the NFPA chemists detected no microbial growth and determined that the
foods were as safe to eat as they had
been when canned more than 100 years
earlier.

The nutrient values varied depending
upon the product and nutrient. NFPA
chemists Janet Dudek and Edgar Elkins
report that significant amounts of vitamins C and A were lost. But protein levels remained high, and all calcium values
"were comparable to today's products."

NFPA chemists also analyzed a 40-
year-old can of corn found in the base-
ment of a home in California. Again, the
canning process had kept the corn safe
from contaminants and from much nutrient loss. In addition, Dudek says, the
kernels looked and smelled like recently
canned corn.

The canning process is a product of the
Napoleonic wars. Malnutrition was ram-
pant among the 18th century French
armed forces. As Napoleon prepared for
his Russian campaign, he searched for a
new and better means of preserving food
for his troops and offered a prize of
12,000 francs to anyone who could find
one. Nicolas Appert, a Parisian candy
maker, was awarded the prize in 1809.

Although the causes of food spoilage
were unknown at the time, Appert was
an astute experimenter and observer. For
instance, after noting that storing wine in
airtight bottles kept it from spoiling, he
filled widemouth glass bottles with food,
carefully corked them, and heated them
in boiling water.

The durable tin can—and the use of
pottery and other metals—followed
shortly afterwards, a notion of English-
man Peter Durand. Soon, these "tinned"
foods were used to feed the British army
and navy.

21 Billion Cans a Year

Canned foods are more than a relic
dug from the past. They make up 12 percent of grocery sales in the United
States. More than 1,500 food products
are canned—including many that aren't
available fresh in most areas, such as el-
derberry, guava, mango, and about 75
different juice drinks. Consumers can
buy at least 130 different canned vegetable products—from artichokes and as-
paragus to turnips and zucchini. More
than a dozen kinds of beef are canned,
including beef burgers and chopped,
corned and barbecued beef.

According to a recent study cospon-
sored by the U.S. Department of Agriculture and NFPA, canned foods provide
the same nutritional value as fresh grocery produce and their frozen counter-
parts when prepared for the table. NFPA
researchers compared six vegetables in
three forms: home-cooked fresh, warmed
canned, and prepared frozen.

"Levels of 13 minerals, eight vitamins,
and fiber in the foods were similar," says

 Reprinted from *FDA Consumer,* Vol. 24, No. 7, September 1990, pp. 14, 16-18, by permission.

Dudek. In fact, in some cases the canned product contained high levels of some vitamins that in fresh produce are destroyed by light or exposure to air.

The Canning Process

Food-spoiling bacteria, yeasts and molds are naturally present in foods. To grow, these microorganisms need moisture, a low-acid environment (acid prevents bacterial growth), nutrients, and an appropriate (usually room) temperature.

Dennis Dignan, Ph.D., chief of FDA's food processing section, explains that foods are preserved from food spoilage by controlling one or more of the above factors. For instance, frozen foods are stored at temperatures too low for microorganisms (bacteria, yeasts and molds) to grow. When foods are dried, sufficient moisture is not available to promote growth.

It is the preservation process that distinguishes canned from other packaged foods. During canning, the food is placed in an airtight (hermetically sealed) container and heated to destroy microorganisms. The hermetic seal is essential to ensure that microorganisms do not contaminate the product after it is sterilized through heating, says Dignan. Properly canned foods can be stored unrefrigerated indefinitely without fear of their spoiling or becoming toxic.

Canning for a New Age

Dignan also notes that foods packaged in materials other than metal cans are considered "canned" by food processing specialists if the food undergoes the canning preservation process. Thus, today a canned food may be packaged in a number of other types of containers, such as glass jars, paperboard cans, and plastics that can be formed into anything from pouches to soup bowls to serving trays.

For example, FDA consumer safety officer Tom Gardine, holding up a small, plastic container of half-and-half for his morning coffee, says, "This is a canned food." He explains that the coffee creamer was heated to destroy bacteria and sealed to prevent microorganisms from entering the sterile container. Until it is opened, the creamer is intended to be stored on the shelf, not in the refrigerator.

Meals for today's U.S. military come in plastic pouches—a new version of the heavier C-rations in metal cans. Such flexible pouches aren't as popular with American civilians as they are with Eu-

ropeans. Many Americans, instead, are buying their canned foods in plastic containers that come with a peel-off metal top and plastic lid—ready for the microwave. Barriers (made of sophisticated synthetic materials) that provide an airtight seal are sandwiched in these plastic layered containers. They are used for applesauce, pudding, and other foods that can be stored on supermarket or home shelves for years.

Then there are containers made of new transparent plastic materials like polyethylene terephthalate—used for peanut butter and catsup. Packages made of paperboard layers have been designed in the shape of boxes to contain such foods as fruit juices, tomato sauce, and even milk.

Even the tin can is changing. For years, the three-piece can (made from a top, a bottom, and a body formed from a plate soldered into a cylinder) was the only can around. Now there are two-piece cans, which eliminate the side seam and one seamed end. These cans are made by feeding metal into a press that forms the can body and one end into a single piece.

In the traditional three-piece cans, a welded side seam has replaced the lead-soldered side seam in all but 3.7 percent of American cans, says NFPA official Roger Coleman. The welding process uses electrodes that apply pressure and electric current to overlapping edges at the side seam. These new seams eliminate concern about lead leaching into metal canned foods. In the 3.7 percent of U.S. cans where lead still is used, it is often for dry foods (such as coffee) packaged in cans, according to Coleman. Leaching is not a concern here.

Many imported cans, however, still bear lead-soldered side seams. To tell whether a can has been soldered with lead, first peel back the label to expose the seam. The edges along the joint of a lead-soldered seam will be folded over. Silver-gray metal will be smeared on the outside of the seam. A welded seam is flat, with a thin, dark, sharply defined line along the joint.

Turning Up the Heat

Foods with a naturally high acid content—such as tomatoes, citrus juices, pears, and other fruits—will not support the growth of food poisoning bacteria. In tests, when large numbers of food poisoning bacteria are added to these foods, the bacteria die within a day. (The exact

amount of time depends upon the bacteria and amount of acidity.) Foods that have a high acid content, therefore, do not receive as extreme a heat treatment as low-acid foods. They are heated sufficiently to destroy bacteria, yeasts and molds that could cause food to spoil.

Canners and food safety regulators are most concerned about foods with low acid content, such as mushrooms, green beans, corn, and meats. The deadly *Clostridium botulinum* bacterium, which causes botulism poisoning, produces a toxin in these foods that is highly heat-resistant. The sterilization process that destroys this bacteria also kills other bacteria that may poison or spoil food.

Low-acid canned foods receive a high dose of heat—usually 107 degrees Celsius (250 degrees Farenheit) for at least three minutes. (The amount of time the food is heated, though, depends upon the size of the container and the product.) The canned food is heated in a retort, a kind of pressure cooker.

The coffee creamer on Gardine's desk, however, was packaged differently. Although both the half-and-half and plastic container were sterilized with heat, they were heated separately and then brought together in a sterile environment where the container was filled and sealed. The advantage of this "aseptic processing," a type of canning, is that higher temperatures with reduced heating times prevent deterioration in the quality of the food.

Aseptic processing is the "wave of the present and the future," says Gardine. It is now used for liquids, and scientists are on the way to perfecting the method for canning stews and chowders. However, says Gardine, because solid foods may be more difficult to keep sterile during the filling and sealing period, FDA is being especially cautious in approving uses for aseptic processing.

Finessing the Attack on Food Spoilers

Another critical element in the canned food process is sealing products in airtight containers. It is essential that air be removed from the container before sealing. Air could cause the can to expand during heating, perhaps damaging the seals or seams of the container.

A telltale sign of loss of this vacuum—and a possibly contaminated product—is a can with bulging ends. (See box.) If a seal is not airtight, bacteria may enter the can, multiply, and contaminate the product.

The hermetic seal finesses the canning

How to Recognize Can Defects

"Never eat food from a tin can with bulging ends" was a maxim many grew up with. Bulging was one of several clues that might indicate contamination of food packaged in metal cans. Guidelines have been adapted for recognizing defects in cans made of plastic and other materials, as well. The guidelines are:

Metal Cans
• an obvious opening underneath the double seam on the top or bottom of the can
• a can with bulging ends
• a fracture in the double seam
• a pinhole or puncture in the body of the can
• an unwelded portion of the side seam
• a leak from anywhere in the can

Plastic Cans
• any opening or non-bonding in the seal
• a break in the plastic
• a fractured lid
• a swollen package

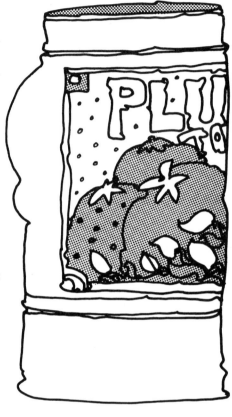

Paperboard Cans
• a patch in the seal where bonding or adhesive is missing
• a slash or slice in the package
• a leak in a corner of the package
• a swollen package

Glass Jars
• a pop-top that does not pop when opened (indicating loss of the vacuum)
• a damaged seal
• a crack in the glass of the jar

Flexible Pouches
• a break in the adhesive across the width of the seal
• a slash or break in the package
• a leak at a manufactured notch used for easy opening
• a swollen package

(Taken from a chart for retailers developed by FDA and NFPA and published by the Association of Official Analytical Chemists.)

—D.B.

process. The bacteria in a food and container are killed through heating, and at the same time new bacteria are kept from contaminating the food.

The distinction between the canning process and food handling before processing is an important one for food processors and regulators. Last February, 22 students at Mississippi State University became ill after eating omelets made with canned mushrooms imported from China. Similar outbreaks followed in New York and Pennsylvania, affecting more than 100 people. FDA identified the culprit as staphylococcal enterotoxin, a poison produced by the bacteria *Staphylococcus aureus.*

FDA's investigation suggests that poor sanitation caused the problem, and that the mushrooms were contaminated with staphylococcal enterotoxin even before they were canned. The canning process did not destroy the substance because food preservation processes are not normally designed to destroy staphylococcal enterotoxin, a highly heat-resistant toxin.

Since this incident, FDA and the Peoples Republic of China have been working together to determine the source of the contamination. However, FDA authorities still are preventing mushrooms canned in China from entering the United States. And, says Gardine, FDA is focusing attention on sanitation procedures in imported foods.

Surpassing Napoleon

The canned food principle that won Nicolas Appert his prize of 12,000 francs has endured over the years. What might surprise Appert, however, is how his discovery is making food shopping and storing easier for the 20th century consumer.

Those who order coffee at fast food restaurants now also are served canned half-and-half, which has been transported and stored without concern about refrigeration. Hikers can take flexible pouches of canned food on backpacking trips without having to worry about saving water to reconstitute freeze-dried meals. And, in this society of microwave owners, Americans who don't have time to prepare a well-balanced meal can pick up a plastic container filled with a canned, nutritious dinner.

The Unwelcome Dinner Guest

Preventing Food-Borne Illness

Annabel Hecht

Annabel Hecht is a a freelance writer who lives in Silver Spring, Md.

"It must be something I ate," is often the explanation people give for a bout of home-grown "Montezuma's Revenge" (acute diarrhea) or some other unwelcome gastrointestinal upset.

Despite the fact that America's food supply is the safest in the world, the unappetizing truth is that what we eat can very well be the vehicle for food-borne illnesses that can cause a variety of unpleasant symptoms and may be life-threatening to the less healthy among us. Tens of millions of cases of food-borne diarrheal disease occur in the United States every year, at a cost to the economy of an estimated $1 billion to $10 billion.

The Food and Drug Administration has given high priority to combating microbial contamination of the food supply. But the agency can't do the job alone. Part of the responsibility for preventing food-borne illness lies with consumers, for 30 percent of all such illness results from unsafe handling of food at home.

The prime causes of food-borne illness are a collection of bacteria with tongue-twisting names: *Campylobacter jejuni, Salmonella, Staphylococcus aureus, Clostridium perfringens, Vibrio vulnificus,* and *Shigella.* The protozoa *Giardia lamblia* and *Entamoeba histolytica* (amoebic protozoa) and hepatitis A virus round out the list.

These organisms can become unwelcome guests at the dinner table. They're in a wide range of foods, including meat, milk and other dairy products, coconut, fresh pasta, spices, chocolate, seafood, and even water.

Egg products, tuna, potato and macaroni salads, and cream-filled pastries harboring these pathogens also are implicated in food-borne illnesses, as are vegetables grown in soil fertilized with contaminated manure.

Poultry is the food most often contaminated with disease-causing organisms. It's been estimated that 60 percent or more of raw poultry sold at retail probably carries some disease-causing bacteria.

Bacteria such as *Listeria monocytogenes, Vibrio vulnificus,* and *Staphylococcus aureus* have been found in raw seafood. Oysters, clams, mussels, scallops, and cockles may be carriers of the hepatitis A virus.

Careless food handling sets the stage for the growth of disease-causing "bugs." For example, hot or cold foods left standing too long at room temperature provide an ideal climate for bacteria to grow. Improper cooking also plays a role in food-borne illness.

Foods may be cross-contaminated when cutting boards and kitchen tools that have been used to prepare a contaminated food, such as raw chicken, are not cleaned before being used for another food such as vegetables.

Symptoms

Common symptoms of food-borne illness include diarrhea, abdominal cramping, fever, sometimes blood or pus in the stools, headache, vomiting, and severe exhaustion. However, symptoms will vary according to the type of bacteria and by the amount of contaminants eaten.

Symptoms may come on as early as a half hour after eating the contaminated food or they may not develop for several days or weeks. They usually last only a day or two, but in some cases can persist a week to 10 days. For most healthy people, food-borne illnesses are neither long-lasting nor life-threatening. However, they can be severe in the very young, the very old, and those who are already ill or whose immune systems are suppressed. (See "Food Safety Crucial for People with Lowered Immunity" in the July-August 1990 *FDA Consumer.*)

When symptoms are severe, the victim should see a doctor or get emergency help. This is especially important for those who are most vulnerable (see accompanying chart). For mild cases of food poisoning, liquid intake should be maintained to replace fluids lost through vomiting and diarrhea.

Unlike most food-borne illnesses, the symptoms of botulism are neurological and can be fatal. Emergency care is essential.

Prevention Tips

The idea that the food on the dinner table can make someone sick may be disturbing, but there are many steps you can take to protect your families and dinner guests. It's just a matter of following basic rules of food safety.

Prevention of food poisoning starts

with your trip to the supermarket. Pick up your packaged and canned foods first. Don't buy food in cans that are bulging or dented or in jars that are cracked or have loose or bulging lids. Look for any expiration dates on the labels and never buy outdated food. Likewise, check the "use by" or "sell by" date on dairy products such as cottage cheese, cream cheese, yogurt, and sour cream and pick the ones that will stay fresh longest in your refrigerator.

If you have a health problem, especially one that may have impaired your immune system, don't eat raw shellfish and use only pasteurized milk and cheese.

Choose eggs that are Grade A or better and that are refrigerated in the store. Before putting them in your cart, open the carton and make sure that none are cracked or leaking.

Save to the last frozen foods and perishables such as meat, poultry or fish. Always put these products in separate plastic bags so that drippings don't contaminate other foods in your shopping cart.

Check for cleanliness at the meat or fish counter and the salad bar. For instance, cooked shrimp lying on the same bed of ice as raw fish could become contaminated.

When shopping for shellfish, buy from markets that get their supplies from state-approved sources; stay clear of vendors who sell shellfish from roadside stands or the back of a truck. And if you're planning to harvest your own shellfish, heed posted warnings about the safety of the water.

Take an ice chest along to keep frozen and perishable foods cold if it will take more than an hour to get your groceries home.

Safe Storage

The first rule of food storage in the home is to refrigerate or freeze perishables right away. Refrigerator temperature should be 40 to 45 degrees Fahrenheit, and the freezer should be zero. Check both "fridge" and freezer periodically with a good thermometer.

Poultry and meat heading for the refrigerator may be stored as purchased in the plastic wrap for a day or two. If only part of the meat or poultry is going to be used right away, it can be wrapped loosely for refrigerator storage. Just make sure juices can't escape to contaminate other foods. Wrap tightly foods destined for the freezer. Leftovers should be stored in tight containers. Store eggs in their carton in the refrigerator itself rather than on the door, where the temperature is warmer.

Seafood should always be kept in the refrigerator or freezer until preparation time.

Don't crowd the refrigerator or freezer so tightly that air can't circulate. Check the leftovers in covered dishes and storage bags daily for spoilage. Anything that looks or smells suspicious should be thrown out.

A sure sign of spoilage is the presence of mold, which can grow even under refrigeration. While not a major health threat, mold can make food unappetizing.

Mold is deceptive in that only a small part is visible. The larger part extends below the surface of the food. However, it is possible to save a part of the food by cutting off and discarding the visible blemish along with a large section of the food around it.

Many items besides fresh meats, vege-

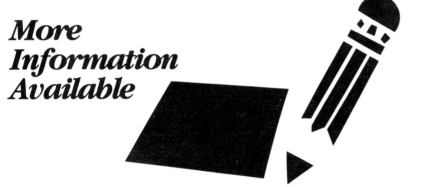

More Information Available

For additional information on food safety, write to:

Food and Drug Administration
• For general information, write to "Food Safety," Consumer Affairs Office (HFE-88), Food and Drug Administration, 5600 Fishers Lane, Rockville, Md. 20857.
• For information on shellfish, write for "For Oysters and Clam Lovers, the Water Must Be Clean," a reprint from *FDA Consumer,* available from FDA's Office of Public Affairs (HFI-40), 5600 Fishers Lane, Rockville, Md. 20857.
• For information on food safety for people with AIDS, write for "Eating Defensively: Food Safety Advice for Persons with AIDS," a brochure and videotape, available from AIDS Information Clearinghouse, P.O. Box 6003, Rockville, Md. 20850. Brochure is free; videotape is $8.95.

Food Marketing Institute
• For a brochure on refrigerator and freezer storage, pantry and dry storage, and foods that need special care, send 50 cents and a legal-sized stamped, self-addressed envelope to: "The Food Keeper," Food Marketing Institute, 1750 K St. N.W., Washington, D.C. 20006.

Orders for 11-49 copies are discounted 15 percent; 50-99 copies, discounted 25 percent; 100-999 copies, discounted 40 percent; and 1,000 copies are discounted 50 percent.

U.S. Department of Agriculture
• For information on the proper handling of meat and poultry, call USDA's Meat and Poultry Hotline at the toll-free number 800-535-4555, between 10 a.m. and 4 p.m. on weekdays. Write to "The Meat and Poultry Hotline," USDA-FSIS, Room 1165-S, Washington, D.C. 20250 for a new booklet, "A Quick Consumers Guide to Safe Food Handling."

tables, and dairy products need to be kept cold. For instance, mayonnaise and ketchup should go in the refrigerator after opening. Some spices keep best when refrigerated. Always check the labels on cans or jars to determine how the contents should be stored. If you've neglected to refrigerate items, it's usually best to throw them out.

For foods that can be stored at room temperature, some precautions will help make sure they remain safe. Potatoes and onions should not be stored under the sink, because leakage from the pipes can damage the food. Potatoes don't belong in the refrigerator either. Store them in a cool, dry place. Don't store foods near household cleaning products and chemicals.

When you're putting canned goods away, move the older ones to the front of the shelf and put the new cans in the back row so you'll be sure to use the older ones first. Check all cans to see if any are sticky on the outside. This may indicate a leak. Newly purchased cans that appear to be leaking should be returned to the store, which should notify FDA.

Keep It Clean

The first cardinal rule of safe food preparation in the home is: Keep everything clean.

The cleanliness rule applies to the areas where food is prepared and, most importantly, to the cook. It's plain common sense to wash hands thoroughly be-

fore starting to prepare a meal and after handling raw meat or poultry. Cover long hair with a net or scarf, and be sure that any open sores or cuts on the hands are completely covered. If the sore or cut is infected, stay out of the kitchen. And if you must smoke, don't do it while you're cooking.

Keep the work area clean and uncluttered. Always use clean utensils and wash them between cutting different foods. Plastic or glass cutting boards are preferable to wooden ones because cuts in the wood can harbor bacteria. As with utensils, clean the board thoroughly after each use.

Wash the lids of canned foods before opening to keep dirt from getting into the food. Also, clean the blade of the can opener after each use. Food processors and meat grinders should be taken apart and cleaned as soon as possible after they are used.

Do not put cooked meat on an unwashed plate or platter that has held raw meat.

Wash fresh fruits and vegetables thoroughly.

Keep Temperature Right

The second cardinal rule of home food preparation is: Keep hot foods hot and cold foods cold.

Use a thermometer to ensure that meats are completely cooked. For instance, beef and lamb should be cooked to at least 60 degrees Celsius (140 degrees Fahrenheit), pork to 66 C (150 F), and poultry to 74 C (165 F). Don't eat poultry that is pink inside.

Eggs should be cooked until the white is firm and the yolk begins to harden.

Seafood should be thoroughly cooked. Fish is done when the thickest part becomes opaque and the fish flakes easily when poked with a fork. Shrimp can be simmered three to five minutes or until the shells turn red. Clams and mussels are steamed over boiling water until the shells open (5 to 10 minutes). Oysters should be sautéed, baked or boiled until plump, about five minutes.

Protect seafood from cross-contamination after cooking, and eat it promptly.

Cooked foods should not be left standing on the table or kitchen counter for more than two hours. Disease-causing bacteria grow in temperatures between 40 and 140 F. Cooked foods that have been in this temperature range for more than two hours should not be eaten.

If a dish is to be served hot, get it from

How Long Will It Keep?

Following is a rundown of storage guidelines for some of the foods that are regulars on America's dinner tables.

Product	Storage Period	
	In Refrigerator	In Freezer
Fresh Meat:		
Beef: Ground	1–2 days	3–4 months
Steaks and roasts	3–5 days	6–12 months
Pork: chops	3–5 days	3–4 months
Ground	1–2 days	1–2 months
Roasts	3–5 days	4–8 months
Cured meats:		
Lunch meat	3–5 days	1–2 months
Sausage	1–2 days	1–2 months
Gravy	1–2 days	3 months
Fish:		
lean (such as cod)	1–2 days	up to 6 months
fatty (such as blue, perch, salmon)	1–2 days	2–3 months
Chicken: whole	1–2 days	12 months
parts	1–2 days	9 months
giblets	1–2 days	3–4 months
Dairy Products:		
Swiss, brick, processed cheese	3–4 weeks	*
Milk	5 days	1 month
Eggs: fresh in shell	3–5 weeks	–
hard-boiled	1 week	–

* Cheese can be frozen, but freezing will affect the texture and taste.

(Sources: Food Marketing Institute for fish and dairy products, USDA for all other foods.)

Food Safety 'Musts'

- Get perishable foods into the refrigerator as quickly as possible after buying them.
- Wash raw vegetables thoroughly.
- Keep your kitchen or food preparation areas clean.
- Wash your hands before preparing food.
- Keep hot foods hot and cold foods cold after they are prepared.

the stove to the table as quickly as possible. Reheated foods should be brought to a temperature of at least 165 F. Keep cold foods in the refrigerator or on a bed of ice until serving. This rule is particularly important to remember in the summer months.

After the meal, leftovers should be refrigerated as soon as possible. (Never mind that scintillating dinner table conversation!) Meats should be cut in slices of three inches or less and all foods should be stored in small, shallow containers to hasten cooling. Be sure to remove all the stuffing from roast turkey or chicken and store it separately. Giblets should also be stored separately. Leftovers should be used within three days.

And here are just a few more parting tips to keep your favorite dishes safe. Don't thaw meat and other frozen foods at room temperature. Instead, move them from the freezer to the refrigerator for a day or two; or defrost in cold water (changing the water every 30 minutes), in the microwave oven, or during the cooking process. Never taste any food that looks or smells "off," or comes out of leaking, bulging or severely damaged cans or jars with leaky lids.

Though all these do's and don'ts may seem overwhelming, remember, if you want to stay healthy, when it comes to food safety, the old saying "rules are made to be broken" does not apply!

(Please see following chart for more food safety information.)

Organisms That Can Bug You

Disease and Organism That Causes It	Source of Illness	Symptoms
Bacteria		
Botulism Botulinum toxin (produced by *Clostridium botulinum* bacteria)	Spores of these bacteria are widespread. But these bacteria produce toxin only in an anerobic (oxygenless) environment of little acidity. Found in a considerable variety of canned foods, such as corn, green beans, soups, beets, asparagus, mushrooms, tuna, and liver paté. Also in luncheon meats, ham, sausage, stuffed eggplant, lobster, and smoked and salted fish.	Onset: Generally 4–36 hours after eating. Neurotoxic symptoms, including double vision, inability to swallow, speech difficulty, and progressive paralysis of the respiratory system. **Get Medical Help Immediately. Botulism Can Be Fatal.**
Campylobacteriosis *Campylobacter jejuni*	Bacteria on poultry, cattle, and sheep can contaminate meat and milk of these	Onset: Generally 2–5 days after eating. Diarrhea, abdom-

Disease and Organism That Causes It	Source of Illness	Symptoms
	animals. Chief food sources: raw poultry, meat, and unpasteurized milk.	inal cramping, fever, and sometimes bloody stools. Lasts 7–10 days.
Listeriosis *Listeria monocytogenes*	Found in soft cheese, unpasteurized milk, imported seafood products, frozen cooked crab meat, cooked shrimp, and cooked surimi (imitation shellfish). The *Listeria* bacteria resist heat, salt, nitrite, and acidity better than many other microorganisms. They survive and grow at low temperatures.	Onset: From 7–30 days after eating, but most symptoms have been reported 48–72 hours after consumption of contaminated food. Fever, headache, nausea, and vomiting. Primarily affects pregnant women and their fetuses, newborns, the elderly, people with cancer, and those with impaired immune systems. Can cause fetal and infant death.
Perfringens food poisoning *Clostridium perfringens*	In most instances, caused by failure to keep food hot. A few organisms are often present after cooking and multiply to toxic levels during cool down and storage of prepared foods. Meats and meat products are the foods most frequently implicated. These organisms grow better than other bacteria between 120–130 F. So gravies and stuffing must be kept above 140 F.	Onset: Generally 8–12 hours after eating. Adominal pain and diarrhea, and sometimes nausea and vomiting. Symptoms last a day or less and are usually mild. Can be more serious in older or debilitated people.
Salmonellosis	Raw meats, poultry, milk and other dairy	Onset: Generally 6–48 hours after

(Continued on next page)

Organisms That Can Bug You *(Continued)*

Disease and Organism That Causes It	Source of Illness	Symptoms
Salmonella bacteria	products, shrimp, frog legs, yeast, coconut, pasta, and chocolate are most frequently involved.	eating. Nausea, abdominal cramps, diarrhea, fever, and headache. All age groups are susceptible, but symptoms are most severe for elderly, infants and infirm.
Shigellosis (bacillary dysentery) *Shigella* bacteria	Found in milk and dairy products, poultry, and potato salad. Food becomes contaminated when a human carrier does not wash hands and then handles liquid or moist food that is not cooked thoroughly afterwards. Organisms multiply in food left at room temperature.	Onset: 1–7 days after eating. Abdominal cramps, diarrhea, fever, sometimes vomiting, and blood, pus or mucus in stools.
Staphylococcal food poisoning Staphylococcal enterotoxin (produced by *Staphylococcus aureus* bacteria)	Toxin produced when food contaminated with the bacteria is left too long at room temperature. Meats, poultry, egg products, tuna, potato and macaroni salads, and cream-filled pastries are good environments for these bacteria to produce toxin.	Onset: Generally 30 minutes–8 hours after eating. Diarrhea, vomiting, nausea, abdominal pain, cramps, and prostration. Lasts 24–48 hours. Rarely fatal.
Vibrio infection *Vibrio vulnificus*	The bacteria live in coastal waters and can infect humans either through open wounds or through consumption of contaminated seafood. The bacteria	Onset: Abrupt. Chills, fever, and/or prostration. At high risk are people with liver conditions, low gastric

Disease and Organism That Causes It	Source of Illness	Symptoms
	are most numerous in warm weather.	(stomach) acid, and weakened immune systems.
Protozoa		
Amebiasis *Entamoeba histolytica*	Exist in the intestinal tract of humans and are expelled in feces. Polluted water and vegetables grown in polluted soil spread the infection.	Onset: 3–10 days after exposure. Severe crampy pain, tenderness over the colon or liver, loose morning stools, recurrent diarrhea, loss of weight, fatigue, and sometimes anemia.
Giardiasis *Giardia lamblia*	Most frequently associated with consumption of contaminated water. May be transmitted by uncooked foods that become contaminated while growing or after cooking by infected food handlers. Cool, moist conditions favor organism's survival.	Onset: 1–3 days. Sudden onset of explosive watery stools, abdominal cramps, anorexia, nausea, and vomiting. Especially infects hikers, children, travelers, and institutionalized patients.
Virus		
Hepatitis A virus	Mollusks (oysters, clams, mussels, scallops, and cockles) become carriers when their beds are polluted by untreated sewage. Raw shellfish are especially potent carriers, although cooking does not always kill the virus.	Onset: begins with malaise, appetite loss, nausea, vomiting, and fever. After 3–10 days patient develops jaundice with darkened urine. Severe cases can cause liver damage and death.

Burgers: never say "rare"

Should the rare hamburger become a thing of the past? Unfortunately, yes. The burger that's pink inside should probably be banned, especially for small children, the elderly, and those likely to be most seriously affected by food poisoning because of an impaired immune system. It's possible that new methods of meat inspection, under study by the Department of Agriculture, will make pink burgers safer. But for the foreseeable future, better say "well done."

Last winter in Washington state—in one of the worst food-poisoning outbreaks ever to occur in the U.S.—contaminated hamburgers made 450 people sick and were fatal to at least one toddler. (Two other small children died, but it's not certain that the tainted hamburgers were responsible.) The contaminant was a rare strain of E. coli, a very common bacterium that normally inhabits the intestines and feces of humans and other animals without harm to the host. If these fecal bacteria contaminate food and are eaten, however, diarrhea may result. This strain, designated E. coli 0157:H7, can cause bloody diarrhea and abdominal cramps, as well as the more serious hemolytic uremic syndrome (HUS), which affects the kidneys and the blood clotting system. There's no cure for the disease, which has to run its course; hospitalization is usually necessary. Most people can expect to recover completely, though HUS is sometimes fatal, especially for kids.

A problem irradiation can't fix

How can future outbreaks be prevented? An overhaul of our meat inspection system may soon be underway. The contaminated hamburger was improperly handled at the slaughterhouse, as well as being insufficiently cooked at the restaurant. Irradiation is also being promoted as a means to rid meats and other foods of bacteria. But the levels of irradiation approved by the government for meats (only poultry and pork have been approved, though as yet neither is being irradiated) are too low to kill all bacteria. Some bacteria would survive and could multiply. Even with improved handling and inspection methods, and even with irradiation, meat (especially ground meats) would still have to be well cooked. That's the only sure way to kill E. coli and other dangerous bacteria.

Heat above 155° Fahrenheit kills E. coli. Jack-in-the-Box, the restaurant that served the tainted burgers, cooked them only to 140°. The federal government, as well as many states, now recommends that all ground meats be cooked to 155°, well past the pink stage. Ground meats are most dangerous because grinding equipment may be a source of contaminants and because ground meat offers microorganisms more surfaces on which to multiply. Steaks, roasts, and other whole cuts pose much less risk.

Six tips

■ Cook ground meat until well-done: the center should look gray or brown, and the juices should run clear, not pink or red. In restaurants, check small children's portions before they eat.

■ Don't depend on the sniff test. Meat contaminated with E. coli does not smell bad.

■ At home, keep utensils and working surfaces clean. Wash them and your hands thoroughly with soap and warm water after you've handled raw meat.

■ Thaw frozen ground meats in the refrigerator, and cook them right away. Don't let them sit outside the refrigerator.

■ Don't drink raw milk or eat raw-milk products. Unpasteurized milk can be a source of E. coli.

■ Don't eat steak tartare or other raw-meat dishes.

Reprinted by permission from *University of California at Berkeley Wellness Letter,* June 1993, pp. 1-2. Copyright © 1993 by the Health Letter Associates.

SALMONELLA ENTERITIDIS

From the Chicken to the Egg

Dale Blumenthal

Dale Blumenthal is a staff writer for FDA Consumer.

White, shining, unmarred—a Grade A mystery now lies in the uncracked egg. Is it safe to eat?—9,999 times out of 10,000, yes. But . . .

• In May 1989, six nursing home patients in Pennsylvania died from *Salmonella enteritidis* poisoning after eating stuffing that contained undercooked eggs.

• In July, 21 guests at a baby shower in New York became ill after eating a pasta dish made with a raw egg. One victim was 38 weeks pregnant and delivered her baby while ill. The newborn infant developed *Salmonella enteritidis* blood poisoning and required lengthy hospitalization.

• Last August, a healthy 40-year-old man died, and 14 others were hospitalized, after eating egg-based custard pie contaminated with *Salmonella enteritidis,* which was served at a company party in Pennsylvania. The list goes on.

Public health officials are concerned. More than 49 outbreaks of *Salmonella enteritidis* poisoning took place in nine states and Puerto Rico last year, resulting in at least 13 deaths and more than 1,628 illnesses. According to the Jan. 5, 1990, issue of the Centers for Disease Control's *Morbidity and Mortality Weekly Report,* from January 1985 through October 1989, 189 *Salmonella enteritidis* outbreaks in the United States caused 6,604 illnesses and 43 deaths. Many more illnesses probably went unreported, says Joseph Madden, Ph.D., deputy director of FDA's division of microbiology.

Health investigators suspect that contaminated shell eggs caused nearly half of these outbreaks. The egg connection in these cases was determined by tracing the food eaten by the victims and taking cultures both from patients and foods.

Especially at risk for *Salmonella* poisoning are the elderly, the very young,

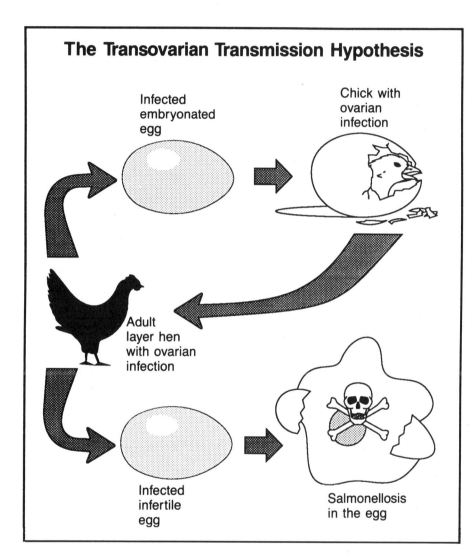

The Transovarian Transmission Hypothesis

Infected embryonated egg

Chick with ovarian infection

Adult layer hen with ovarian infection

Infected infertile egg

Salmonellosis in the egg

pregnant women (because of risk to the fetus), and people already debilitated by serious illness, malnutrition, or weakened immune systems. Symptoms of *Salmonella enteritidis* infection usually include diarrhea, vomiting, abdominal pain, chills, fever, and headache. The bacteria can invade organs outside the gastrointestinal tract, causing complications that require lengthy hospitalization, even in healthy people.

Symptoms usually develop 12 to 36 hours after eating the contaminated food. The initial illness also can bring about serious chronic complications.

In 1985, in an incident in Chicago, more than 16,000 people contracted food poisoning from low-fat milk contaminated with *Salmonella* bacteria. Within two weeks, about 2 percent of these patients developed a chronic reactive arthritis condition linked to the infection. Although the *Salmonella* bacteria that made these people ill was not *Salmonella enteritidis,* researchers have found that rats infected with *Salmonella enteritidis* may develop the same arthritic condition. Researchers are concerned that *Salmonella enteritidis* may also cause this complication in humans.

Reprinted from *FDA Consumer,* April 1990, pp. 7-10, by permission.

5. FOOD SAFETY

Since 1976, says Robert Tauxe, M.D., a CDC expert on the spread of the disease, the reported rate for *Salmonella enteritidis* infections from food "has increased more than sixfold in the northeastern part of the United States." First noted in the New England states, the infections also appeared in the mid-Atlantic region by 1983, and now have become a problem in the south Atlantic states as well. Recently, outbreaks were reported in Minnesota, Ohio and Nevada.

The problem also has become an international egg to crack. "The U.S. *Salmonella* epidemic," says Tauxe, "is dwarfed by dramatic increases that have been reported from Yugoslavia, Finland, Sweden, Norway, and the United Kingdom." In Britain alone, the number of confirmed *Salmonella enteritidis* cases reported for January through July 1988 (4,424 cases) was more than double the number (2,000) for the same period in 1987.

Source: Intact Eggs

At first, says Tauxe, "we did not have an explanation for this striking increase." The first real clue that intact eggs were a source of the problem came in 1983, when CDC traced a large outbreak caused by *Salmonella enteritidis* to a commercial stuffed pasta product made with raw eggs.

Investigators then reviewed reports of past outbreaks and determined that at least since 1973, *Salmonella enteritidis* outbreaks appeared to be caused by the bacteria in clean, uncracked, Grade A eggs.

"In the 1960s," Tauxe says, "salmonellosis [the disease caused by the *Salmonella* bacteria] associated with chicken eggs was epidemic in the United States. At that time it was determined that eggs were being contaminated by *Salmonella* in chicken feces on the *outside* of the egg shell, which penetrated into the eggs through cracks in the shell." That led to strict rules, established and enforced by the U.S. Department of Agriculture, for washing and sanitizing shells of commercial eggs.

But this new epidemic is associated with *Salmonella enteritidis* in inspected, uncracked and sanitized Grade A eggs. "The infected egg may appear normal," says Tauxe. The contamination comes from the *inside,* not the outside, of the egg.

How Does Contamination Occur?

No one knows how some intact eggs become contaminated with *Salmonella enteritidis.* Poultry researchers, how-

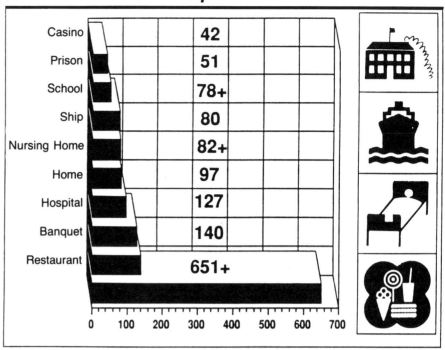

Where People Got Infected

Location	Cases
Casino	42
Prison	51
School	78+
Ship	80
Nursing Home	82+
Home	97
Hospital	127
Banquet	140
Restaurant	651+

ever, suggest that the egg yolk becomes infected before the shell forms.

In fact, Charles Benson, Ph.D., of the University of Pennsylvania, says that in his experiments the bacteria were found not in the white, as when organisms penetrate the egg shell, but only in the yolk. This occurred even though Benson added iron to the white to encourage the bacteria to grow in the albumen, which has antibacterial properties.

Madden believes that in the past 10 years a new strain of *Salmonella enteritidis* that can live in chickens may have evolved. Other researchers are finding that *Salmonella enteritidis* bacteria migrate from the yolk to the white of the egg, where they can survive up to 12 hours. However, it is in the yolk where the bacteria multiply and thrive.

These and other findings, such as ovarian infections in egg-laying chickens, have led to the concept of "transovarian transmission." According to this theory, the infection occurs first in the chicken and is transferred to the egg before the shell is formed.

Researchers also speculate that the infection may be passed from bird to bird in the same flock. For instance, Madden notes that several birds might pick up *Salmonella enteritidis* from the droppings of rodents and sparrows (known carriers of the organism) and spread it among the others. There are also reported cases, Madden adds, of workers picking up the bacteria on their clothing and transmitting *Salmonella* from one chicken house to another.

Only after scientists understand how *Salmonella* is transmitted will they know how to control it. Right now the proposed solution is a long-range plan to prevent spread of the disease by testing flocks and replacing infected ones.

The Voluntary Model State Program

The Northeastern Conference on Avian Diseases in 1987 proposed a voluntary model state program, which FDA and USDA then modified. The program calls for state agriculture, veterinary and health officials to work together to test the poultry flocks in their states for *Salmonella enteritidis.*

Under the voluntary plan, eggs from infected flocks are to be pasteurized (broken and heat processed) to destroy the bacteria. There is no evidence that *Salmonella enteritidis* survives pasteurization. Pasteurized eggs are used in many commercial food products, such as baked goods.

Making Testing Mandatory

The effectiveness of the voluntary program depends upon producers' willingness to test and, if necessary, replace infected flocks. However, according to Madden, the increase and spread of the problem suggest that producers and states are not following the program.

USDA responded to the increasing concern over the *Salmonella enteritidis* problem by passing an interim rule on

Feb. 16. The regulation, which allows for a 60-day comment period but went into effect immediately, makes testing of primary and multiplier flocks mandatory. Much of the work will be done through NPIP.

Backing of Law

FDA also has the backing of law to attack the *Salmonella enteritidis* problem. The Public Health Service Act authorizes FDA to take steps to "prevent the introduction, transmission, or spread of communicable diseases." Under this provision, the agency can issue regulations requiring flock testing and certification before the eggs can be shipped in interstate commerce.

Another law supports the mandatory program. Under the Food, Drug, and Cosmetic Act, the agency can seize products of a diseased animal. If an egg producer does not want the eggs destroyed, FDA can request a court order requiring that the eggs be pasteurized.

67 Billion Eggs

Despite the hard times egg producers are facing, eggs continue to be an inexpensive and important source of protein. According to UEP, the average American eats 250 eggs a year. A survey from the market research group Technical Assessment Systems finds that 90 percent of the population eat eggs in some form each day. (This includes eggs contained in foods like baked items and egg noodles.)

Nearly 5 percent of Americans surveyed said they either ate raw eggs daily or could not specify whether the egg consumed was raw or cooked. Raw and lightly cooked contaminated eggs are causing the illness. Thorough cooking kills the bacteria.

According to Madden, a person can become ill after eating only a small amount of a contaminated egg. For instance, he says, one New York incident involved a family who cooked three eggs sunny side up. The yolk of one egg broke onto the other eggs during cooking, and all three family members became ill.

Madden explains that one broken egg was probably responsible for all three illnesses, as it is extremely unlikely that more than one egg per container would be contaminated. In fact, only 1 in 200 eggs from an infected flock may be contaminated. The risk is even lower for all eggs—only 1 in 10,000 eggs on the supermarket shelves are likely to be contaminated with *Salmonella enteritidis*.

Salmonella enteritidis grows quickly,

Safety Tips

Egg Cooking

The elderly, patients already weakened by serious illness, and people with weakened immune systems (such as persons with AIDS) are at high risk for death or serious illness from *Salmonella enteritidis*. Nursing home, hospital, and other food institutions serving those in high-risk groups should *strictly* follow these safe egg guidelines, which also apply to all home preparation.

You can't tell a good egg from a bad egg by the way it smells, tastes or looks. But, these precautions can help minimize risks:

• Review recipes and consider using pasteurized eggs instead of shell eggs whenever possible.

• Avoid serving raw eggs and foods containing raw eggs. Caesar salad, Hollandaise sauce, homemade ice cream, homemade eggnog, and homemade mayonnaise are possible carriers of *Salmonella enteritidis*.

• Lightly cooked foods containing eggs, such as soft custards and French toast, may be risky for those in high-risk groups.

• Cook eggs thoroughly until both the yolk and white are firm, not runny. These cooking times are now recommended by researchers at Cornell University:

Scrambled—1 minute at 250 degrees Fahrenheit

Poached—5 minutes in boiling water

Sunnyside—7 minutes at 250 F or cook covered 4 minutes at 250 F

Fried, over easy—3 minutes at 250 F for one side, then turn the egg and fry for another minute on the other side

Boiled—7 minutes in boiling water.

Handling Practices

• Wash hands with hot, soapy water, and wash and sanitize utensils, equipment (such as blenders), and work areas before and after they come in contact with eggs and uncooked egg-rich foods.

• Use only Grade A or better eggs. Avoid eggs that are cracked or leaking.

• Discard the egg if any shell falls into the egg.

• Leave eggs in their original carton, and store them in the main section of the refrigerator—not the egg section in the door, as the temperature in the door is higher.

• Never leave eggs or egg-containing foods at room temperature for more than two hours, including preparation and serving (but not cooking) times.

• When refrigerating a large amount of a hot egg-rich dish or leftover, divide it into several small shallow containers so it will cool quickly.

• Cook scrambled eggs in batches no larger than three quarts. Hold for serving at 140 F or hotter, such as on a steam table. Do not add a batch of just-cooked scrambled eggs to leftover eggs held on a steam table. —D.B.

---

presenting another danger for spread of the disease when a contaminated egg is mixed with clean eggs, such as when eggs are pooled to make scrambled eggs for a group of people. One organism can multiply into millions in an egg stored at 60 degrees for two days. Eggs should always be stored in the refrigerator and only taken out just before use.

Scientists around the country are trying to find out what refrigeration temperatures are most effective for stopping the growth of *Salmonella enteritidis* in eggs. They are also investigating the cooking times and

temperatures required to destroy the bacteria.

FDA and USDA officials are conducting a public health campaign to spread information on what they know so far about safe cooking and handling of eggs. Over 50,000 bulletins have been distributed to consumers, food service establishments, and institutions that take care of people particularly vulnerable to *Salmonella enteritidis* infections. For copies of the materials, contact USDA, Agricultural Marketing Service/Information Staff, P.O. Box 96456, Washington, D.C. 20090-6456.

Health Claims

Quackery has no such friend as credulity.

—C. Simmons

In ancient Rome, Cato the Elder prescribed cabbages to cure "everything that ails you" and continued to do so even though his wife died from the fevers. London pharmacists in 1632 believed that bananas were so important to health that only trained druggists should administer them. Early in the history of this country, Elisha Perkins claimed vinegar was the cure for yellow fever; yet he died of this disease. Twenty years ago, Adelle Davis was the high priestess of nutrition, promising that you would not age if you ate right. All were sincere but wrong. Yet almost any product, device, or regimen that promises the moon and five miles more will have an attentive audience and many purchasers.

The Food and Drug Administration identifies quackery as misinformation about health. Promoters of fallacies are fond of making such statements as "The American food supply is worthless because it is grown on depleted soil," "Everybody needs vitamin supplements," and "Natural sugar in honey is better than table sugar." Such misinformation may be easier to find than facts. For example, popular talk shows provide a good promotional forum for misinformation, since their need to capture a large audience is met by sensationalism. In despair, nutritionists have said that most nutrition information appearing in the popular press, paperback books, and talk shows is at the least an exaggeration and often blatantly false.

But, you say, anyone interested enough to read this book, much less take a nutrition course, is also alert and smart enough to avoid being taken in by quackery. Right? Wrong! At one time or another, most of us have been victims. Perpetrators of quackery have changed with the times, but their characteristics are the same. For this reason, it is critical to understand how they manipulate the buyer. Only then will consumers be armed to defend themselves. Toward that end several articles in this unit were chosen.

"How Quackery Sells" will help you to understand the strategies of promoters who have fine-tuned the art of selling to an exquisitely high level. They know how to manipulate the emotions of the vulnerable, easily influenced customer so that he or she chooses to buy even though some small voice advises against it. Some promoters operate in multilevel marketing schemes, the topic of "The Multilevel Mirage." This type of selling has become so commonplace that it is easily accepted as an unquestioned part of today's marketing infrastructure. Everybody knows a distributor for something. Unfortunately, many such companies promote worthless or harmful products.

Headlines and feature stories in newspapers, television, and periodicals often reflect good news/bad news on the latest dietary findings. Sometimes they contradict each other. What should you believe? When should you believe? "Food News Blues" contains an exercise to assist in viewing nutrition news items critically. "You've got to take everything with a grain of salt until the last word comes in. I hate to tell people I don't believe everything I read, but the fact is anybody who believes everything they read is nuts," says a newspaper editor quoted in this article.

Whom to believe is another trap for the unwary. Of the 22 million Americans who take aerobic dance classes, many apparently rely on their instructors for nutrition advice, yet these instructors have been shown to know little if any more than their students. Other people turn to health food stores and promoters, an equally unsound solution. Then, too, the unsuspecting purchaser may be misled by bogus credentials. I once received a letter requesting a weight reduction diet because the writer "was tired of teaching and wanted to be a nutrition consultant." In actuality the term "nutritionist" means nothing, since its use is not regulated in any way. To have significance it must be supported by appropriate and bona fide credentials from accredited institutions. A number of unaccredited schools provide nutrition certifications and degrees, even doctorates, upon the receipt of a healthy fee and the completion of a few courses, workbooks, or open book exams covering highly questionable material (see article 56).

Unfortunately, we must also be alert in places we might never suspect. Consumers sometimes assume that health care personnel have nutrition knowledge and training that they do not have or that they will apply the good but limited knowledge they have. Article 55 shows that this may be an unwarranted assumption. This article describes the promotion of nutritional supplements by chiropractors. According to a spokesperson for one of the 50 companies that market their products through chiropractors, about 65 percent regularly dispense supplements to patients. And, in a survey of San Francisco Bay area chiropractors, a significant percentage were found to use hair analysis for nutritional assessment, a method which has been proven to be invalid.

While it is impossible in this volume to address all of the misinformation commonly subscribed to, article 57 contains a good summary of fads in weight loss diets, dietary misinformation about diseases, mythology regarding herbals, and a brief section on food faddism in pediatrics. The reader should check the topic guide for articles in other units that also will be helpful, such as article 20 in unit 2 on vitamin C and colds.

Two additional articles address topics that continue to be relevant. Diet pill ingredients as addressed in "FDA Bans Diet Pill Ingredients After Nearly 20 Years," have been a concern of nutritionists and the FDA for many years. Now the FDA has banned 111 commonly used ingredients. Finally, in the last unit article, there is a discussion of athletes and supplements. It is not hard to understand why athletes are always looking for the competitive edge, but the place to look is within themselves, not in a bottle or box.

Victor Herbert has said that consumers with misinformation about nutrition typically fall into two categories: the deceived and the deluded. The deceived, he says, will respond to education, while the deluded are adamant—even fanatical—about their beliefs and will refuse to consider good scientific data or a logical presentation. This unit is offered to readers who are either already informed or are among the deceived searching for answers.

Looking Ahead: Challenge Questions

Why do you think people are so vulnerable to quackery?

Identify three fallacies that you believe are the most dangerous to nutritional health.

Watch a television talk show when a guest discusses some aspect of nutrition, or find nutrition articles in your local newspaper. How accurate are they?

List three statements you commonly make about food or eating. To what extent are they true?

Make a list of characteristics you would look for in a *reliable* information source.

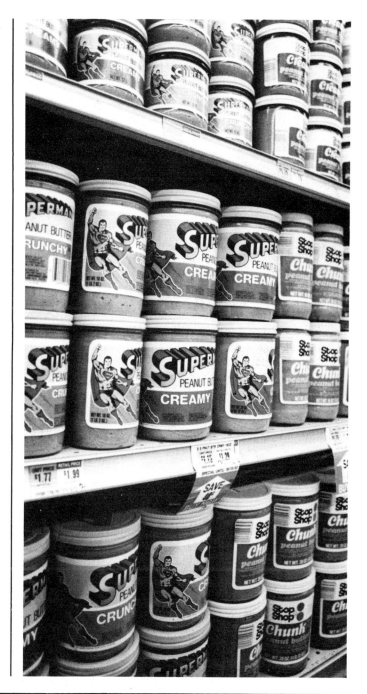

HOW QUACKERY SELLS

William T. Jarvis, Ph.D.
Stephen Barrett, M.D.

Dr. Jarvis is a professor in the Department of Preventive Medicine at Loma Linda University and president of the National Council Against Health Fraud.

Dr. Barrett, who practices psychiatry in Allentown, Pennsylvania, is a board member of the National Council Against Health Fraud. In 1984 he received the FDA Commissioner's Special Citation Award for Public Service in fighting nutrition quackery.

Modern health quacks are supersalesmen. They play on fear. They cater to hope. And once they have you, they'll keep you coming back for more . . . and more . . . and more. Seldom do their victims realize how often or how skillfully they are cheated. Does the mother who feels good as she hands her child a vitamin think to ask herself whether he really needs it? Do subscribers to "health food" publications realize that articles are slanted to stimulate business for their advertisers? Not usually.

Most people think that quackery is easy to spot, but it is not. Its promoters wear the cloak of science. They use scientific terms and quote (or misquote) scientific references. On talk shows, they may be introduced as "scientists ahead of their time." The very word "quack" helps their camouflage by making us think of an outlandish character selling snake oil from the back of a covered wagon—and, of course, no intelligent people would buy snake oil nowadays, would they?

Well, maybe snake oil isn't selling so well, lately. But acupuncture? "Organic" foods? Mouthwash? Hair analysis? The latest diet book? Megavitamins? "Stress" formulas? Cholesterol-lowering teas? Homeopathic remedies? Nutritional "cures" for AIDS? Or shots to pep you up? Business is booming for health quacks. Their annual take is in the *billions!* Spot reducers, "immune boosters," water purifiers, "ergogenic aids," systems to "balance body chemistry," special diets for arthritis. Their product list is endless.

What sells is not the quality of their products but their ability to influence their audience. To those in pain, they promise relief. To the incurable, they offer hope. To the nutrition-conscious, they say, "Make sure you have enough." To a public worried about pollution, they say, "Buy natural." To one and all, they promise better health and a longer life. Modern quacks can reach people emotionally, on the level that counts the most. This article shows how they do it.

Appeals to Vanity

An attractive young airline stewardess once told a physician that she was taking more than 20 vitamin pills a day. "I used to feel run-down all the time," she said, "but now I feel really great!"

"Yes," the doctor replied, "but there is no scientific evidence that extra vitamins can do that. Why not take the pills one month on, one month off, to see whether they really help you or whether it's just a coincidence. After all, $300 a year is a lot of money to be wasting."

"Look, doctor," she said. "I don't care what you say. I KNOW the pills are helping me."

How was this bright young woman converted into a true believer? First, an appeal to her curiosity persuaded her to try and see. Then an appeal to her vanity convinced her to disregard scientific evidence in favor of personal experience—to *think for herself.* Supplementation is encouraged by a distorted concept of *biochemical individuality*—that everyone is unique enough to disregard the Recommended Dietary Allowances (RDAs). Quacks will not tell you that scientists deliberately set the RDAs high enough to allow for individual differences. A more dangerous appeal of this type is the suggestion that although a remedy for a serious disease has not been shown to work for other people, *it still might work for you. (You are extraordinary!)*

A more subtle appeal to your vanity underlies the message of the TV ad quack: *Do it yourself—be your own doctor.* "Anyone out there have 'tired blood'?" he used to wonder. (Don't bother to find out what's wrong with you, however. Just try my tonic.) "Troubled with irregularity?" he asks. (Pay no attention to the doctors who say you don't need a daily movement. Just use my laxative.) "Want to kill germs on contact?" (Never mind that mouthwash doesn't prevent colds.) "Trouble sleeping?" (Don't bother to solve the underlying problem. Just try my sedative.)

Turning Customers Into Salespeople

Most people who think they have been helped by an unorthodox method enjoy sharing their success stories with their

From *Nutrition Forum,* Vol. 8, No. 2, March/April 1991, pp, 9-13. Reprinted with permission from *Nutrition Forum Newsletter,* now published by Stephen Barrett, M.D., P. O. Box 1747, Allentown, PA 18105.

friends. People who give such *testimonials* are usually motivated by a sincere wish to *help their fellow humans.* Rarely do they realize how difficult it is to evaluate a "health" product on the basis of personal experience. Like the airline stewardess, the average person who feels better after taking a product will not be able to rule out coincidence— or the placebo effect (feeling better because he thinks he has taken a positive step). Since we tend to believe what others tell us of personal experiences, testimonials can be powerful persuaders. Despite their unreliability, they are the cornerstone of the quack's success.

Multilevel companies that sell nutritional products systematically turn their customers into salespeople. "When you share our products," says the sales manual of one such company, "you're not just selling. You're passing on news about products you believe in to people you care about. Make a list of people you know; you'll be surprised how long it will be. This list is your first source of potential customers." A sales leader from another company suggests, "Answer all objections with *testimonials.* That's the secret to *motivating* people!"

Don't be surprised if one of your friends or neighbors tries to sell you vitamins. More than a million Americans have signed up as multilevel distributors. Like many drug addicts, they become suppliers to support their habit. A typical sales pitch goes like this: "How would you like to look better, feel better and have more energy? Try my vitamins for a few weeks." People normally have ups and downs, and a friend's interest or suggestion, or the thought of taking a positive step, may actually make a person feel better. Many who try the vitamins will mistakenly think they have been helped—and continue to buy them, usually at inflated prices.

Faked endorsements are being used to promote anti-aging products and other nostrums sold by mail. The literature, which resembles a newspaper page with an ad on one side and news on the other, contains what appears to be a handwritten note from a friend (identified by first initial). "Dear Anne," it might say, "This really works. Try it! B." Although both the product and the "newspaper page" are fakes, many recipients wonder who among their acquaintances might have signed the note.

The Use of Fear

The sale of vitamins has become so profitable that some otherwise reputable manufacturers are promoting them with misleading claims. For example, for many years, Lederle Laboratories (makers of *Stresstabs*) and Hoffmann-La Roche advertised in major magazines that stress "robs" the body of vitamins and creates significant danger of vitamin deficiencies. Another slick way for quackery to attract customers is the *invented disease.* Virtually everyone has symptoms of one sort or another—minor aches or pains, reactions to stress or hormone variations, effects of aging, etc. Labeling these ups and downs of life as symptoms of disease enables the quack to provide "treatment."

Reactive hypoglycemia" is one such diagnosis. For decades, talk show "experts" and misguided physicians have preached that anxiety, headaches, weakness, dizziness, stomach upset, and other common reactions are often caused by "low blood sugar." But the facts are otherwise. Hypoglycemia is rare. Proper administration of blood sugar tests is required to make the

diagnosis. A study of people who thought they had hypoglycemia showed that half of them had symptoms during a glucose tolerance test even though their blood sugar levels remained normal.

"Yeast allergy" is another favorite quack diagnosis. Here the symptoms are blamed on a "hidden" infection that is treated with antifungal drugs, special diets, and vitamin concoctions.

Food safety and environmental protection are important issues in our society. But rather than approach them logically, the food quacks exaggerate and oversimplify. To promote "organic" foods, they lump all additives into one class and attack them as "poisonous." They never mention that natural toxicants are prevented or destroyed by modern food technology. Nor do they let on that many additives are naturally occurring substances.

Sugar has been subject to particularly vicious attacks, being (falsely) blamed for most of the world's ailments. But quacks do more than warn about imaginary ailments. They sell "antidotes" for real ones. Care for some vitamin C to reduce the danger of smoking? Or some vitamin E to combat air pollutants? See your local supersalesman.

Quackery's most serious form of fear-mongering has been its attack on water fluoridation. Although fluoridation's safety is established beyond scientific doubt, well-planned scare campaigns have persuaded thousands of communities not to adjust the fluoride content of their water to prevent cavities. Millions of innocent children have suffered as a result.

Hope for Sale

Since ancient times, people have sought at least four different magic potions: the love potion, the fountain of youth, the cure-all, and the athletic superpill. Quackery always has been willing to cater to these desires. It used to offer unicorn horn, special elixirs, amulets, and magical brews. Today's products are vitamins, bee pollen, ginseng, *Gerovital,* "glandular extracts," and many more. Even reputable products are promoted as though they are potions. Toothpastes and colognes will improve our love life. Hair preparations and skin products will make us look "younger than our years." And Olympic athletes tell us that breakfast cereals will make us champions.

False hope for the seriously ill is the cruelest form of quackery because it can lure victims away from effective treatment. Even when death is inevitable, however, false hope can do great damage. Experts who study the dying process tell us that while the initial reaction is shock and disbelief, most terminally ill patients will adjust very well as long as they do not feel abandoned. People who accept the reality of their fate not only die psychologically prepared, but also can put their affairs in order. On the other hand, those who buy false hope can get stuck in an attitude of denial. They waste financial resources and, worse yet, their remaining time.

The choice offered by the quack is not between hope and despair but between false hope and a chance to adjust to reality. Yet hope springs eternal. The late Jerry Walsh was a severe arthritic who crusaded coast-to-coast debunking arthritis quackery on behalf of the Arthritis Foundation. After a television appearance early in his career, he received 5,700 letters. One hundred congratulated him for blasting the quacks, but 4,500 were from arthritis victims who asked where they could obtain the very fakes he was exposing!

Clinical Tricks

The most important characteristic to which the success of quacks can be attributed is probably their ability to exude confidence. Even when they admit that a method is unproven, they can attempt to minimize this by mentioning how difficult and expensive it is to get something proven to the satisfaction of the FDA these days. If they exude *self-confidence* and enthusiasm, it is likely to be contagious and spread to patients and their loved ones.

Because people like the idea of making choices, quacks often refer to their methods as *"alternatives."* Correctly used, it can refer to aspirin and Tylenol as alternatives for the treatment of minor aches and pains. Both are proven safe and effective for the same purpose. Lumpectomy can be an alternative to radical mastectomy for breast cancer. Both have verifiable records of safety and effectiveness from which judgments can be drawn. Can a method that is unsafe, ineffective or unproven be a genuine alternative to one that is proven? Obviously not.

Quacks don't always limit themselves to phony treatment. Sometimes they offer legitimate treatment as well—the quackery is promoted as *something extra.* One example is the "ortho-molecular" treatment of mental disorders with high dosages of vitamins in addition to orthodox forms of treatment. Patients who receive the "extra" treatment often become convinced that they need to take vitamins for the rest of their life. Such an outcome is inconsistent with the goal of good medical care, which should be to discourage unnecessary treatment.

The *one-sided coin* is a related ploy. When patients on combined (orthodox and quack) treatment improve, the quack remedy (e.g., laetrile) gets the credit. If things go badly, the patient is told that he arrived too late, and conventional treatment gets the blame. Some quacks who mix proven and unproven treatment call their approach *complementary therapy.*

Quacks also capitalize on the natural healing powers of the body by *taking credit* whenever possible for improvement in a patient's condition. One multilevel company—anxious to avoid legal difficulty in marketing its herbal concoction—makes no health claims whatsoever. "You take the product," a spokesperson suggests on the company's introductory videotape, "and tell me what it does for you." An opposite tack—*shifting blame*—is used by many cancer quacks. If their treatment doesn't work, it's because radiation and/or chemotherapy have "knocked out the immune system."

To promote their ideas, quacks often use a trick where they bypass an all-important basic question and *ask a second question* which, by itself, is not valid. An example of a "second question" is "Why don't the people of Hunza get cancer?" The quack's answer is "because they eat apricot pits" (or some other claim). The first question should have been "Do the people of Hunza get cancer?" The answer is "Yes!" Every group of people on earth gets cancer. So do all animals (vegetarians and meat-eaters alike) and plants. Another common gambit is the question, "Do you believe in vitamins?" The real question should be, "Does the average person eating a well balanced diet need to take supplements?" The answer is no.

Another selling trick is the use of *weasel words.* Quacks often use this technique in suggesting that one or more items on a list is reason to suspect that you *may* have a vitamin deficiency, a yeast infection, or whatever else they are offering to fix.

The *money-back guarantee* is a favorite trick of mail-order quacks. Most have no intention of returning any money—but even those who are willing know that few people will bother to return the product.

Another powerful persuader—*something for nothing*—is standard in advertisements promising effortless weight loss. It is also the hook of the telemarketer who promises a "valuable free prize" as a bonus for buying a water purifier, a 6-month supply of vitamins, or some other health or nutrition product. Those who bite receive either nothing or items worth far less than their cost. Credit card customers may also find unauthorized charges to their account.

The willingness to believe that a stranger can supply unique and valuable "inside" information—such as a tip on a horse race or the stock market—seems to be a universal human quirk. Quacks take full advantage of this trait in their promotion of *secret cures.* True scientists don't keep their breakthroughs secret. They share them with all mankind. If this were not so, we would still be going to private clinics for the vaccines and other medications used to conquer smallpox, polio, tuberculosis, and many other serious diseases.

Seductive Tactics

The practice of healing involves both art and science. The art includes all that is done for the patient psychologically. The science involves what is done about the disease itself. If a disease is psychosomatic, art may be all that is needed. The old-time doctor did not have much science in his little black bag, so he relied more upon the art (called his "bedside manner") and everyone loved him. Today, there is a great deal of science in the bag, but the art has been relatively neglected.

In a contest for patient satisfaction, art will beat science nearly every time. Quacks are masters at the art of delivering health care. The secret to this art is to make the patient believe that he is cared about as a person. To do this, quacks *lather love lavishly.* One way this is done is by having receptionists make notes on the patients' interests and concerns in order to recall them during future visits. This makes each patient feel special in a very personal sort of way. Some quacks even send birthday cards to every patient. Although seductive tactics may give patients a powerful psychological lift, they may also encourage over-reliance on an inappropriate therapy.

Handling the Opposition

Quacks are involved in a constant struggle with legitimate health care providers, mainstream scientists, government regulatory agencies, and consumer protection groups. Despite the strength of this orthodox opposition, quackery manages to flourish. To maintain their credibility, quacks use a variety of clever propaganda ploys. Here are some favorites:

"They persecuted Galileo!" The history of science is laced with instances where great pioneers and their discoveries were met with resistance. Harvey (nature of blood circulation), Lister (antiseptic technique), and Pasteur (germ theory) are notable examples. Today's quack boldly asserts that he is another

example of someone ahead of his time. Close examination, however, will show how unlikely this is. First of all, the early pioneers who were persecuted lived during times that were much less scientific. In some cases, opposition to their ideas stemmed from religious forces. Second, it is a basic principle of the scientific method that the burden of proof belongs to the proponent of a claim. The ideas of Galileo, Harvey, Lister, and Pasteur overcame their opposition because their soundness could be demonstrated.

A related ploy, which is a favorite with cancer quacks, is the charge of *"conspiracy."* How can we be sure that the AMA, the FDA, the American Cancer Society, and others are not involved in some monstrous plot to withhold a cancer cure from the public? To begin with, history reveals no such practice in the past. The elimination of serious diseases is not a threat to the medical profession—doctors prosper by curing diseases, not by keeping people sick. It should also be apparent that modern medical technology has not altered the zeal of scientists to eliminate disease. When polio was conquered, iron lungs became virtually obsolete, but nobody resisted this advancement because it would force hospitals to change. Neither will medical scientists mourn the eventual defeat of cancer.

Moreover, how could a conspiracy to withhold a cancer cure hope to be successful? Many physicians die of cancer each year. Do you believe that the vast majority of doctors would conspire to withhold a cure for a disease that affects them, their colleagues, and their loved ones? To be effective, a conspiracy would have to be worldwide. If laetrile, for example, really worked, many other nations' scientists would soon realize it.

Organized quackery poses its opposition to medical science as a philosophical conflict rather than a conflict about proven versus unproven or fraudulent methods. This creates the illusion of a "holy war" rather than a conflict that could be resolved by examining the facts.

Quacks like to charge that *"Science doesn't have all the answers."* That's true, but it doesn't claim to have them. Rather, it is a rational and responsible process that can answer many questions—including whether procedures are safe and effective for their intended purpose. It is quackery that constantly claims to have answers for incurable diseases. The idea that people should turn to quack remedies when frustrated by science's inability to control a disease is irrational. Science may not have all the answers, but quackery has no answers at all! It will take your money and break your heart.

Many treatments advanced by the scientific community are later shown to be unsafe or worthless. Such failures become grist for organized quackery's public relations mill in its ongoing attack on science. Actually, "failures" reflect a key element of science: its willingness to test its methods and beliefs and abandon those shown to be invalid. True medical scientists have no philosophical commitment to particular treatment approaches, only a commitment to develop and use methods that are safe and effective for an intended purpose.

When a quack remedy flunks a scientific test, its proponents merely reject the test. Science writer John J. Fried provides a classic description of this in his book, *Vitamin Politics:*

> Because vitamin enthusiasts believe in publicity more than they believe in accurate scientific investigation, they use the media to perpetuate their faulty ideas without ever having to face up to the fallacies of their nonsensical theories. They announce to the world that horse manure, liberally rubbed into the scalp, will

cure, oh, brain tumors. Researchers from the establishment side, under pressure to verify the claims, will run experiments and find that the claim is wrong. The enthusiasts will not retire to their laboratories to rethink their position. Not at all. They will announce to the world that the establishment wasn't using enough horse manure, or that it didn't use the horse manure long enough, or that it used horse manure from the wrong kind of horses. The process is never-ending. . . . The public is the ultimate loser in this charade.

Promoters of laetrile were notorious for shifting their claims. First they claimed that laetrile could cure cancer. Then they said it could not cure but could prevent or control cancer. Then they claimed laetrile was a vitamin and that cancer was a disease caused by a vitamin deficiency. Today they say that laetrile alone is not enough—it is part of "metabolic therapy," which includes special diet, supplement concoctions, and other modalities that vary from practitioner to practitioner.

The *disclaimer* is a related tactic. Instead of promising to cure your specific disease, some quacks will offer to "cleanse" or "detoxify" your body, balance its chemistry, release its "nerve energy," bring it in harmony with nature, or do other things to "help the body to heal itself." This type of disclaimer serves two purposes. Since it is impossible to measure the processes the quack describes, it is difficult to prove him wrong. In addition, if the quack is not a physician, the use of nonmedical terminology may help to avoid prosecution for practicing medicine without a license.

Books espousing unscientific practices typically suggest that the reader consult a doctor before following their advice. This disclaimer is intended to protect the author and publisher from legal responsibility for any dangerous ideas contained in the book. Both author and publisher know full well, however, that most people will not ask their doctor. If they wanted their doctor's advice, they probably would not be reading the book in the first place. Sometimes the quack will say, "You may have come to me too late, but I will try my best to help you." That way, if the treatment fails, you have only yourself to blame. Patients who see the light and abandon quack treatment may also be blamed for stopping too soon.

"Health Freedom"

If quacks cannot win by playing according to the rules, they try to change the rules by switching from the scientific to the political arena. In science, a medical claim is treated as false until proven beyond a reasonable doubt. But in politics, a medical claim may be accepted until proven false or harmful beyond a reasonable doubt. This is why proponents of laetrile, chiropractic, orthomolecular psychiatry, chelation therapy, and the like, take their case to legislators rather than to scientific groups.

Quacks use the concept of *"health freedom"* to divert attention away from themselves and toward victims of disease with whom we are naturally sympathetic. "These poor folks should have the freedom to choose whatever treatments they want," cry the quacks—with crocodile tears. They want us to overlook two things. First, no one wants to be cheated, especially in matters of life and health. Victims of disease do not demand quack treatments because they want to exercise their "rights," but because they have been deceived into thinking that they offer hope. Second, the laws against worthless nostrums are not directed against the victims of disease but at the promoters who attempt to exploit them.

Any threat to freedom strikes deeply into American cultural values. But we must also realize that complete freedom is appropriate only in a society in which everyone is perfectly trustworthy—and no such society exists. Experience has taught us that quackery can even lead people to poison themselves, their children, and their friends.

It is because of the vulnerability of the desperately ill that consumer protection laws have been passed. These laws simply require that products offered in the health marketplace be both safe and effective. If only safety were required, any substance that would not kill you on the spot could be hawked to the gullible.

Some people claim we have too much government regulation. But the issue should be one of quality, not quantity. We can always use good regulatory laws. Our opposition should be toward bad regulations that stifle our economy or cramp our lifestyles unnecessarily. Consumer protection laws need to be preserved.

Unfortunately, some politicians seem oblivious to these basic principles and expound the "health freedom" concept as though they are doing their constituents a favor. In reality, "health freedom" constitutes a hunting license for quackery, with open season declared on the sick, the frightened, the alienated, and the desperate. It represents a return to the law of the jungle in which the strong feed upon the weak.

How to Avoid Being Tricked

The best way to avoid being tricked is to stay away from tricksters. Unfortunately, in health matters, this is no simple task. Quackery is not sold with a warning label. Moreover, the dividing line between what is quackery and what is not is by no means sharp. A product that is effective in one situation may be part of a quack scheme in another. (Quackery lies in the promise, not the product). Practitioners who use effective methods may also use ineffective ones. For example, they may mix valuable advice to stop smoking with unsound advice to take vitamins. Even outright quacks may relieve some psychosomatic ailments with their reassuring manner.

This article illustrates how adept quacks are at selling themselves. Sad to say, in most contests between quacks and ordinary people, the quacks still are likely to win.

THE MULTILEVEL MIRAGE

Stephen Barrett

Stephen Barrett, M.D., practices psychiatry in Allentown, PA, edits Nutrition Forum Newsletter, *and is co-author/editor of 25 books.*

Don't be surprised if a friend or acquaintance tries to sell you vitamins, herbs, homeopathic remedies, weight-loss powders, or other health-related products. Millions of Americans have signed up as distributors for multilevel companies that market such products from person to person. Often they have tried the products, concluded that they work, and become suppliers to support their habit.

Multilevel marketing (also called network marketing) is a form of direct sales in which independent distributors sell products, usually in the customers' home or by telephone. In theory, distributors can make money not only from their own sales but also from those of the people they recruit.

Becoming a distributor is easy. It usually involves completing a one-page application and spending $25 to $50 for a distributor kit. Kits typically include a sales manual, product literature, order forms, and a subscription to a magazine or newsletter published by the company. Distributors buy products "wholesale," sell them "retail," and recruit other distributors who do the same. When enough distributors have been enrolled, the recruiter is eligible to collect a percentage of their sales. Companies suggest that this process provides a great money-making opportunity. It is unlikely, however, that people who don't join during the first few months of operation, or become one of the early distributors in their community, can build enough of a sales pyramid to do well.

DUBIOUS CLAIMS

Most multilevel companies that market health products claim that their products can prevent or cure a wide range of diseases. A few companies merely suggest that people will feel better, look better, or have more energy if they supplement their diet with extra nutrients. When clear-cut therapeutic claims are made in product literature, the company is an easy target for government enforcement action. Some companies run this risk, hoping that the government will not take action until their customer base is well established. Other companies make no claims in their literature but rely on testimonials, encouraging people to try their products and credit them for any improvement that occurs.

Most multilevel companies tell distributors not to make claims for the products except for those found in company literature. (That way the company can deny responsibility for what distributors say.) However, many companies hold sales meetings at which people are encouraged to tell their story to others in attendance. Some companies sponsor telephone conference calls during which leading distributors describe their financial success, give sales tips, and describe their personal experiences with the products. Testimonials also may be published in company magazines, audiotapes or videotapes. Testimonial claims can trigger enforcement action, but since it is time-consuming to collect evidence of their use, few government agencies bother to do so.

6. HEALTH CLAIMS

Government enforcement action against multilevel companies has not been vigorous. These companies are usually left alone unless their promotions become so conspicuous and their sales volume so great that an agency feels compelled to intervene. Even then, few interventions have substantial impact once a company is well established.

CURRENT PROMOTIONS

During the past ten years, I have investigated more than forty multilevel companies marketing health products. Here are some recent examples:

• Enrich International, Pleasant Grove, Utah, markets more than 150 herbal, homeopathic, and supplement products. Its products have included *Tummy Gum,* for appetite control, *Increase,* claimed to be a homeopathic product that can correct all types of baldness problems; *Cataract,* "to aid for any eye and vision problems, cataracts being the most severe"; and *Co-Q10,* claimed to improve angina pectoris, congestive heart failure, high blood pressure, diabetes and gum disease. Distributors are given *The Mini Herb Guide,* which tells which products to use for 70 different health problems. A disclaimer says that the information "should not be used for diagnosing and prescribing" and "is not intended as a substitute for medical care." In October 1990, the FDA asked the company to recall 19 product information sheets that contained misleading and unapproved therapeutic claims. Subsequently, Woodland Books, Provo, Utah, which publishes books about herbs and "alternative" health care methods, sent a mailing to distributors with a message on the envelope: "Here are the tools to help sell your Enrich products." Inside the mailing was a catalog, a similar message from Enrich Corporation's president, and flyer stating that "Woodland's books help create markets for your products." One book is *The Little Herb Encyclopedia,* by Jack Ritchason, one of Enrich's leading distributors.

• Omnitrition International, Inc., of Carrollton, Texas, markets supplement products based on formulations by Durk Pearson and Sandy Shaw, authors of *Life Extension.* One product is *WOW!,* "a nutritional alternative to coffee," which contains 80 mg of caffeine and various amounts of vitamins, minerals and amino acids. Another product, *Be Your Best,* is promoted as a bodybuilding aid. Another product is *Omni IV,* a liquid multivitamin/vitamin mineral product for "anyone who is tired of troublesome pills and tablets as a source of nutritional supplementation." (The retail cost is $2.18 per day, about 100 times the cost of equivalent pills.) Omnitrition's sales manual suggests approaching prospects by offering to show how to double and even triple their current income over the next 12 months. The manual also advises distributors to promote the products by telling how much they like them rather than focusing on ingredients.

• Matol Botanical International, a Canadian firm, markets *Km,* a foul-tasting extract of 14 common herbs. Company literature states that no therapeutic claims can be made for *Km* in the United States. However, I have received many reports that distributors are making such claims. A *Km* brochure describes alleged uses of the herbs in centuries past. For example, celery seed is said to contain compounds which "have been found to be gently calming," while passion flower was believed to "quiet and soothe the body and assure peaceful rest." *Km* was originally marketed in Canada as *Matol,* which was claimed effective for ailments ranging from arthritis to cancer, as well as rejuvenation. Canada's Health Protection Branch took action that resulted in an order to advertise only its name, price and contents. In 1988, the FDA attempted to block importation of *Matol* into the United States. However, the company evaded the ban by adding an ingredient and changing the product's name.

• Sunrider International, of Torrance, California, markets herbal products with claims that they can help "regenerate" the body. Although some of the ingredients can exert pharmacological effects on the body, there is little evidence they can cure major diseases or that Sunrider distributors are qualified to advise people how to use them properly. During the mid-1980s, the FDA took several regulatory actions to stop false and misleading health claims for several Sunrider products. In 1989, the company signed a consent agreement pledging to pay $175,000 to the state of California and to stop representing that its products have any effect on disease or medical conditions. The company toned down its literature but continued to make therapeutic claims in testimonial tapes included in its distributor kits.

• Light Force, of Santa Cruz, California, markets Spirulina products with claims that they can suppress appetite, boost immunity, and increase energy. Company sales materials claim that Spirulina is a "superfood" and "works to cleanse and detoxify the body." Its magazine, *The Enlightener,* has carried reports about users who lost weight or recovered from arthritis, cancer, multiple sclerosis and serious injuries while taking Light Force products.

MOTIVATION: POWERFUL BUT MISGUIDED

The "success" of network marketing lies in the enthusiasm of its participants. Most people who think they have been helped by an unorthodox method enjoy sharing their success stories with their friends. People who give such testimonials are usually motivated by a sincere wish to help their fellow humans. Since people tend to believe what others tell them about personal experiences, testimonials can be powerful persuaders. Despite their unreliability, they are the cornerstone of quackery's success.

Perhaps the trickiest misconception about quackery is that personal experience is the best way to tell whether something works. When someone feels better after having used a product or procedure, it is natural to give credit to whatever was done. However, this is unwise. Most ailments are self-limiting, and even incurable conditions can have sufficient day-to-day variation to enable bogus methods to gain large followings. In addition, taking action often produces temporary relief of symptoms (a placebo effect). For these reasons, scientific experimentation is almost always necessary to establish whether health methods are really effective. Instead of testing their products, multilevel companies urge customers to try them and credit them if they feel better.

Another factor in gaining devotees is the emotional impact of group activities. Imagine, for example, that you have been feeling lonely, bored, depressed or tired. One day a friend tells you that "improving your nutrition" can help you feel better. After selling you some products, the friend inquires regularly to find out how you are doing. You seem to feel somewhat better. From time to time you are invited to interesting lectures where you meet people like yourself. Then you are asked to become a distributor. This keeps you busy, raises your income, and provides an easy way to approach old friends and make new ones—all in an atmosphere of enthusiasm. Some of your customers express gratitude, giving you a feeling of accomplishment. People who increase their income, their social horizons, or their self-esteem can get a psychological boost that not only can improve their mood but also may alleviate emotionally based symptoms.

Multilevel companies refer to this process as "sharing" and suggest that everyone involved is a "winner." That simply isn't true. The entire process is built on a foundation of deception. The main winners are the company's owners and the small percentage of distributors who become sales leaders.

Do you think that multilevel participants are qualified to judge whether prospective customers need supplements—or medical care? Even though curative claims are forbidden by the written policies of each company, the sales process encourages customers to experiment with self-treatment. It may also promote distrust of legitimate health professionals and their treatment methods.

Some people would argue that the apparent benefits of "believing" in the products outweigh the risks involved. Do you think that people need false beliefs in order to feel healthy or succeed in life? Would you like to believe that something can help you when in fact it is worthless? Should our society support an industry that is trying to mislead us? Can't Americans do something better with the billion or more dollars being wasted each year on multilevel "health" products?

RECOMMENDATIONS

Consumers would be wise to avoid multilevel products altogether. Those that have nutritional value (such as vitamins and low-cholesterol foods) are invariably overpriced and may be unnecessary as well. Those promoted as remedies are either unproven, bogus, or intended for conditions that are unsuitable for self-medication.

Government agencies should police the multilevel marketplace aggressively, using undercover investigators and filing criminal charges when wrongdoing is detected.

FOOD NEWS BLUES

*Grapefruit peel lowers cholesterol? Coffee's dangerous again? Here's
how to separate the sense from the nonsense in your morning paper.*

Anthony Schmitz

Anthony Schmitz is a contributing editor.

Note long ago I set a coffee cup on the table and opened the newspaper to a piece of good news. "New Study Finds Coffee Unlikely to Cause Heart Ills," read the headline. One less thing to worry about, I thought, until I remembered a story from a few weeks before. That morning the headline warned, "Study: Heart Risk Rises on 4, More Cups Coffee Daily." My paper—yours too, most likely—does this all the time. Concerning the latest dietary findings, it flips and flops like a fish thrown to shore.

"Medical research," it declared one Wednesday, "repeatedly has linked the soluble fiber in oats with reductions in serum cholesterol." By Thursday of the next week all that had changed. "Studies Cast Doubt on Benefits From Oat Bran," the headline cried. Once again the paper offered its readers a familiar choice. Which story to believe? This week's, last week's, or none at all?

The paper in question is the *St. Paul Pioneer Press.* It's a respectable provincial daily, not unlike the papers in Houston, Detroit, and dozens of other cities. One day recently the news editor, Mike Peluso, said he'd take a crack at explaining his paper's flip-flops.

Peluso is compact, graying, more grave than jocular. He met me at the newsroom door. "You want a cup of coffee?" he asked, pointing at a vending machine. No, I said, trying to recall whether this week coffee was good or bad. Peluso shrugged and headed for his cluttered cubicle. Beyond its flimsy walls reporters jabbered into phones.

I arranged the coffee and oat bran clip-pings on a paper-strewn table. Peluso examined them one by one. He grimaced. He sighed. He swallowed black coffee from a paper cup.

"How do you reconcile the conflicting claims?" he asked himself. "One month coffee can't hurt you, the next month quit coffee and your heart will tick forever."

Exactly.

Peluso shook his head. "I don't know. I don't have any answers for that. You've got to talk about the real world here."

For Peluso, the real world looks something like this: News of a hot nutrition study gets beamed into the newsroom from wire services such as Associated Press, the *New York Times,* or the *Baltimore Sun.* Peluso and his staff poke at the story, trying to find flaws that argue against putting it in the paper. By and large it's a hamstrung effort. Never mind that the reporter who wrote the piece is thousands of miles away. She'd defend the story anyway. The paper's own health reporter is scant help; he's been on the beat two months.

Meanwhile, Peluso knows that his competitors—another daily paper, plus radio and television news—won't spend a week analyzing the study. They'll run it today. Which is to say Peluso will, too. But the story the reader sees won't be as detailed as the piece that came over the wire. Compared to the *New York Times* or the *Washington Post,* the *Pioneer Press* is something of a dwarf. Stories get trimmed to fit. Subtleties and equivocations—the messy business of research—don't always make the cut.

"Look," said Peluso, "we're not medical authorities. We're just your normal skeptics. And it's not like we're inventing this research. We're simply reporting on it. We present what's there and let people draw their own conclusions."

"So what should readers make of all the contradictory advice you offer them?"

Peluso sighed again. "I don't know," he said. "You've got to take everything with a grain of salt until the last word comes in. I hate to tell people I don't believe everything I read, but the fact is anybody who believes everything they read is nuts."

RESEARCHERS WHOSE WORK makes news soon learn that the match between science and journalism wasn't made in heaven. Richard Greenberg, a microbiologist who directs the office of scientific and public affairs at the Institute of Food Technologists, has watched what happens when the scientific method collides with journalistic technique.

"The first thing you've got to remember," says Greenberg, "is that science is not fact. It is not truth. It is not holy scripture. It's a compendium of information. You try to put all the research together and come to a consensus. Just because somebody runs a study that comes to a particular conclusion doesn't change everything that's gone before."

Scientists don't generally reach consensus in time for the next deadline. After 30 years of study, coffee's link to heart disease remains an open question. Four-plus cups a day may slightly increase the risk, though some research suggests only decaf is linked to heart problems. Similarly, a decade's worth of oat bran experiments have served only to get a good argument going. Some studies suggest oat bran isn't any better at lowering cholesterol than white bread. If you eat enough of either, the message goes, you won't have room for fatty food. Others say oat bran has innate—though so far inexplicable—cholesterol-lowering properties.

While on their way to answering the big questions about fat or cholesterol or fiber, researchers often pause and dicker merrily about the design flaws in one study or the dicey statistical analysis in another. "Among ourselves," says one epidemiologist, "we're more interested in the detail of how things are done than in saying right now whether oat bran's good for you."

For journalists it's exactly the opposite. The arcana of statistical analysis and research design are boring at best, baffling at worst. The big question is whether oat bran will keep your heart ticking.

"The reporter and headline writer are trying to distill the meaning of the latest piece of research," says Greenberg. "They're trying to grab the eye of the reader. They're searching for absolutes where there are no absolutes. And this is what happens: One day you read caffeine is bad. Then you read that if you take caffeine out, coffee is okay. Then you hear the solvent that takes out the caffeine is dangerous. Then you find out the caffeine isn't dangerous after all. It so confuses the public they don't know who to believe. And the truth is, there wasn't really any

news in any of these studies. Each of them was just another micromillimeter step toward scientific consensus."

For Greenberg, news exists in those rare moments when scientists weigh the evidence and agree to agree—when the American Heart Association, the National Cancer Institute, or the National Academy of Sciences pronounces that you ought to eat less fat, or more vegetables.

But by the terms of journalism, scientific consensus is a dead-letter file. If everybody agrees, there's no conflict. If there's no conflict, there's no news. In comparison, debates such as those about coffee or oat bran are a newsroom gold mine. Contradictions and conflict abound. Better still, almost everyone has oatmeal or coffee in the cupboard.

"You can't convince an editor not to run this stuff," says Howard Lewis, editor of the newsletter *Science Writers.* "My advice is that they do it for the same reason they run the comic strips and the astrology columns. But I feel it's all a hoax. Usually they're not accomplishing anything except sowing panic or crying wolf."

A Purdue communications professor raised a stir a few years back when he suggested that research news might be more harmful than helpful. Writing in the journal *Science, Technology, and Human Values,* Leon Trachtman observed that some 90 percent of the new drugs touted in newspaper reports never reached the market or were driven from it because they were ineffective, too toxic, or both. Readers relying on this information would have made wrong choices nine times out of ten.

So who's served, Trachtman asked, by publicizing these drugs before there's a scientific consensus on them? "When there's no consensus, why broadcast contradictory reports?" Ultimately, he said, readers are paralyzed by the pros and cons. He asked whether the result will be contempt for research, followed by demands to stop wasting money on it.

Not surprisingly, Leon Trachtman got blasted for implying that a scholastic elite ought to be making decisions for us. Among the critics was David Perlman, science editor for the *San Francisco Chronicle,* who writes regularly about health and nutrition. Often, Perlman says, research leads to public debates. Will avoiding fatty foods really lengthen your life? Should government experts try convincing people to change their eating habits? It's debatable. But citizens can hardly take

part if they're capable of nothing more than numbly accepting expert advice. "To abdicate an interest in science," says Perlman, citing mathematician Jacob Bronowski, "is to walk with open eyes toward slavery." Perlman trusts people's ability to sort through well-written news.

"It's not just the masses who are confused," says Trachtman. "It's the same for well-trained scientists once they're out of their field. I think people ought to establish a sensible, moderate course of action and then not be deflected from it every morning by what they read in the paper."

> "You've got to take everything with a grain of salt until the last word comes in. I hate to tell people , I don't believe everything I read, but the fact is anybody who believes everything they read is nuts."
>
> — A NEWSPAPER EDITOR

> "The public doesn't know what to believe anymore. And the truth is, there wasn't really any news on coffee in any of these studies. Each of them was just another micromillimeter step toward scientific consensus."
>
> — A FOOD RESEARCHER

BUT LET'S FACE FACTS: Do you have the resolve to ignore a headline that declares, "Sugar, Alzheimer's Linked"? If you can't help but play the game, you can at least try to defend yourself from nonsense by following these rules:

COUNT THE LEGS. First, ask if the group studied bears any relation to you. Don't let research done only on four-legged subjects worry you. Pregnant rats, for instance, are more likely to bear offspring with missing toes after getting extremely high jolts of caffeine. What's this mean for humans? Probably nothing. There's no evidence that drinking moderate amounts

1. Study: Eating Citrus Can Help Against Cholesterol

Associated Press

MIAMI—Eating citrus can reduce cholesterol plaque in clogged arteries and help reverse atherosclerosis, a leading cause of heart attacks and strokes, researchers said Wednesday.

2. A two-year experiment with pigs found that citrus pectin—the sticky substance that's used to make jelly—reduces the formation of fatty plaque in coronary arteries, said Dr. Sigurd Normann of the University of Florida.

3. "The practical impact of our investigation is that we can tell a patient with severe atherosclerosis all is not lost," said fellow researcher Dr. James Cerda. "Based on this research, I would advise my patients with high cholesterol levels to eat a low-fat diet, get some exercise, and eat at least one grapefruit or several fresh oranges every day."

4. The researchers emphasized that citrus juice doesn't have the same beneficial effects because pectin is found only in the rind and in the pulp.

5. Normann, chief of cardiac pathology at the university's college of medicine, presented the study Thursday to the Federation of American Societies of Experimental Biology in Atlanta.

6. The primary grant for the research came from the Florida Citrus Commission, a state-appointed, industry-funded panel, but the commission played no role in reviewing the results, university officials said.

Normann said the study used pigs because their arteries and susceptibility to atherosclerosis are similar to humans.

7. Dr. Margo Denke, a specialist with the Center for Human Nutrition at the University of Texas's Southwestern Medical Center in Dallas, said she was impressed with the research. The findings fit in with previous studies showing pectin, a type of soluble fiber, can reduce cholesterol levels.

"They saw the change in a very short period of time, which is quite dramatic," she said. "But I think that more research is going to need to be done, and we might not expect such a dramatic effect in humans."

The study indicated as little as one grapefruit a day was enough to show results, but Denke said some other research has suggested that higher amounts might be necessary.

Dr. George Lumb, a scholar in residence at Duke Medical School who has conducted research on heart disease for 30 years, questioned whether people would be willing to eat that much fresh citrus fruit every day. He said his research team is conducting studies on 24 volunteers with high cholesterol levels to test the effects of pectin-enriched fruit punch.

Reprinted by permission of Associated Press.

HOW TO SPOT FRONT-PAGE FALLACIES

Your newspaper probably prints some type of food news every day. It may be important, it may be meaningless. Don't count on the paper's editors knowing the difference. You can defend yourself against half-baked findings and wild advice—if you read carefully. Here's how to pick apart a food news piece, one that hit the pages of the *Minneapolis Star Tribune* on April 26, 1991.

1. The bold, beckoning words at a newspaper story's top are usually cranked out by a special headline writer whose familiarlity with the subject can be measured in minutes. If eating citrus can help against cholesterol, your first questions should be: How much citrus? Whom does it help?

2. Now you know they're talking about pigs. Even if you have four legs and a snout, you shouldn't go for the pectin quite yet. The writer left out the study size—seven control pigs, seven pigs on pectin—which is too small to make the results widely applicable *even for pigs*. For humans, the conclusions are shakier still. That's not to say the research is irrelevant. Human arteries harden about the same way pigs' do. But the story doesn't say what else the pigs ate. Pigs are more sensitive to food's cholesterol; we're more sensitive to fat. Animal studies alone can't prove anything about human nutrition and health.

3. Did the pigs eat an amount of pectin that a reasonable pig, or a reasonable person, might eat? The answer (not that it's here) is no. Researchers fed 60-pound Yucatan micropigs half an ounce of pure pectin a day. Changes are you weigh two or three times more than a micropig. To have any hope of a cholesterol drop like that of the pigs you'd have to eat at least *two dozen* grapefruits a day.

4. Great news if you eat grapefruit *rind*. Most people don't.

5. There's a big difference between papers delivered at a conference, such as this one, and papers published in the *Journal of the American Medical Association*, the *New England Journal of Medicine*, *Science*, *Nature*, and the like. Journal articles are usually reviewed by experts who help editors toss out the scientific chaff. Presentations at conferences aren't as carefully winnowed and shouldn't be taken as seriously.

6. If the bills are paid by the citrus industry, wouldn't the researchers inevitably find *something* good to say about grapefruits and oranges? Maybe, maybe not. Quaker Oats, for example, recently funded research that showed oat bran has no special cholesterol-lowering effect. But a study of the debate over the drug tolbutamide (a diabetes treatment linked to heart attacks) found that doctors who got drug company funding were four times more likely than were their peers to say that people should keep on using the dangerous drug. You can't jump to conclusions about bias, warns *Washington Post* science writer Victor Cohn. Some crooked researchers *do* get money from corporations, he notes. "But the peddler of a biased point of view is as likely to be an anti-establishment crusader or an academic ladder-climber as a corporate darling." You have to judge each study on its own merits.

7. The last paragraphs are often more helpful than the first. This is usually where outside experts comment, putting the findings in perspective. In this case Margo Denke, a member of the American Heart Association's nutrition committee, makes three good points: This study confirms others showing that soluble fiber lowers cholesterol. Humans, however, aren't the same as pigs. And there ought to be more research done before anyone warms up the citrus bandwagon.

"If you don't like grapefruit," Denke says, "you shouldn't make yourself eat it."

—*A.S.*

of caffeine causes human birth defects.

If research subjects have two legs, read closely to see if they're anything like you. Early research that helped launch the oat bran fad involved only men, most of whom were middle-aged. All had dangerously high blood cholesterol, which reportedly fell after they ate a daily cup-plus of oat bran—enough for a half-dozen muffins. Fine, unless you're female, have low cholesterol already, or can't stand the thought of eating half a dozen bran muffins every day.

CHECK FOR PERSPECTIVE. Even if you're a match for the group being studied, don't assume the results are significant. "Check if the journalist gets the perspective of other people in the field," says Harvard epidemiologist Walter Willett. "People who've watched the overall flow of information are in a good position to say, 'Well, this really nails it down,' or, 'That's interesting, but it needs confirmation.'"

ASK HOW MANY GUINEA PIGS. Quaker Oats research manager Steven Ink, who's written a guide to nutrition studies, says the best research uses at least 50 subjects. By this standard, we should look askance at the recent study showing that eating 17 tiny meals a day lowers cholesterol: Only seven people took part. But rules of thumb don't always work. A small number *can* be meaningful if the effect observed is large and consistent. You don't need to feed 50 people cyanide to figure out that it's going to be bad for everyone.

What's more, Ink advises, subjects shouldn't be fed quantities of food that no one in his right mind would eat. One example is the recent study showing that trans fatty acids such as those in margarine may be bad for your heart. Subjects ate three times more trans fatty acids than the average American.

Finally, any group tested should be compared to a similar group. Early studies that linked coffee to heart disease were skewed because coffee drinkers differed greatly from the control group: The coffee drinkers were more likely to smoke and to eat a high-fat, high-cholesterol diet. Both habits carry bigger heart risks than does drinking coffee.

WAIT FOR CONFIRMATION. "Don't let one study change your life," says Jane Brody, the *New York Times* health writer. She waits for three types of food research to agree before changing her eating habits:

First, she looks for studies of large groups that show a link between a food and good or bad health—Italy's big appetite for olive oil and its low rate of heart disease, for instance. Then she watches for lab evidence in test animals that suggests how the food causes its effect in people. Finally, she considers human experiments in which two groups are compared—one eating the food, the other not eating it, with neither group knowing which is which.

Applying this rule to her own meals, Brody skimps on butter and favors olive oil. She eats plenty of fruits and vegetables, lots of potatoes, rice, beans, and pasta, and modest amounts of lean meat. "This plan won't make you sick, has a good chance of keeping you well, and is immune to these fads that are here today and gone tomorrow," Brody says.

HUNT FOR HOLES. No matter how carefully you read, you'll have to rely on the information your newspaper chooses to supply. If the big mattress ad on an inside page gets dropped at the last minute, the editors may suddenly have room for an exhaustive treatment of the latest coffee study. But if a candidate for national office gets caught with his pants down, the space required for a thorough exposé may mean the coffee piece gets gutted.

When editors at the *St. Paul Pioneer Press* got hold of a wire service report debunking oat bran, they found room for the first two-thirds. The third that didn't fit held a stern critique by other experts. They charged that the study contained too few people (20 female dietitians), didn't control the rest of what they ate, and started with subjects who had unusually low cholesterol.

"The reader really has to be skeptical," says Frank Sacks, the Harvard researcher whose oat bran study was under attack. "Take my case, for instance. The reporter really ought to say that this is a new finding, that it needs to be replicated. This is a warning sign that you have to wait a while. Reporters hate that when you say it. They call it waffling. But the truth is your hot new finding might not be confirmed down the line. You hate it when that happens, but it happens time and again.

"The real conservative advice is not to take any of this stuff in the newspaper with a whole lot of credence," says Sacks. "You could just wait for the conservative health organizations like the American Heart Association to make their recommendations and then follow their advice."

"WE DON'T HAVE an opinion," said John Weeks somewhat plaintively. I'd called the American Heart Association to get its line on oat bran and coffee.

"We get calls every day from the media," said Weeks. "They want to know what we think about every new study that comes out. And we don't have an opinion. We don't try to assimilate every new study. Our dietary guidelines would be bouncing all over the place if we did. Once the evidence is there, we move on it. Until then, we don't."

The Heart Association is sticking with the same dietary advice it's dispensed since 1988, when it last revised its model diet. Eat less fat. Eat more grains, vegetables, and fruit. The evidence that oat bran lowers cholesterol is so limited that the association makes no specific recommendation about it. Concerning coffee, the group has nothing to say.

Weeks's advice for whipsawed newspaper readers has a familiar ring. "What people need to keep in mind," he said, "is that one study does not a finding make."

"You mean," I asked, quoting Mike Peluso's newsroom wisdom, "I'm nuts to believe everything I read?"

Said Weeks, "That's exactly correct."

VITAMIN PUSHERS AND FOOD QUACKS

Victor Herbert, M.D., J.D.

Victor Herbert, M.D., J.D., is professor of medicine at Mt. Sinai School of Medicine in New York City and chief of the Hematology and Nutrition Laboratory at the Sinai-affiliated Bronx VA Medical Center. He is a board member of the National Council Against Health Fraud and a member of the American Cancer Society's Committee on Questionable Methods. He has served on the Food and Nutrition Board of the National Academy of Sciences and its Recommended Dietary Allowances (RDA) Committee. He has written more than 650 scientific articles and received several national awards for his nutrition research. His books include *The Mount Sinai School of Medicine Complete Book of Nutrition* and *Genetic Nutrition: Designing a Diet Based on Your Family Medical History*.

We still are in the midst of a vitamin craze. Nutrition hustlers are cleaning up by stoking our fears and stroking our hopes. With their deceptive credentials, they dominate air waves and publications. Talk show hosts love them because their false promises of superhealth draw huge audiences. The situation now appears even worse than it was more than twenty-five years ago, when FDA Commissioner George P. Larrick stated:

> The most widespread and expensive type of quackery in the United States today is the promotion of vitamin products, special dietary foods, and food supplements. Millions of consumers are being misled concerning the need for such products. Complicating this problem is a vast and growing "folklore" or "mythology" of nutrition which is being built up by pseudoscientific literature in books, pamphlets and periodicals. As a result, millions of people are attempting self-medication for imaginary and real illnesses with a multitude of more or less irrational food items. Food quackery today can only be compared to the patent medicine craze which reached its height in the last century.

"Health food" rackets cost Americans billions of dollars a year. The major victims of this waste are the elderly, the pregnant, the sick, and the poor.

The Fundamentals of Good Nutrition

Have you been brainwashed by vitamin pushers? Do you believe you should supplement your diet with extra nutrients? Do you believe that, "If some is good, more is better"? Do you believe extra nutrients can't hurt"? Or that they provide "nutrition insurance"? If you believe any of these things, you have been misled.

The fundamentals of good nutrition are simple: To get the amounts and kinds of nutrients your body needs, eat moderate amounts of food from each of the food groups designated by the U.S. Department of Agriculture's Daily Food Guide, choosing a wide variety within each category. (For detailed instructions send $1 for USDA's *Food Guide Pyramid* booklet [Publication No. HG 249] to the Consumer Information Center, Pueblo, CO 81009.) This food plan provides for adequate quantities of all vitamins, minerals, and protein components. Actually, normal people eating a balanced variety of foods are likely to consume *more* nutrients than they need. Of course, health hucksters won't tell you this because their income depends upon withholding that truth. Unlike responsible practitioners, they do not make their living by trying to keep you healthy, but rather by tempting you with false claims. These claims raise their personal appearance fees, sell their books and magazine articles, and sell the products of companies in which (unknown to you) they may have a financial interest.

The Dangers of Excess Vitamins

When on the defensive, quacks are quick to demand, "How do you know it doesn't help?" The reply to this is "How do you know it doesn't *harm?*" Many substances that are harmless in small or moderate doses can be harmful either in large doses or by gradual build-up over many years. Just because a substance (such as a vitamin) is found naturally in food does not mean it is harmless in large doses.

When scientists speak of "excess" vitamins, they mean dosages in excess of the "Recommended Dietary Allowances (RDAs)" set by the Food and Nutrition Board of the National Research Council, National Academy of Sciences. The RDAs are the "levels of intake of essential nutrients considered, in the judgment of the Food and Nutrition Board on the basis of available scientific knowledge, to be adequate to meet the known nutritional needs of practically all healthy persons." RDAs should not be confused with "requirements." They are more than most people require. They are set not only to meet body needs, but to allow substantial storage to cover periods of reduced intake or increased need. Amounts higher than the RDAs serve no vitamin function in the body. They should be considered *drugs* and can be an invitation to trouble.

There are two situations in which the use of vitamins in excess of the RDAs is legitimate. The first is the treatment of

From *Nutrition Forum*, March/April 1993, pp. 9-15. Reprinted with permission of Stephen Barrett, M.D., Publishers, P.O. Box 1747, Allentown, PA 18105.

medically diagnosed deficiency states—conditions that are rare except among alcoholics, persons with intestinal malabsorption defects, and the poor, especially those who are pregnant or elderly. The other use is in the treatment of certain conditions in which vitamins are used for their chemical (non-vitamin) actions. None of these situations is suitable for self-treatment.

How can vitamin pushers and food quacks be identified? The following behavior should make you suspicious.

They use anecdotes and testimonials to support their claims.

We all tend to believe what others tell us about personal experiences. But separating cause and effect from coincidence can be difficult. If people tell you that product X has cured their cancer, arthritis, or whatever, be skeptical. They may not actually have had the condition. If they did, their recovery most likely would have occurred without the help of product X. Most single episodes of disease recover with just the passage of time, and most chronic ailments have symptom-free periods. Establishing medical truths requires careful and repeated investigation—with well-designed experiments, not reports of coincidences misperceived as cause-and-effect. That's why testimonial evidence is forbidden in scientific articles and usually is inadmissible in court.

Never underestimate the extent to which people can be fooled by a worthless remedy. During the early 1940s, many thousands of people became convinced that "glyoxylide" could cure cancer. Yet analysis showed it was simply distilled water!

Symptoms that are psychosomatic (bodily reactions to tension) are often relieved by anything taken with a suggestion that it will work. Tiredness and other minor aches and pains may respond to any enthusiastically recommended nostrum. For these problems, even physicians may prescribe a placebo. A placebo is a substance that has no pharmacological effect on the condition for which it is used, but is given to satisfy a patient who supposes it to be a medicine. Vitamins (such as B_{12}) are commonly used in this way.

Placebos act by suggestion. Unfortunately, some doctors swallow the advertising hype or become confused by their own observations and "believe in vitamins" beyond those supplied by a good diet. Those who share such false beliefs do so because they confuse coincidence or placebo action with cause and effect. Homeopathic believers make the same error.

Talk show hosts give quacks a boost when they ask "What do all the vitamins you take do for you personally?" Then thousands or even millions of viewers are treated to the quack's talk of improved health, vigor and vitality—with the implicit point: "It did this for me. It will do the same for you." A most revealing testimonial experience was described during a major network show that hosted several of the world's most prominent promoters of nutritional faddism. While the host was boasting that his new eating program had cured his "hypoglycemia," he mentioned in passing that he was no longer drinking twenty to thirty cups of coffee a day. Neither the host nor any of his "experts" had the good sense to tell their audience how dangerous it can be to drink so much coffee. Nor did any of them

recognize that the host's original symptoms were probably caused by excess caffeine.

They promise quick, dramatic, miraculous cures.

The promises are usually subtle or couched in "weasel words"—so they can deny making them when the feds close in. Such promises are the quacks' most immoral practice. They don't seem to care how many people they break financially or in spirit—by elation over their claims of quick cure followed by deep depression when the claims prove false. Nor do quacks keep count—while they fill their bank accounts—of how many people they lure away from effective medical care into disability or death.

They use disclaimers couched in pseudomedical jargon.

Instead of promising to cure your disease, some quacks will promise to "detoxify" your body, "balance" its chemistry, release its "nerve energy," bring it in harmony with nature, "stimulate" or "strengthen" your immune system, or "support" various organs in your body. (Of course they never identify or make valid before-and-after measurements of any of these processes.) These disclaimers serve two purposes. Since it is impossible to measure the processes they allege, it may be difficult to prove them wrong. Moreover, if a quack is not a physician, the use of nonmedical terminology may help to avoid prosecution for practicing medicine without a license—although it shouldn't.

They display credentials not recognized by responsible scientists or educators.

The backbone of educational integrity in America is a system of accreditation by agencies recognized by the U.S. Secretary of Education and/or the Council on Postsecondary Accreditation. "Degrees" from unaccredited schools are rarely worth the paper they are printed on. In the health field, there is no such thing as a reliable school that is not accredited. Since quacks operate outside of the scientific community, they also tend to form their own "professional" organizations.

In some cases, the only membership requirement is payment of a fee. My office wall displays fancy "professional member" certificates for Charlie Herbert (a cat) and Sassafras Herbert (a dog). Each was acquired simply by submitting the animal's name, our address, and a check for $50. Don't assume that all groups with scientific-sounding names are respectable. Find out whether their views are scientifically based.

Unfortunately, possession of an accredited degree does not guarantee reliability. Some schools that teach unscientific methods (chiropractic, naturopathy, and acupuncture) have achieved accreditation. Worse yet, a small percentage of individuals trained in reputable institutions (such as medical or dental schools or accredited universities) have strayed from scientific thought.

Some quacks are promoted with superlatives like "the world's foremost nutritionist" or "America's leading nutrition expert." There is no law against this tactic, just as there is none against calling oneself the "World's Foremost Lover." However, the scientific community recognizes no such title.

They encourage patients to lend political support to their treatment methods.

A century ago, before scientific methodology was generally accepted, valid new ideas were hard to evaluate and were sometimes rejected by a majority of the medical community, only to be upheld later. But today, treatments demonstrated as effective are welcomed by scientific practitioners and do not need a group to crusade for them. *Quacks seek political endorsement because they can't prove that their methods work.* Instead, they may seek to legalize their treatment and force insurance companies to pay for it. Judges and legislators who believe in caveat emptor (let the buyer beware) are natural allies for quacks.

They say that most disease is due to faulty diet and can be treated with "nutritional" methods.

This simply isn't so. Consult your doctor or any recognized textbook of medicine. They will tell you that although diet is a factor in some diseases (most notably coronary heart disease), most diseases have little or nothing to do with diet. Common symptoms like malaise (feeling poorly), tiredness, lack of pep, aches (including headaches) or pains, insomnia and similar complaints are usually the body's reaction to emotional stress. The persistence of such symptoms is a signal to see a doctor to be evaluated for possible physical illness. It is not a reason to take vitamin pills.

Some quacks seem to specialize in the diagnosis and treatment of problems considered rare or even nonexistent by responsible practitioners. Years ago hypothyroidism and adrenal insufficiency were in vogue. Today's "fad" diagnoses are "hypoglycemia," "mercury amalgam toxicity," "candidiasis hypersensitivity," and "environmental illness." Quacks are also jumping on the allergy bandwagon, falsely claiming that huge numbers of Americans are suffering from undiagnosed allergies, "diagnosing" them with worthless tests, and prescribing worthless "nutritional" treatments.

They recommend a wide variety of substances similar to those found in your body

The underlying idea—like the wishful thinking of primitive tribes—is that taking these substances will strengthen or rejuvenate the corresponding body parts. For example, according to a health food store brochure:

> Raw glandular therapy, or "cellular therapy" ... seems almost too simple to be true. It consists of giving in supplement form (intravenous or oral) those specific tissues from animals that correspond to the "weakened" areas of the human body. In other words, if a person has a weak pancreas, give him raw pancreas substance; if the heart is weak, give raw heart, etc.

Vitamins and other nutrients may be added to the various preparations to make them more marketable. When taken by mouth, such concoctions are no better than placebos. They usually don't do direct harm, but their allure may steer people away from competent professional care. Injections of raw animal tissues, however, can cause severe allergic reactions to their proteins. Some preparations have also caused serious infections.

Proponents of "tissue salts" allege that the basic cause of disease is mineral deficiency—correction of which will enable the body to heal itself. Thus, they claim, one or more of twelve salts are useful against a wide variety of diseases, including appendicitis (ruptured or not), baldness, deafness, insomnia, and worms. Development of this method is attributed to a nineteenth-century physician named W.H. Schuessler.

Enzymes for oral use are another rip-off. They supposedly aid digestion and "support" many other functions within the body. The fact is, however, that enzymes taken by mouth are digested into their component amino acids by the stomach and intestines and therefore don't function as enzymes within the body. Oral pancreatic enzymes have legitimate medical use in diseases involving decreased secretion of one's own pancreatic enzymes. Anyone who actually has a pancreatic enzyme deficiency probably has a serious underlying disease requiring competent medical diagnosis and treatment.

When talking about nutrients, they tell only part of the story.

They tell you all the wonderful things that vitamins and minerals do in your body and/or all the horrible things that can happen if you don't get enough. But they conveniently neglect to tell you that a balanced diet can provide all the nutrients you need, and that the USDA Pyramid Food Guide system makes balancing your diet simple. Unfortunately, it is legal to lie in a publication or lecture or on a talk show as long as the claims are not connected to selling a specific product. Many supplement manufacturers use subtle approaches. Some simply say "Buy our product X ... It contains nutrients that help promote healthy eyes (or hair, or whatever organ you happen to be concerned about)." Others distribute charts saying what each nutrient does and the signs and symptoms of deficiency disease. This encourages supplementation with the hope of enhancing body functions and/or avoiding the troubles described.

Another type of fraudulent concealment is the promotion of "supplements" and herbal extracts based on incomplete information. Many health food industry products are marketed with claims based on faulty extrapolations of animal research and/or unconfirmed studies on humans. The most notorious such product was L-tryptophan, an amino acid. For many years it was promoted for insomnia, depression, premenstrual syndrome and overweight, even though it had not been proven safe or effective for any of these purposes. In 1989, it triggered an outbreak of eosinophilia-myalgia syndrome, a rare disorder characterized by severe muscle and joint pain, weakness, swelling of the arms and legs, fever, skin rash, and an increase of eosinophils (certain white blood cells) in the blood. Over the next year, more than 1,500 cases and 28 deaths were reported.

The out-break was traced to a manufacturing problem at the plant of a wholesale supplier. The naked truth is that L-tryptophan should not have been marketed to the public in the first place because—like most single-ingredient amino acids—it had not been proven safe for medicinal use. In fact, the FDA had issued a ban during the mid-1970s, but had not enforced it.

They claim that most Americans are poorly nourished.

This is an appeal to fear that is not only untrue, but ignores the fact that the main forms of bad nourishment in the United States are undernourishment among the poverty-stricken and overweight in the population at large, particularly the poor. Poor people can ill afford to waste money on unnecessary vitamin pills. Their food money should be spent for nourishing food. With one exception, food-group diets contain all the nutrients that people need. The exception involves the mineral iron. The average American diet contains barely enough iron to meet the needs of infants, fertile women, and, especially, pregnant women. This problem can be solved simply by cooking in a "Dutch oven" or any iron pot or eating iron-rich foods such as soy beans, liver, and veal muscle.

It is falsely alleged that Americans are so addicted to "junk" foods that an adequate diet is exceptional rather than usual. It is true that some snack foods are mainly "naked calories" (sugars and/or fats without other nutrients). But it is not necessary for every morsel of food we eat to be loaded with nutrients. No normal person following the USDA's food group system is in any danger of vitamin deficiency.

They tell you that if you eat badly, you'll be OK if you take supplements.

This is the "Nutrition Insurance Gambit." The statement is not only untrue but encourages careless eating habits. The remedy for eating badly is a well balanced diet. If in doubt about the adequacy of your diet, write down what you eat for several days and see whether your daily average is in line with the USDA's guidelines. If you can't do this yourself, your doctor or a registered dietitian can do it for you.

They allege that modern processing methods and storage remove all nutritive value from our food.

It is true that food processing can change the nutrient content of foods. But the changes are not so drastic as the quack, who wants you to buy supplements, would like you to believe. While some processing methods destroy some nutrients, others add them. A balanced variety of foods will provide all the nourishment you need.

Quacks distort and oversimplify. When they say that milling removes B-vitamins, they don't bother to tell you that enrichment puts them back. When they tell you that cooking destroys nutrients, they omit the fact that only a few nutrients are sensitive to heat. Nor do they tell you that these few nutrients are easily obtained from a portion of fresh uncooked fruit, vegetable, or fresh or frozen fruit juice each day.

They claim that fluoridation is dangerous.

Curiously, quacks are not always interested in real deficiencies. Fluoride is necessary to build decay-resistant teeth and strong bones. The best way to obtain adequate amounts of this essential nutrient is to augment community water supplies so their fluoride concentration is about one part fluoride for every million parts of water. But quacks are usually opposed to water fluoridation, and some advocate water filters that remove fluoride. It seems that when they cannot profit from something, they may try to make money by opposing it.

They oppose pasteurization of milk.

One of the strangest aspects of nutrition quackery is its embrace of "raw" (unpasteurized) milk. Public health authorities advocate pasteurization to destroy any disease-producing bacteria that may be present. Health faddists and quacks claim that it destroys essential nutrients. Although about 10 percent of the heat-sensitive vitamins (vitamin C and thiamine) are destroyed during pasteurization, milk would not be a significant source of these nutrients anyway. Raw milk, whether "certified" or not, can be a source of harmful bacteria that cause dysentery and tuberculosis. The FDA has banned the interstate sale of raw milk and raw-milk products packaged for human consumption. In 1989, a California Superior Court judge ordered the nation's largest raw milk producer to stop advertising that its raw milk products are safe and healthier than pasteurized milk and to label its products with a conspicuous warning.

They claim that soil depletion and the use of "chemical" fertilizers result in less nourishing food.

These claims are used to promote the sale of so-called "organically grown" foods. If a nutrient is missing from the soil, a plant just does not grow. Chemical fertilizers counteract the effects of soil depletion. Plant vary in mineral content, but this is not significant in the American diet. Quacks also lie when they claim that plants grown with natural fertilizers (such as manure) are nutritionally superior to those grown with synthetic fertilizers. Before they can use them, plants convert natural fertilizers into the same chemicals that synthetic fertilizers supply.

They claim that under stress, and in certain diseases, your need for nutrients is increased.

Many vitamin manufacturers have advertised that "stress robs the body of vitamins." One company has asserted that, "if you smoke, diet, or happen to be sick, you may be robbing your body of vitamins." Another has warned that "stress can deplete your body of water-soluble vitamins . . . and daily replacement is necessary." Other products are touted to fill the "special needs of athletes."

While it is true that the need for vitamins may rise slightly under physical stress and in certain diseases, this type of advertising is fraudulent. The average American—stressed or not—is not in danger of vitamin deficiency. The increased needs to which the ads refer almost never rise above the RDAs and can be met by proper eating. Someone who is really in danger of deficiency as a result of illness would be a very ill person who needs medical care, probably in a hospital. But these promotions are aimed at average Americans who certainly don't need vitamin supplements to survive the common cold, a round of golf, or a jog around the neighborhood! Athletes get more than enough vitamins when they eat the food needed to meet their caloric requirements.

Many vitamin pushers suggest that smokers need vitamin C supplements. While it is true that smokers in North America have somewhat lower blood levels of this vitamin, these levels are still far above deficiency levels. In America, cigarette smoking is the leading cause of death preventable by self-discipline. Rather than seeking false comfort by taking vitamin C, smokers who are concerned about their health should stop smoking. Moreover, since doses of vitamin C high enough to acidify the urine speed up excretion of nicotine, they may even cause some smokers to smoke more to avoid symptoms of nicotine withdrawal. Suggestions that "stress vitamins" are helpful against emotional stress are also fraudulent.

They claim you are in danger of being "poisoned" by ordinary food additives and preservatives.

This is a scare tactic designed to undermine your confidence in food scientists and government protection agencies. Quacks want you to think they are out to protect you. They hope that if you trust them, you will buy what they recommend. The fact is that the tiny amounts of additives used in food pose no threat to human health. Some actually protect our health by preventing spoilage, rancidity, and mold growth.

Two examples illustrate how ridiculous quacks can get about food additives, especially those found naturally in food. Calcium propionate is used to preserve bread and occurs naturally in Swiss cheese. Quacks who would steer you toward (higher-priced) bread made without preservatives are careful not to tell you that a one-ounce slice of "natural" Swiss cheese contains the same amount of calcium propionate used to retard spoilage in two one-pound loaves of bread. Similarly, those who warn about monosodium glutamate (MSG) don't tell you that the wheat germ they hustle as a "health food" is a major natural source of this substance.

Also curious is their failure to warn that many plant substances sold in health food stores are potentially toxic and can cause disability or death. The April 6, 1979, *Medical Letter* listed more than thirty such products, most of them used for making herbal teas.

They claim that "natural" vitamins are better than "synthetic" ones.

This claim is a flat lie. Each vitamin is a chain of atoms strung together as a molecule. Molecules made in the "factories" of nature are identical to those made in the factories of chemical companies. Does it makes sense to pay extra for vitamins extracted from foods when you can get all you need from the foods themselves?

They claim that sugar is a deadly poison.

Many vitamin pushers would have us believe that sugar is "the killer on the breakfast table" and is the underlying cause of everything from heart disease to hypoglycemia. The fact is, however, that when sugar is used in moderation as part of a normal, balanced diet, it is a perfectly safe source of calories and eating pleasure. In fact, if you ate no sugar, your liver would make it from protein and fat because your brain needs it.

They recommend that everybody take vitamins or "health foods" or both.

Food quacks belittle normal foods and ridicule the food-group systems of good nutrition. They may not tell you that they earn their living from such pronouncements—via public appearance fees, product endorsements, sale of publications, or financial interests in vitamin companies, health food stores, or organic farms.

The very term "health food" is a deceptive slogan. All food is health food in moderation; any food is junk food in excess. Did you ever stop to think that your corner grocery, fruit market, meat market, and supermarket are also health food stores? They are—and they generally charge less than stores that use the slogan.

Many vitamin pushers make misleading claims for bioflavonoids, rutin, inositol, paraaminobenzoic acid (PABA), and other such food substances. These substances are not needed in the diet, and the FDA forbids nutritional claims for them on product labels.

By the way, have you ever wondered why people who eat lots of "health foods" still feel they must load themselves up with vitamin supplements?

They suggest that hair analysis can be used to determine the body's nutritional state.

"Health food" stores and various unscientific practitioners suggest this test. For $25 to $50 plus a lock of your hair, you can get an elaborate computer printout of vitamins and minerals you supposedly need. Hair analysis has limited value (mainly in forensic medicine) in the diagnosis of heavy metal poisoning, but it is worthless as a screening device to detect nutritional problems. In fact, a deficiency in the body may be accompanied by an *elevated* hair level. If a hair analysis laboratory recommends supplements, you can be sure that its computers are programmed to recommend them to everyone.

Several years ago Dr. Stephen Barrett sent hair samples from two healthy teenagers under different assumed names to thirteen commercial hair analysis laboratories. The reported levels of most minerals varied considerably between identical samples sent to the same laboratory and from laboratory to laboratory. The labs also disagreed about what was "normal" or "usual" for many of the minerals. So even if hair analysis could be useful in nutritional practice, there's no assurance that commercial laboratories perform it accurately.

They suggest that a questionnaire can be used to indicate whether you need dietary supplements.

No questionnaire can do this. A few entrepreneurs have devised lengthy computer-scored questionnaires with questions about symptoms that could be present if a vitamin deficiency exists. But such symptoms occur much more frequently in conditions unrelated to nutrition. Even when a deficiency actually exists, the tests don't provide enough information to discover the cause so that suitable treatment can be recommended. That requires a physical examination and appropriate laboratory tests. Many responsible nutritionists use a computer to help evaluate their clients' diet. But this is done to make *dietary* recommendations, such as reducing fat content or increasing fiber content. Supplements are seldom useful unless the person is unable (or unwilling) to consume an adequate diet.

Be wary, too, of brief questionnaires purported to provide a basis for determining whether supplements may be needed. Responsible questionnaires compare the individual's average daily consumption with the recommended numbers of servings from each food group. The safest and best way to get nutrients is generally from food, not pills. So even if a diet is deficient, the most prudent action is usually diet modification rather than supplementation with pills.

They tell you it is easy to lose weight.

Diet quacks would like you to believe that special pills or food combinations can cause "effortless" weight loss. But the only way to lose weight is to burn off more calories than you eat. This requires self-discipline: eating less, exercising more, or preferably doing both. There are 3,500 calories in a pound of body weight. To lose one pound a week (a safe amount), you must eat an average of 500 fewer calories per day than you burn up. The most sensible diet for losing weight is one that is nutritionally balanced in carbohydrates, fats and proteins. Most fad diets "work" by producing temporary weight loss—as a result of calorie restriction. But they are invariably too monotonous and are often too dangerous for long-term use. Unless a dieter develops and maintains better eating and exercise habits, weight lost on a diet will soon return.

They offer phony "vitamins."

With vitamins so popular, why not invent some new ones. Ernst T. Krebs, M.D., and his son Ernst T. Krebs, Jr., invented two of them. In 1949 they patented a substance that they later named pangamate and trade-named "vitamin B-15." The Krebs' also developed the quack cancer remedy, laetrile, which was marketed as "vitamin B-17."

To be properly called a vitamin, a substance must be an organic nutrient that is necessary in the diet, and deficiency of the substance must be shown to cause a specific disease. Neither pangamate nor laetrile is a vitamin. Pangamate is not even a single substance. Different sellers put different synthetic ingredients in the bottle. Laetrile contains six percent of cyanide by weight and has poisoned people.

They warn you not to trust your doctor.

Quacks, who want you to trust them, suggest that most doctors are "butchers" and "poisoners." For the same reason, quacks also claim that doctors are nutrition illiterates. This, too, is untrue.

The principles of nutrition are those of human biochemistry and physiology, courses required in every medical school. Some medical schools don't teach a separate required course labeled "nutrition" because the subject is folded into other courses, at the points where it is most relevant. For example, nutrition in growth and development is taught in pediatrics, nutrition in wound healing is taught in surgery, and nutrition in pregnancy is covered in obstetrics. In addition, many medical schools do offer separate instruction in nutrition.

A physician's training, of course, does not end on the day of graduation from medical school or completion of specialty training. The medical profession advocates lifelong education, and some states require it for license renewal. Physicians can further their knowledge of nutrition by reading medical journals and textbooks, discussing cases with colleagues, and attending continuing education courses. Most doctors know what nutrients can and cannot do and can tell the difference between a real nutritional discovery and a piece of quack nonsense. Those who are unable to answer questions about dietetics (meal planning) can refer patients to someone who can—usually a registered dietitian.

Like all human beings, doctors sometimes make mistakes. However, quacks deliver mistreatment most of the time.

They claim they are being persecuted by orthodox medicine and that their work is being suppressedl.

They may also claim that the American Medical Association is against them because their cures would cut into the incomes that doctors make by keeping people sick. Don't fall for such nonsense! Reputable physicians are plenty busy. Moreover, many doctors engaged in prepaid health plans, group practice, full-time teaching, and government service receive the same salary whether or not their patients are sick—so keeping their patients healthy reduces their workload, not their income.

Quacks claim there is a "controversy" about facts between themselves and "the bureaucrats," organized medicine, or "the establishment." They clamor for medical examination of their claims, but ignore any evidence that refutes them.

Any physician who found a vitamin or other preparation that could cure sterility, heart disease, arthritis, cancer, or the like, could make an enormous fortune. Patients would flock to such a doctor (as they now do to those who *falsely* claim to cure such problems), and colleagues would shower the doctor with awards—including the $700,000+ Nobel Prize! And don't forget, doctors get sick, too. Do you believe they would conspire to suppress cures for diseases that also afflict them and their loved ones?

The Bottom Line

Food quacks benefit only themselves, collecting large fees for public appearances, publications, or "consultant" status to vitamin and health food companies which they sometimes control. Their victims are not only milked financially (for billions of dollars each year), but may also suffer serious harm from vitamin overdosage and from seduction away from proper medical care.

There is nutritional deficiency in this country, but it is found primarily among the poor, particularly among those who are elderly, are pregnant or are small children. These groups need improved diets. Their problems will not be solved by the phony panaceas of hucksters, but by better dietary practices. The best way to get vitamins and minerals is in the packages provided by nature: foods that are contained in a balanced and varied diet. If humans needed to eat pills for nutrition, pills would grow on trees.

The basic rule of good nutrition is moderation in all things. Contrary to the claim that "It may help," the advice of food quacks may harm—both your health and your pocketbook. They will continue to cheat the American public, however, until the communications industries develop sufficient concern for the public interest to attack their quackery instead of promoting it. And if the media cannot develop adequate social conscience on their own, they should be forced to do so by stronger laws and more vigorous law enforcement.

I don't mean to imply that everyone who promotes quack ideas is deliberately trying to mislead people. One reason why quackery is so difficult to spot is that most people who spread health misinformation hold sincere beliefs. For them nutrition is not a science but a religion—with quacks as their gurus. But where health is concerned, sincerity is not enough!

CHIROPRACTORS AND NUTRITION: THE "SUPPLEMENT UNDERGROUND"

Stephen Barrett, M.D.

Stephen Barrett, M.D., a practicing psychiatrist and consumer advocate, edits Nutrition Forum Newsletter and is co-author/ editor of 31 books, including Health Schemes, Scams, and Frauds *[Consumer Reports Books, 1990]. He has been investigating the chiropractic marketplace for more than 20 years.*

Many companies market supplement concoctions to chiropractors with claims that would be illegal on product labels. Although this marketing channel poses considerable danger to consumers, government enforcement agencies have been reluctant to explore it.

About 50 companies market supplements through chiropractic offices, where they typically are sold for at least twice their wholesale cost. Many of these products are intended for the treatment of disease even though they are unproven and lack FDA approval for this use. Since it is illegal to place an unproven therapeutic claim on a product label, claims of this type are conveyed separately through product literature distributed at chiropractic meetings, company-sponsored seminars, and by mail.

The percentage of chiropractors engaging in unscientific nutrition practices is unknown, but several reports suggest that it is substantial. In 1988, 74% of about 2400 chiropractors who responded in a survey by the leading chiropractic newspaper reported using nutritional supplements in their practices. Not long afterward, researchers from San Jose State University's Department of Nutrition and Food Science mailed a survey to 438 members of the San Francisco Bay Area Chiropractic Society. Of the 100 who responded, 60% said that they routinely provide nutrition information to their patients, 38% said they provide it on request, 60% claimed that they treat patients for nutritional deficiencies, 19% said they use hair analysis, and 9% indicated that they use "applied kinesiology" for nutritional assessment [Journal of the American Dietetic Association 89:939–943, 1989]. Neither hair analysis nor applied kinesiology are valid for nutritional assessment of patients. . . .

TYPICAL CHIROPRACTIC BELIEFS

. . . Chiropractors who give nutritional advice typically recommend vitamin supplements that are unnecessary or are not appropriate for treatment of the patient's health problem. Some chiropractors have charged thousands of dollars for treatment programs involving diagnostic evaluations, vitamins, adjustments, and massage over a period of several months.

ACA COUNCIL ON NUTRITION

The American Chiropractic Association's Council on Nutrition, which was founded in 1974, holds symposiums and seminars and publishes a quarterly journal (*Nutritional Perspectives*) and a monthly newsletter. The journal states that the council is "dedicated to the health of mankind on the premise that proper nutrition is a major factor in promoting and maintaining good health and preventing disease." During the past year, the journal has contained editorials, letters to the editor, abstracts of scientific reports, and reprints from *FDA Consumer* and other publications. Recent issues have contained 28 to 32 pages, of which about 35% are ads by supplement manufacturers. The title page states that ads "are initially screened" by a committee of the council, but that neither the council or its personnel are responsible for the advertising and that publication of the ads does not imply approval or endorsement by the journal or the council.

Recent issues of the councils' newsletter have supported the (bogus) idea that mercury-amalgam fillings are dangerous and opposed pending legislation to strengthen the FDA. One issue was accompanied by a form letter asking the FDA to lift its ban on L-tryptophan supplements.

The Council on Nutrition also appoints the American Chiropractic Board of Nutrition, which sets standards and administers a certifying examination for chiropractors. To become certified, chiropractors must take 300 hours of approved courses and pass an examination in

From *Nutrition Forum*, July/August 1992, pp. 25-27. Reprinted with permission of Stephen Barrett, M.D., Publishers, P.O. Box 1747, Allentown, PA 18105.

basic and clinical nutrition. According to the council's correspondence secretary, 42 of the council's 300 members are certified. . . .

In 1991, the American Chiropractic Association passed the following resolution, which was co-authored by the executive director of the ACA Council on Nutrition:

> The ACA's Council holds the position that it is appropriate for a doctor of chiropractic to recommend the use of vitamins, minerals, and food supplements to the extent that this is not in conflict with state statutes and regulations. A nutritional assessment should be made of the patient prior to the use of nutritional supplements. The recommendation of nutritional supplements should include a nutritional assessment of the patient. The practitioner shall record the rationale for the supplements in the patient's charts. The doctor should attempt to determine that the products being recommended are not experimental.

A similar resolution was passed regarding weight-control programs. Commenting on these resolutions, the newsletter's editor said:

> Save and memorize these resolutions! Their importance cannot be overstated. Before these resolutions were passed, there was no official "opinion" or direction by the ACA regarding this area. With these resolutions, we have, for the first time, something in writing; a part of the American Chiropractic Association that says YES WE CAN use nutrition. . . . Now we have the clout and the backing of the American Chiropractic Association behind us.

MARKETING STRATEGIES

Under federal law, "drugs" are defined as any articles (except devices) "intended for use in the diagnosis, cure, mitigation, treatment, or prevention of disease" and "articles (other than food) intended to affect the structure or function of the body." All drugs must be labeled with adequate directions for their intended uses. Drugs not generally recognized as safe and effective by experts are "new" drugs. It is a federal crime to market a "new" drug in interstate commerce without FDA approval or without adequate directions for use. To gain FDA approval substantial evidence must be presented to the FDA that the product is safe and effective for its intended use.

Chiropractic suppliers are marketing thousands of unapproved nutritional products intended for the treatment of disease. The manufacturers seldom advertise openly what the products are for. Some companies make therapeutic claims through seminars, exhibits at chiropractic

conventions, and material provided by "independent" regional distributors. Some companies provide their own product literature, which may or may not provide complete directions for use. Some companies provide copies of articles from the popular press or health food magazines that mention or promote substances contained in their products. A few companies distribute elaborate manuals listing the diseases their products can supposedly treat. . . .

Several chiropractors and naturopaths have written manuals suggesting specific products for large numbers of diseases. Those that I have collected within the past few years contain a disclaimer that nothing should be construed as a claim or representation that any of the products mentioned constitutes or is intended for use as a cure, palliative or ameliorative for nay of the conditions noted. . . .

In December 1991 *The Chiropractic Journal* (a newspaper distributed free-of-charge to chiropractors) published an ad from Physiologics, of Boulder, Colorado, which said:

> Are you ignoring a major income source? Spend 5 seconds per patient and increase your profits $53,000 or more per year. According to national studies, over 50% of the population could benefit from some type of nutritional support therapy. Of those individuals who use supplements, the average purchase is 1.5 supplements per visit. That means if you see an average of 30 patients per day, you will have the opportunity to provide 15 of them with nutritional supplements. Our studies show your average profit margin per patient equals $13.75 . . . = $53,625 gross profit per year. . . .

THE BOTTOM LINE

It is clear that the entire communication system between supplement manufacturers and their chiropractic clients is set up with the hope of "distancing" illegal claims from their product labels. Although some chiropractors may give rational nutrition advice to their patients, their journals contain little or no discussion of how such advice is given, or should be given. Although I am aware of several cases in which patients were seriously harmed by vitamin megadoses prescribed by chiropractors, I have seen no case reports in chiropractic journals or warnings that high doses can be toxic. Worst of all, however, despite the many problems described in this article, no prominent chiropractor or chiropractic organization has openly suggested that there is anything wrong with the way chiropractors "practice nutrition."

Diploma Mills Grind Out Self-Styled Nutritionists Dispensing Bad Advice

Although Mrs. G. had been assured by competent medical practitioners that her stomach distress was nothing to be concerned about, she continued to worry. Seeking the advice of a nutritionist, she visited Dr. Gary Pace, a Long Island practitioner. Mrs. G. was charged an exorbitant fee ($300), given two unproven diagnostic tests (saliva and hair analysis), a computerized questionnaire—which no matter how she answered would indicate she was suffering from a nutritional deficiency—and was prescribed 36 dietary supplements and 65 drops of liquid herbs daily.

Dr. Pace was no doctor at all, but a former electrical engineer with a phony Ph.D. in nutrition from Deonsbach University, a now-defunct California diploma mill. Mrs. G. selected him "because he had the biggest ad in the Yellow Pages."

In 1985, Pace was indicted by the New York State Attorney General for "inducing hundreds of customers to pay . . . for improper physical examinations, worthless laboratory tests, bogus nutritional advice and unnecessary vitamins, minerals and herbal supplements."

This vignette, reported in *New York Newsday*, is strong evidence that when it comes to seeking out a nutrition counselor, the rule is "buyer beware." There are a whole array of self-styled "nutritionists" offering advice that is less than reliable and sometimes dangerous. They range from nontraditional practitioners such as homeopaths, naturopaths, iridologists and multilevel

marketing salespeople from companies like Shaklee Corporation to health food store workers and nutrition counselors with bogus degrees.

Armed with dubious credentials, nutrition advisors on the fringe misrepresent themselves as being legitimate nutritionists. Some use their questionable degrees to present themselves as experts on radio and television talk shows or in newspapers and magazines. Others even have their own television programs and magazine columns. Often, they recommend unnecessary and expensive supplements, perform worthless diagnostic tests to detect nonexistent nutritional deficiencies or allergies, and offer phony cures and treatments.

Diploma Mill Experts. In 1985, a Congressional panel estimated that 500,000 Americans possess fraudulent mail-order credentials or diploma mill degrees, leading one Congressional member of the panel to warn that "every American can have cause for concern in the search for a bona fide professional."

In their book, *Diploma Mills: Degrees of Fraud,* (Macmillan Publishing Co., 1988) David Stewart and Henry Spille state that nutrition is "especially fertile as an arena for diploma mill and related fraud."

In the past decade, thousands of "degrees" in nutrition have been issued by a number of unaccredited correspondence schools. Kurt Donsbach, founder of one of the most infamous nutrition diploma mills, Donsbach University, claimed that his

"school" graduated over 1,000 people before it closed its doors. Donsbach University was sold to Jacob Shilling, Ph.D., a Donsbach "graduate" in 1987. Its name was then changed to the International University for Nutrition Education (see chart).

Weak education laws in some states have allowed diploma mills to flourish. Most "schools" that currently offer questionable nutrition credentials operate in California. Though California has tried to clean house in recent years, it is still a haven for such institutions.

These schools are free to advertise widely. "Advertising is the lifeblood of the diploma mill business," according to Stewart and Spille. Advertisements for nutrition diploma mills appear in supermarket tabloids, health food store publications such as *Let's Live* and *Bestways* and even in well-known and respected magazines like *Cooking Light.*

Obtaining a Bachelor's, Master's or even a Ph.D. in nutrition or a health-related field from one of these institutions may take an average of a year or less and range in price from $1,500 to $3,000, as opposed to the four years or more and tens of thousands of dollars from an accredited university or college. Certificates can take one to three months, costing anywhere from $100 to $1,000. Bernadean University, one of the California diploma mills will make you a "Certified Nutritionist" or a "Certified Cancer Researcher" for a mere $100 . . .

—Ira Milner, R.D.

QUESTIONABLE NUTRITION CREDENTIALS
(Some are no longer available)

SCHOOL	LOCATION	CERTIFICATE OR DEGREE	DEGREE REQUIREMENTS
American Holistic College of Nutrition	Birmingham, Alabama	B.S./M.S./Ph.D. in Nutrition	B.S. requires only 6 courses including one on the legal aspects of the holistic health practice. M. S. requires an additional 3 courses including psycho-dietetics and one focusing on detoxification. Ph. D. requires 3 more courses.
American College of Nutripathy (Biological Immunity Research Institute)	Scottsdale, Arizona	B.S./M.S. in Nutripathic Science, Ph.D. in Nutripathic Philosophy, D.N. Doctor of Nutripathy	*Nutrition Forum,* Sept. 1987 enrolled a writer in the college and found that it was possible to get a degree "as quickly as you can pass the open book tests." The college emphasizes hair analysis, reflexology, saliva analysis and food combining.
American Nutrimedical University & Affiliated Schools (John F. Kennedy Center for Academic Research)	Gary, Indiana	B.S./M.S. in Nutrimedicine, L.C. Licentiate of Chiropathy, N.M.D. Doctor of Nutrimedicine	According to brochures, "Several courses are required to get a Doctor of Nutrimedicine. If you have no B.S., the university offers one after you complete 12 lessons.
American Nutrition Consultants Association, School of Nutritional Science	Pasadena, California	Certificate of Completion or Diploma in the Science of Nutritional Consultation	The only requirements to enter are "a professed interest in the science of dietetics and nutrition and the desire to become a nutrition consultant. All required textbooks are written by the president of the school. Course length is 6 months or less.
Bernadean University	Van Nuys, California	N.D. Doctor of Naturopathy, P.M.D. Doctor of Preventive Medicine (Also offers doctorates in homeopathy, acupuncture, reflexology, herbalism and iridology). Other degrees include "Certified Nutritionist" and "Cancer Researcher"	A bachelor's degree is not required to go into the Ph.D. program. To become a "cancer researcher" all that is required is completion of a textbook written by the president of the school and to pass an open book test.
Clayton School of Natural Healing (same operation as American Holistic College of Nutrition)	Birmingham, Alabama	D.Sc. in Nutrition, N.D. Doctor of Naturopathy, H.H.D. Doctor of Holistic Health	Doctorate of Naturopathy is given after completing only 8 courses including herbology, massage and homeopathy. Average time to completion is 4 to 6 months. No degree is required to enter the program.
Columbia Pacific University	San Rafael, California	B.S./M.S./Ph.D. in Health Sciences	Course credit is given for "life and work experience." Courses are passed by completion of workbooks. A Ph.D. can be obtained in 12 months.
Institute of Nutritional Sciences	San Ysidro, California	B.S./M.S./Ph.D. in Nutritional Science	Self paced program for B.S., M.S. or Ph.D. Requires a high school diploma. Mental nutrition, homeopathy, herbology and medical limitations of orthodox medicine are among the required courses. A 14-day residence at a bogus cancer treatment center in Mexico is required of all graduates.
International Correspondence Schools, School of Fitness & Nutrition	Scranton, Pennsylvania	Diploma in Fitness and Nutrition	No prerequisites to enter program. According to school brochures "The course is designed to start you from the beginning with no previous experience, special talent or special schooling required." Eleven courses with open book exams can get enrollees a degree in less than a year.
International University of Nutrition Education (Formerly Donsbach University)	Chula Vista, California	B.S./M.S./Ph.D. in Clinical Nutrition. Ph.D.'s could specialize in Therapeutic Nutrition, Nutri-Medical Eye & Visual Health Care, Nutri-Medical Dentistry, Nutri-Sports Medicine or Nutri-Medical Homeopathy	The current president is a Donsbach graduate. Little specific information is available unless you enroll in the program. But brochures say in fine print "IUNE and its degree programs are not accredited by any accrediting commission recognized by the United States Department of Education."
LaSalle University	Mandeville, Louisiana	B.S./M.S./Ph.D. in Nutrition/Holistic Healthcare	A high school diploma is not required. Work and life experience count as college credits and are enough to get you into the Ph.D. program. Courses include herbology, massage, and iridology.
Health Excellence Systems (formerly Life Sciences Institute, College of Health Science, College of Life Science, American College of Health Science, American College of Life Science)	Manchaca, Texas	Ph.D. in Nutritional Science	No prerequisites for entering the Ph.D. program. Program usually consists of about 100 lessons of a few pages each after which enrollees must answer a 25 to 50 question test at home. Courses include application of food combining and fasting.
Nutritionists Institute of America	Kansas City, Missouri	Certification as Assistant Nutritionist, Associate Nutritionist or Nutritional Consultant	No prerequisites except that students must be able to read at a high school level. An assistant nutritionist's certificate can be obtained in 3 months or less.

Information included in this chart was obtained from school catalogs, brochures, pamphlets and advertisements placed in publications.

Nutrition Myths & Misinformation

MISINFORMATION
• • •
Weight Reduction Fads

Fad Diets and Weight Reduction

Fergus M. Clydesdale PhD • Professor of Food Science and Nutrition • University of Massachusetts • Amherst

Weight reduction is of great concern to a large part of the U.S. population. Many Americans are trying to lose anywhere from 2 to 400 lbs, in any number of ways, from the sensible to the bizarre. Weight reduction has helped to spawn an industry whose size has been estimated to be in the tens of billions of dollars. The reason for this is obesity—which not only increases the risk of cancer, diabetes, high blood pressure, and other health-related conditions but also causes psychological insecurity and untold social agony in its victims.

A visitor to this planet, on the basis of observation, would decide that to lose weight, one needed only to buy a book or a magazine with a new diet in it. They might wonder, though, if these books or magazines contain any useful information, because if they did, there would be no need for a new one every month. Therefore, these visitors would conclude that weight reduction must involve the act of purchasing these books and not the act of reading or following the diets they contain.

Gimmicks and 'amazing logic'

Unfortunately, like the consumers who buy these diets, these visitors would find that just buying books and magazines doesn't reduce weight, and often that even reading them and attempting to follow their advice is a futile endeavor. The types of diets which are most often advocated vary in complexity and merit. They all offer quick, easy weight loss—usually with a gimmick.

Some diets even offer amazing logic, such as that in the Beverly Hills Diet book, which tells readers that "As long as food is fully digested, fully processed through the body, you will not gain weight. It's only the undigested food, food that is 'stuck' in your body, for whatever reason, that accumulates and becomes fat."

I have even had students tell me that they lost 10 lbs in two weeks on a diet which suggested that one "grab a mate instead of a plate." Unfortunately, examination of the thermodynamics involved suggests a level of activity which even Superman might find difficult to achieve.

Four categories of diets

Due to the number of diets involved and the rate at which new diets are published, it is impossible to discuss all of them. At least a half-dozen new 'miracle' diets will have appeared after this article is submitted for publication, and thus could not have been included. I have decided, therefore, to categorize weight reduction schemes into four groups, so that readers might better judge for themselves the worthiness of each new diet.

These categories of weight reduction schemes are:
1. Caloric restriction of a balanced food intake
2. Caloric intake controlled through manipulation of diet or use of a 'special food,' such as a homogenate
3. Caloric intake minimized and a 'pill' emphasized
4. An imbalance of carbohydrate, protein, or fat recommended, along with either caloric freedom or caloric restriction

Balanced caloric restriction

Any number of diets would fall into the first category and as long as they meet nutritional needs and the energy balance is reasonable they may be used.

Weight Watchers is such a plan and recommends nutritionally adequate diets which can be achieved without the use of their products. Similarly, Richard Simmons talks of moderation and a balanced diet which, if followed, is also nutritionally adequate.

Manipulated caloric intake

The Pritikin program and the recent F-Plan diet, both of which recommend high-fiber intake, fall into the second category, along with those advocating purchase of special high-fiber homogenates.

The presumption that dietary fiber may prevent obesity involves the belief that fiber-rich foods are filling but contain fewer calories, and also that such foods promote rapid intestinal passage and thus fewer calories can be absorbed. However, the use of a high-fiber diet in the treatment of obesity has yet to be fully evaluated (*Obesity*, Technomic Publishing Co., 1980).

Emphasis on a 'pill'

A cursory glance at any magazine will illustrate the 'magic pill' diets in the third category. Some of the pills are vitamin supplements with a little sugar, while others may contain anorectic drugs like phenylpropanolamine which the FDA has warned may increase blood pressure if misused.

All of us have seen advertisements claiming that their product "burns away more body fat each day than 15 hours of non-stop exercise," followed by many seemingly unquestionable endorsements. However, tucked away in one corner there is generally a statement which says "This program involves a high-speed crash-loss diet that lowers caloric intake, essential to the reduction of body weight. Such results cannot be achieved solely through the use of the tablets."

Dietary imbalance

The fourth category is based on the physiological response to dietary restriction. Diets which are low in both carbohydrate and fat are ketogenic. These are dangerous dietary regimens which should be considered only under strict medical supervision.

A high-protein ketogenic diet (900-1500 kcal/day) has no particular advantage over a balanced non-ketogenic diet in sparing protein or inducing fat loss. Its major appeal is the diuretic effect during the first 10 to 14 days, which provides a striking but transient weight loss. The body quickly rehydrates and people talk with amazement about the 5 lbs they put on over a weekend on a 'normal' diet.

Quite different from this ketogenic diet is the protein-sparing fast. In this program, caloric restriction is limited to 300-400 kcal/day of a high-protein supplement. After its glucose stores are depleted during a fast, the body adapts to make ketones from fat (which the brain can use in a fasted state) rather than to provide glucose from glucogenic amino acids. Thus lean body mass is conserved while weight reduction is achieved.

This fast, however, may be hazardous and it is essential to provide sufficient supplemental potassium to prevent hypokalemia, as well as other nutrients. A number of deaths, apparently due to ventricular arrhythmias, have occurred in the U.S. and Canada in people who used "liquid protein diets."

In spite of this, a weight loss program called the Cambridge Diet has gained some popularity. This program, involving a powder that is mixed with water to provide 330 kcal/day, is sold to consumers by sales 'counselors.' The American Council on Science and Health has stated, "This is an extremely low-calorie diet. Health authorities, including ACSH, recommend that people not try this type of extreme diet except under close medical supervision. This type of regimen is usually used only as a last resort; it certainly isn't appropriate for people who have only a few pounds to lose."

Other diets have different combinations of macronutrients, such as the one described in the recent book by J.J. Wurtman titled "The Carbohydrate Craver's Diet," but evidence is very limited as to their efficacy. However, as long as they provide an adequate level of nutrients they are a 'safe' diet, but their weight reduction efficacy has yet to be proved.

Realities of weight loss

Despite all the weight reduction diets, the social and health pressures, and the use of supportive therapy, the failure rate for loss and maintenance of weight has been estimated as high as 95%.

I have found that dieters respond best when told how difficult weight reduction is. It is not a moral issue; the overweight are not sinful, but they may not enjoy life as much on a daily basis with extra pounds to carry around. Weight loss cannot be thought of as an interim behavior; rather, a commitment to a new and permanent life style is necessary. Successful dieters do not go on a diet; they *change their way of life.* Yearly as well as daily results are important, and the successful program includes exercise in this new way of life.

It is extremely difficult to lose weight without exercise. This need not be extreme, and walking is an effective form of exercise. Its mood-elevating effects, its beneficial effect on high-density lipoproteins (which have been reported to protect against cardiovascular disease), and its favorable effect on the lean/fat ratio in the body all make exercise an attractive ingredient in a new life style.

Suggested reading

Bray GA: *Obesity: Comparative Methods of Weight Control,* Technomic Publishing Co., Inc., Westport CT, 1980

Garrow JS: *Energy Balance and Obesity in Man* (2nd ed), Elsevier/North Holland Biomedical Press, New York City, 1978

Kissileff HR, Van Itallie TB: Physiology of the control of food intake. *Ann Rev Nutr* 2:371, 1982

Miller RW: EMS: fraudulent flab remover. *FDA Consumer,* May 29, 1983

Rothwell NJ, Stock MJ: Regulation of energy balance. *Ann Rev Nutr* 1:235, 1981

Some Low-Calorie Novelty Diets

Over the last decade, the American public has been tempted by a host of novelty weight reduction diets. Advocates of these diets imply that their particular nutrient, food, or combination of foods will selectively oxidize body fat, inhibit voluntary food intake, remove 'toxic' metabolic products, increase metabolic rate, and result in quick and major weight loss (*Arch Intern Med* 143:1195, 1983).

This report lists the grapefruit or the pineapple diet, the strawberries-and-cream diet, the pumpkin-carrot diet, and the egg and orange diet. All advocate reduced caloric intake, but the initial weight loss is due to immediate water loss. All novelty diets give little attention to the need to include adequate amounts of all known essential nutrients and to develop a long-range nutritional and activity program designed to *maintain* a desirable body weight.

Proponents of the **enzyme catalyst diet** imply that raw fruits, vegetables, seeds, and plant juices are prime sources of enzymes used by the body to trigger mitochondrial function and thereby "to melt accumulated fat cells and to wash them right out of the body." Enzymes present in raw fruits and vegetables are proteins and are hydrolyzed by hydrochloric acid in the stomach and digested by proteolytic enzymes in the intestine.

The **Beverly Hills diet** represents a classic example of a novelty diet, based as it is on unsubstantiated 'enzymatic laws' and such beliefs that undigested food becomes 'stuck' in the body and promotes the development of body fat. In addition to being nutritionally unsound, this diet also promoted binge eating: unlimited french fries could be eaten on one day as long as one ate pineapple the next day. The 'Beverly Hills Diet' is so restrictive that it could not be followed for any length of time.

The **Dolly Parton diet** is a low-protein, low-fat regimen based on the premise that certain food combinations—bananas and skim milk, for example—require more calories to digest than they provide in energy value to the body. On any given day of the diet, the subject can eat unlimited amounts of the foods assigned to that day; if weight loss does occur, it results from reduced calorie intake due to boredom, as well as to the associated diuresis.

The **endocrine disorders diet** for weight reduction was doomed to failure, not only because of its enigmatic name but also because it requires a daily intake of 36 oz of raw goat's milk, shredded wheat biscuits, stewed prunes, vegetable soup, green beans, and white bread. There is no rationale for this type of diet.

The **Zen macrobiotic diet** may have arisen as a result of a misconception of an originally well-balanced vegetarian regimen, transforming it into a nutrient-deficient program. 'Unhealthy' *yang* foods (such as meat, eggs, and fish) and 'unwholesome' *yin* foods (such as sugar, dairy products, fruits, and even vegetables) are gradually limited and eliminated until the diet consists solely of brown rice and tea. Adherence to this diet will indeed induce weight loss...along with severe malnutrition and death.

Diseases and Dietary Misinformation

Scare Talk About Foods and Cancer

Elizabeth M. Whelan ScD MPH • Executive Director • and Kathleen A. Meister MS • Research Associate • American Council on Science and Health • New York City

In her best-selling book *Metropolitan Life*, Fran Leibowitz described a non-dairy coffee whitener as "a combination of vegetable oil and cancer-causing initials." Most of her readers—and your patients—would accept this without question. Ms. Leibowitz merely repeated a prevailing American health myth—that 'chemicals in our food' cause cancer.

Probably 10% of the American public actually think that food additives are the *leading* cause of cancer. But there is little evidence that food additives cause *any* cancer. In their landmark paper on cancer causes (*JNCI* 66:1191, 1981), Richard Doll and Richard Peto attribute "a token proportion of less than one percent" of cancers to food additives.

Why are people so misinformed? We think three factors contribute to the confusion: popular fears, misunderstandings of true statements about food/cancer links, and extensive media coverage of cancer scares.

Popular fears

Two related syndromes are now epidemic: 'cancerophobia' and 'chemicalophobia.' For many people, cancer is *the* most dreaded of all diseases. Many Americans assume that the U.S. has an unusually high cancer rate. Actually, this nation's cancer rate appears to be about average for a technologically developed country.

Distrust of chemicals is almost universal; 'chemical' has become a pejorative word. Many people seem to think that the likelihood that a compound is carcinogenic is directly proportional to the length of its name. Yet, according to Doll and Peto, two fearsome-sounding additives—the antioxidants butylated hydroxyanisole (BHA) and butylated hydroxytoluene (BHT) are actually suspected of helping to *protect* against stomach cancer.

Misunderstandings of food/cancer links

Many popular publications have told their readers that up to 35% of all cancers are related to diet. Scientists consider it plausible. Laymen tend to misunderstand the statement because they assume it refers to food additives, when it really refers to major dietary components.

Overall diet composition may influence the risk of some types of cancer. Obesity apparently increases uterine cancer risk (*Sci Amer* 233:64, 1975). Preliminary studies suggest that people eating a low-fiber, high-fat diet have higher rates of breast, prostate, and colon cancers (*Cancer Res* 35(pt 2):3231, 1975). This evidence is too tentative at this time to justify recommending diet modifications to your patients in an effort to prevent cancer.

Interestingly, the incidence of stomach cancer, which we would expect to be strongly linked to diet, has declined steadily in this country since the 1940s. The U.S. now has the lowest stomach cancer rate in the world.

Media coverage

Any report linking a substance to cancer, no matter how flimsy or tentative, makes headlines. Sometimes, government agencies also contribute to public panic by reacting strongly to preliminary reports of *possible* cancer hazards.

Your patients may ask about the current status of these well-publicized cancer scares:

Saccharin: There is little evidence to indicate that saccharin, at current levels of use, causes cancer in human beings. Doll and Peto described its contribution to the bladder cancer rate as "negligible."

DES in beef: The daily doses of DES given to pregnant women, thought to have caused cancer in some of their daughters, were several million times the amount of DES found in a serving of meat from DES-treated animals. Human exposure to estrogens from non-beef sources, including endogenous synthesis, always far exceeds the greatest possible exposure from beef.

Nitrosamines in beer and bacon: Nitrosamines are carcinogens, but they are not found in significant quantities in alcoholic beverages sold in the U.S. Nitrosamines can, however, be formed in some circumstances if the nitrite preservatives in cured meats combine with other food substances. FDA and the food industry are working to minimize nitrosamine formation in cured meats.

Nitrites: In 1978, the FDA and the Department of Agriculture announced that nitrite itself could cause cancer, and they planned to ban it. Two years later, a careful reexamination of the same data that prompted the ban disclosed no evidence that nitrite was carcinogenic. Plans for the ban were dropped, but many people still retain their fear of nitrite.

6. HEALTH CLAIMS

Coffee: 1981's top cancer scare was based on a preliminary epidemiologic report suggesting a statistical link between coffee consumption and pancreatic cancer (*N Engl J Med* 304:630, 1981). This paper raised an interesting hypothesis but proved very little. Yet, many people mistakenly believe that the report linked caffeine with cancer. In fact, if a definite link between coffee and pancreatic cancer is ever established in the future, it is unlikely that caffeine will be the implicated substance. Tea consumption was not related to pancreatic cancer in this study, and tea, like coffee, contains caffeine.

Present status

These brief reports indicate that, despite widespread cancerophobia among citizens of this country, we have one of the safest food supplies in the world. Certain relationships between food and cancer *have* been identified, but these are carefully monitored by the FDA and public health experts.

Unfortunately, an uninformed public cannot evaluate scientific reports. Too many equally untrained self-appointed nutritionists are only too willing to implicate all processed foods and additives as dangerous to one's health.

Suggested reading

Benarde M: *The Food Additives Dictionary*, Simon & Schuster, New York, 1981 (lots of common sense in a good, inexpensive paperback written by a distinguished scientist).

Barrett S (ed): *The Health Robbers*, George F. Stickley Co., Philadelphia, 1980 (this encyclopedic book on health fraud and misinformation discusses 'the fear of additives' and nutrition myths among many other topics).

Doll R, Peto R: *The Causes of Cancer*, Oxford University Press, New York, 1981 (the landmark paper, now reprinted as a paperback book).

Cranberries and Urinary Infections

Most reports on the value of cranberry juice in urinary tract infections cite the work of D. V. Moen as a reference (*Wisc Med J* 61:282, 1962). Examination of this source, though, shows that it is just a short 'clinical note' reporting the apparent value of 6 oz of 'cranberry juice' twice a day in relieving a 66-year-old woman of the symptoms of chronic pyelonephritis.

Thus are legends born: cranberry juice *must* be good for urinary tract infections, since it contains a precursor of hippuric acid, which has a strong antibacterial action in the urine(*J Nutr* 6:455, 1933).

(Most cranberry juice is sold in the form of 'cranberry cocktail,' consisting of about one-third cranberry juice mixed with water and sugar.)

In one study, 3 of 4 subjects given 1.5 to 4 liters of cranberry cocktail per day did show transient changes in urinary pH, while a fourth subject had sustained lowering of urinary pH (*J Am Diet Assn* 51:251, 1967). On the other hand, Bodel and associates gave 1.2 to 4 liters/day of cranberry cocktail to 5 volunteers and found only slight changes in urine pH (*J Lab Clin Med* 54:881, 1959).

Bodel's group noted that 0.02 M is the minimal concentration of hippuric acid that is bacteriostatic for *E. coli* at pH of 5. Even though 3-4 gm of hippuric acid are usually excreted after ingestions of large amounts of cranberry cocktail, effective urinary concentrations could not be achieved because of the increased urinary volume: 4 liters of cranberry cocktail is a *lot* of cranberry cocktail!

Why not give undiluted cranberry juice? Or cranberry sauce? Pure cranberry juice is not available except on special order from the processor. It is very tart and must be liberally sweetened to be palatable. Cranberry sauce has the same drawback as cranberry cocktail; one must eat a lot of it to achieve noticeable increases in urine acidity.

It appears that, despite their relatively high acidity, cranberry products in palatable quantities cannot be recommended for reliable, sustained, consistent lowering of urinary pH.

Nutrition and Mental Illness

At the 1981 American Psychiatric Association meeting in New Orleans, several teams of investigators reported on their studies of various nutritional aspects of mental illness.

Jeffery A. Mattes of the Long Island Jewish-Hillside Medical Center described his study of the role of artificial food colors and other additives in the genesis of hyperactivity. After review of numerous double-blind cross-over studies, he was unable to find any significant value of the Feingold diet for hyperkinetic children. He feels that the few favorable results with the diet are sporadic, inconsistent, and most likely due to environmental variables other than diet.

Similarly, Morris A. Lipton of the University of South Carolina could find no evidence that autistic children were improved by therapy with vitamin B_6 (pyridoxine) and/or magnesium, as has been advocated.

Heinz A. Lehmann of McGill University, Montreal, has been evaluating the effects of megadose niacin or niacinamide therapy for schizophrenia, as propounded by Dr. Abram Hoffer and others. He repeated Dr. Hoffer's studies, but could duplicate none of Hoffer's favorable results.

The fact that schizophrenic patients have a higher-than-expected incidence of intolerance to cereal grains led to the hypothesis that wheat gluten might be a causal factor in schizophrenia. If so, says Dr. Llewellyn Bigelow of the National Institute of Mental Health, it's a very minor factor; in a thorough investigation, he could find only a few, inconsistent links between gluten and mental illness.

Reviewing the studies of neurotransmitter precursors and brain function, Dr. Alan J. Gelenberg of Harvard found that increasing choline intake (from lecithin) definitely increased brain acetylcholine concentrations. This could benefit patients with tardive dyskinesia (a rare side-effect of psychopharmacotherapy). Choline probably has little role in mood alteration, memory improvement, or therapy of Alzheimer's dementia.

The results of other studies suggest that therapy with two other neurotransmitter precursors—tyrosine and tryptophan—has apparently benefitted patients with depression.

However, this is not necessarily related to increased protein intake or amino acid supplementation. While additional studies are needed, Dr. Gelenberg believes these precursors may have a future role as adjuncts in the treatment of depression.

Cytotoxic Testing for Allergy

From its inception to the present, the cytotoxic test for the diagnosis of food and inhalant allergy has been controversial. The test was introduced by Black in 1956 and modified by Bryan and Bryan in 1958, but interest in its use has increased greatly only in the last few years.

Leukocytotoxic or cytotoxic testing is based on the premise that adding a specific offending food allergen to a sample of a patient's blood results in measurable changes in cellular morphology or destruction of white blood cells (WBCs). Specifically, the patient's WBCs are mixed with a particular food antigen such as yeast, corn, egg, wheat, or milk.

The reaction is then observed under a microscope and the destruction of WBCs subjectively judged as slight, moderate, or severe. Proponents claim that the WBCs will react if the extract is from an offending food, but will remain unaltered if the food is well tolerated.

Initial enthusiasm

Once the incriminating foods are identified, the patient is given a strict diet which eliminates the allergens. Other foods are then gradually reintroduced on a trial-and-error basis, and allergenicity confirmed by the onset of such subjective symptoms as headache, faintness, dizziness, postprandial drowsiness, mucus formation, watery eyes, canker sores, heart palpitations, nausea, diarrhea, flatulence, hives, eczema, and general aches and pains.

According to some of its proponents, "this foolproof test can determine the items in your diet which are causing masked allergies and depriving your body of peak performance" (*Let's Live*, January, 1982).

Psoriasis and the Diet

Can dietary modification help the patient with psoriasis? John M. Douglass reported that his wife's psoriasis improved when she stopped eating fruits (especially citrus fruits), nuts, corn, and milk (*West J Med* 133:450, 1980). Dr. Douglass used a similar program for five patients, and their psoriasis also improved. He also asked them to stop eating acidic foods such as coffee, soda, tomatoes, and pineapple, because empirically he had found that this also helped.

However, UCLA's Marvin Rapaport pointed out that the data obtained on one or a few patients followed subjectively for several years are difficult to interpret when dealing with a disease as complex as psoriasis (*West J Med* 134:364, 1981). Dr. Rapaport suggests that any patient with psoriasis (or, for that matter, any chronic disease) often does well with hospital care and intensive observation.

At this point, the editors of *Nutrition & the M.D.* feel that there are insufficient scientific studies to advise patients with psoriasis to eliminate fruit and milk from their diets.

This may lead to vitamin deficiencies and almost certainly to calcium loss.

Subjective results

S. Allan Boch MD, of the National Jewish Hospital and Research Center, Denver, feels that the test at best is "subjective, with no scientific basis and no normal values." The few studies that have been done on cytotoxic testing, he notes, show no valid separation of the allergic from the non-allergic response, and this is crucial in any subjective test.

Joseph Church MD, an attending physician at Childrens Hospital of Los Angeles Division of Allergy-Clinical Immunology, concurs that the test has "no validity in real science." He also points out some potentially harmful effects: a patient may have a serious medical problem which is neglected due to false confidence in the test results; a highly allergic patient may get erroneous results and ingest foods to which he/she is actually very allergic; elimination of a variety of foods from the diet, without proper nutritional intervention, could easily result in malnutrition.

Further doubts

In 1981, the American Academy of Allergy reported that results of several controlled trials provided no evidence that leukocytotoxic testing is effective for the diagnosis of food and inhalant allergy. The Academy concludes that cytotoxic testing should be reserved for experimental use only in well-designed trials.

'Allergy' was once looked upon with great skepticism, at the time when allergies were blamed for everything from bedwetting to bruxism. Objective diagnostic procedures—such as double-blind food challenges, elimination diets coupled with detailed diet histories, skin tests, and specific IgE tests—can facilitate the diagnosis of specific allergies in many instances.

MYTHOLOGY

Folk Medicine

Russian Cold Remedies

Almost everyone in present-day Russia is an expert on home cures for common wintertime maladies—and in Russia, they have a lot of wintertime. Eliza Klose, a recent Moscow resident, described her experience in *The Washington Post*.

With the advent of autumn, knowledgeable Russians begin to gather their supply of medications—honey, turnips, vitamin-rich cranberries, pomegranates, and especially black currants. Chopped raw and preserved with sugar, these are taken to prevent common colds, just as some

Americans gobble vitamin C. Garlic and onions also seem to keep the cold viruses (and everything else) at a distance.

When a cold does develop, the well-prepared Russian is equipped to treat it. The first step is often tea with raspberry jam added. If there's a fever, a brew of linden leaves with honey is sure to break it. Honey, incidentally, is rarely eaten as a spread in Russia, for the limited supplies are saved for medicinal purposes.

If a sore throat is the problem, it is eased with warm milk with butter or honey. Heated vodka and honey, taken a tablespoon at a time, will conquer any Russian cough. Vodka compresses also relieve swollen lymph nodes.

For a stuffed-up nose, two drops of freshly squeezed onion juice in each nostril will rapidly clear the nasal passages.

Among other popular Russian remedies: chamomile tea brewed with mint and daisies for food poisoning; dried pomegranate skins in hot water for nausea; shelled pumpkin seeds mashed with garlic or honey for intestinal parasites; watermelon seeds or juniper berries for diuresis; and black turnips for any viral diseases.

Sassafras and Comfrey Teas

Generations of pioneer Americans sipped sassafras tea as a mild stimulant—little realizing it contained a potent carcinogen, safrole. When this became known, in 1960 the FDA issued an order banning the use of safrole or sassafras extracts in food. Prior to that time, they had been widely used as flavoring agents, especially in root beer.

Yet, despite these restrictions, sassafras is still widely available today in health food stores and similar outlets. Because of growing interest in natural foods, use of herbal extracts including sassafras tea appears to be increasing.

Recent evidence suggests that sassafras tea has other toxic effects. Safrole inhibits certain liver microsomal enzyme systems. This could lead to secondary toxicity if drugs usually metabolized by these enzymes are given concurrently with sassafras tea (*JAMA* 236:477, 1976).

Furthermore, consumption of herb teas may alter the bioavailability of drugs in other ways. Most herb teas, including sassafras tea, are rich in tannins which can bind, inactivate, or sometimes delay the absorption of certain nutrients and drugs.

A favorite European brew, comfrey tea, is also being widely consumed in this country. The tea, made from both the leaves and the roots of the comfrey herb, contains hepatotoxic pyrrolizidine alkaloids (*Lancet* 1:941, 1981).

Toxicologic studies confirm the chronic effects of these alkaloids in animals, but reliable human data are scarce because chronic poisoning requires several years' exposure before the effects become evident. Still, habitual use of comfrey tea, especially when made from the more toxic root, probably has serious health hazards, and its use should be discouraged.

More Herbal Teas

Herbal teas have been used for centuries and are said to promote good health or to be a remedy for certain ailments. There has recently been a resurgence in the use of these teas, promoted by 'health food' establishments or by those practicing 'natural' health care.

Most of these teas are innocuous, but some are toxic and a few may be lethal. The 'cup of hemlock' drunk by Socrates was, as he knew, a poisonous 'herbal tea.' From before the time of the Greeks to the present, drinking of herbal tea continues, as do reports of its toxicity.

Herbal tea as tonic

Most herbal teas are consumed simply for their pleasant taste—caffeine-free alternatives to coffee and regular tea. Most of these have been time-tested, but some may produce idiosyncratic or allergic reactions. Perhaps the most notable of these is chamomile tea, which reportedly may cause anaphylactic reactions in individuals allergic to ragweed, asters, or chrysanthemums. Such individuals should also avoid tea made from the flowers of goldenrod, marigold, and yarrow.

Some herbal teas can induce bizarre anticholinergic effects. These include those made with burdock, catnip, juniper, hydrangea, and jimson weed. Herbal teas made from senna, aloe, buckthorn, and dock have produced severe diarrhea. Large quantities of licorice tea can cause sodium retention and potassium loss, severe diarrhea, and elevated blood pressure (*Med Lett Drug Ther* 21:29, 1979).

Herbal tea as remedy

By FDA dictum, herbal teas cannot be labeled as having therapeutic value—yet they are widely (but unofficially) heralded as having specific medical benefits. Quack grass and dandelion tea have a mild (and probably harmless) diuretic action. However, diuretic teas made from juniper berries can cause GI irritation, and those made from shave grass or horsetail plants can cause acute neurotoxicity.

A Chinese herbal tea reputed to be a 'cure' for arthritis caused reversible agranulocytosis in a 65-year-old man (*Med J Aust* 2:860, 1977). Analysis of the tea revealed that it contained phenylbutazone, phenacetin, aminopyrine, and mercuric sulfide, with amounts varying widely in different samples. Inadequate labeling and poor standardization of contents are common among herbal teas, and these practices further contribute to the risk of overdose and toxicity from herbal teas.

Herbal tea as toxin

A young woman with irregular menstrual bleeding was found to have greatly reduced serum clotting factors. She denied taking coumarin drugs, but was taking acetaminophen and propoxyphene for backache and severe headache.

A detailed history revealed that she had been drinking large amounts of an herbal tea. The ingredients of the tea included tonka beans, melliot, and woodruff—all containing natural coumarins. These were probably the chief cause of the patient's coagulation defect.

But several other factors may have enhanced this effect, advises the University of Indiana's Redmond P. Hogan III MD, who reports this case (*JAMA* 249:2679, 1983). Prolonged continuous acetaminophen therapy potentiates the effect of oral anticoagulant drugs (*Curr Ther Res* 10:501, 1968). Also, dextropropoxyphene has been reported to potentiate the effect of warfarin (*Br Med J*

1:200, 1976), although no similar reports have implicated the related drug propoxyphene that this patient was taking.

The patient was also consuming 'fairly large doses' of vitamin A, which can reduce the vitamin K-dependent clotting factors (*Fed Proc* 20:989, 1961). Finally, she was self-dosing herself with bromelain, after a friend told her it would remove fatty deposits from her hips. This proteolytic enzyme derived from pineapple is one of many drugs reported to potentiate the effects of coumarin anticoagulants (*Pharm Index* 20:4, 1968).

New LifeStyle Diets

Food Faddism in Pediatrics

Food fads, especially those in the pediatric realm, are not necessarily hazards to health, advises Frank R. Sinatra MD of Los Angeles. Breastfeeding, he points out, was considered a 'fad' not too many years ago; now, it is known to be of proved nutritional benefit (*J Am Coll Nutr* 3:169, 1984).

Moreover, some fads probably have long-term benefits, although they have some limitations in infants and children. Here, Dr. Sinatra is referring primarily to the vegetarian diet, associated with a decreased incidence of both obesity and hypercholesterolemia. Still, the strict vegans' diet may be inadequate in calories, protein, calcium, zinc, iron, and vitamins D and B_{12} and thus not able to support normal growth in infants.

Harmless fad diets

Other fad diets have possible but unproved benefits with minimal nutrition risks. One of these is the Feingold diet— the removal of synthetic colors and flavors and all salicylate-containing foods from the diet in an attempt to control hyperkinetic behavior in school children. Dr. Sinatra believes there are few adverse nutritional consequences of the diet *per se* — unless parents begin to progressively eliminate other foods, as happens when the basic Feingold diet (of unproved efficacy) fails to control hyperkinetic behavior. Also, elimination of fruits from a child's diet can potentially lead to deficiency of vitamin C.

The exclusive use of 'natural' and 'organic' foods and the high-protein 'athletic' diets are other fads that are not particularly harmful, but by the same token, offer no special benefits. High-protein diets increase the body's need for fluids.

Dangerous fad diets

Some pediatric feeding practices not only have no proved benefits but also may result in significant morbidity and even mortality. One of these is the Zen macrobiotic diet, which in the initial stages resembles a vegetarian diet but in the advanced stages is extremely dangerous for growing infants and children. Some investigators have reported that megavitamin therapy in infants with immature metabolic systems may prove life-threatening (*Pediatr Clin North Am* 32:429, 1985).

Another example cited by Dr. Sinatra: the leader of a religious movement recommended a formula made from barley water, corn syrup (or honey) and whole milk, claiming that it was "most like human milk." This appealed to well-intended mothers who elected not to breastfeed their infants, but in some cases the result was hypochromic microcytic anemia, growth retardation, and failure to thrive in their infants.

Similarly, nondairy creamers resemble milk in color, texture, and packaging, and have therefore been unwittingly used as infant formulas both by parents and by physicians (such nondairy creamers are high in calories but nearly devoid of protein content). Some infants given such a formula developed kwashiorkor within a few weeks to months....

CONCLUSION

Coping with Food Faddism

William T. Jarvis, PhD • Loma Linda, CA

People become food faddists for many different reasons. It may result simply from misinformation, from an outgrowth of deeply held philosophical beliefs, or from a health neurosis. Most individuals who are immersed in faddism can be placed into one of two categories—the Deceived and the Deluded. The Deceived mainly need accurate information and perhaps some assistance with logical reasoning. The Deluded require much more effort and may even be beyond help.

The Deceived and Deluded cannot be differentiated on the basis of what they believe or how strongly they *appear* to hold their convictions. The test is how they react when faced with substantive evidence that their beliefs are wrong. The Deceived will change, the Deluded will not. It may take some time to determine which type of person you are dealing with.

Dealing with patients involved in faddism requires skill and tact. Success may depend more on how well one meets their emotional needs than on one's scientific knowledge or academic credentials.

Interpersonal relationships

The prestige represented by professional credentials is important to the doctor/patient relationship. Quacks have always pretended to have expertise in order to enhance their credibility. However, patients are more likely to believe and follow your advice because of personal feelings toward you than because of your professional qualifications.

Patients must recognize that you care more about them personally than you do about information or technology. Careful attention must be given to building a good relationship before seriously challenging their beliefs, attitudes, or behavioral patterns. One must not allow confrontations resulting from the patient's erroneous beliefs to undermine the relationship. Patients should never be made to feel stupid because they have been deceived by faddists' claims. In fact, intelligence per se has little to do with the quality of the beliefs people hold.

6. HEALTH CLAIMS

Be informed on the fads

Being informed on the fads enhances your credibility. If a fad is unfamiliar to you, ask the patient to provide more information. Condemnation of a fad out of ignorance and unwillingness to investigate its claims reinforces the notion of 'establishment bigotry' that faddism has planted in the patient's mind.

Attention must be given to more than just providing nutrition facts. Faddism may be based on beliefs, values and attitudes that are often deeply held by your patients. These include excessive concerns about pollution, 'cancer-phobia,' suspicion of modern technology, and cynicism about 'the establishment.'

Faddists generally couch their claims in 'motherhood and the flag' types of values and symbols. Symbolism is very important to a person's food beliefs. Terms like 'health foods,' 'organic' and 'natural' have no scientific meaning but are important as emotional expressions of health consciousness, wholesomeness, purity and goodness. For instance, honey is generally regarded as natural and good while white sugar (which is very similar nutritionally) is thought to be artificial and 'bad'! When debunking such ideas, credit should be given to the merit that the idea *appears* to have; this avoids the appearance of being *against* these ideals.

Recognize freedom of choice

It should be made clear to patients that the ultimate choices and consequences are their own, and will be honored as such. Benefits the patient expects from a fad-dist regime should be identified, and alternate means of achieving them suggested. When these are balanced against negative factors such as unnecessary cost, long range ineffectiveness and potential harm to health, the decision should be clear to the patient. Patients may still choose unwisely, and if they do, the relationship should be maintained so that communication can continue.

Unless involved in a psychologically disrupting crisis, people generally change their attitudes slowly. Since it is doubtful that "perfect" dietary behavior can be realistically expected, it is imperative that efforts be directed toward these beliefs and practices that pose the greatest potential harm. The most critical of these is the feeling that orthodoxy cannot be trusted.

Be patient and tolerant

The unifying theme which unites all forms of quackery is a paranoid state of mind which promotes the notion that there are conspiracies to withhold cures for disease, to put poisons in our food and water for profit, and to maintain despotic power over the masses. Such thinking is central to the 'health foods' industry, which justifies its existence by fostering the belief that you can't trust the conventional food supply. This philosophy of distrust is a causal factor in practically all cases where people become the victims of serious quackery.

In regard to the Deluded, efforts to alter their beliefs and practices will be fruitless. Under such circumstances the only course of action remaining is to preserve the relationship and to cast the burden of proof for their erroneous beliefs and practices directly onto them.

FDA bans diet pill ingredients after nearly 20 years

After more than 17 years warning, the Food and Drug Administration has announced a final date for banning 111 diet pill ingredients as not generally recognized as safe and effective for over-the-counter (OTC) sales.

The ban includes arginine, kelp, lysine and phenylalanine, often listed in these pages as the ingredients in questionable diet products. Also banned is guar gum which FDA calls a safety hazard. After receiving reports of esophageal obstruction, the agency in July 1990 halted sales of Cal-Ban 3000, and has since taken action against other diet products containing guar gum.

Objections to the ban

Companies promoting the banned ingredients filed five objections to the FDA action. They contend that regulating OTC weight control drug products is unconstitutional, that FDA has no authority to regulate the purchase, sale, manufacture or labeling, and that consumers have the right of freedom of choice and a "health care" right to purchase any of these products.

In reply, FDA said: *Congress has concluded that the absolute freedom to choose an ineffective drug is properly surrendered in exchange for the freedom from the danger to each person's health and well-being from the sale and use of worthless drugs ... the surrender (of freedom to choose) is a rational decision which has resulted in achievement of greater freedom from dangers to health and welfare.*

FDA suggests these companies may reformulate their products or relabel them to delete claims for weight control, while continuing to market them as nutritional supplements. The agency says many companies that use the banned ingredients have their products manufactured and labeled for them by other companies specializing in this.

Monograph possible

Since this is not the long-awaited monograph called for by frustrated FDA agents and the health community, the ban allows the possibility of other ingredients being used, say officials. A monograph states which in-

---

History of ban on OTC diet pills

Aug. 27, 1975 – FDA calls for data on the safety and effectiveness of ingredients used in weight control products.

1982 – FDA publishes recommendations on regulating over-the-counter weight loss products. A total of 113 OTC weight control ingredients are classified. Two (PPA and benzocaine) are listed in **Category 1** – *safe and effective*. Eleven are in **Category 3** – *insufficient data*. The remainder are in **Category 2** – *not safe and effective for OTC use*.

Feb. 16, 1982 – FDA publishes advance notice of a proposal to establish a monograph for OTC weight control drug products.

May 27, 1982 – Deadline for submitting public comments (later extended to July 26).

March 26, 1990 – Congressman Ron Wyden, chairman of the U.S. House Small Business Subcommittee hearings on the weight loss industry, charges that the FDA and other regulatory agencies have abandoned many of their enforcement responsibilities. The proposal begun by FDA "nearly 20 years ago," still languishes at FDA, Wyden said. "We intend to get it dislodged."

May 7, 1990 – FDA announces its intention to propose a ban on more than 100 unproved ingredients used in nonprescription diet or appetite suppression drug products. (Not a monograph.)

October 30, 1990 – Proposal to ban is announced.

August 7, 1991 – FDA announces it will ban 111 diet pill ingredients not generally recognized as safe and effective for OTC sales.

February 10, 1992 – Ban will become effective.

Category I drugs (safe and effective)

1982 – PPA and benzocaine are designated Category I.

April 1, 1991 – FDA announces it is reopening the administrative record on PPA and benzocaine.

May 9, 1991 – FDA convenes a public meeting to discuss safety, effectiveness and abuse of PPA. Comment period remains open.

For further information contact: William E. Gilbertson, Center for Drug Evaluation and Research, FDA, 5600 Fishers Lane, Rockville, MD 20857 (301 295-8000)

OBESITY & HEALTH

Reprinted from *Obesity & Health,* Journal of Research, News and Contemporary Issues, Vol. 6, No. 1, January/February 1992, pp. 10-11. Copyright © 1992 by Health Living Institute, Hettinger, ND.

Nonprescription diet drug products banned

The following 111 ingredients are not generally recognized as safe and effective and are misbranded when present in over-the-counter weight control drug products.

Alcohol	Cnicus benedictus	Iodine	Pepsin	Threonine
Alfalfa	Copper	Isoleucine	Phenacetin	Tricalcium phos-
Alginic acid	Copper gluconate	Juniper, potassium	Phenylalanine	phate
Anise oil	Corn oil	extract	Phosphorus	Tryptophan
Arginine	Corn syrup	Karaya gum	Phytolacca	Tyrosine
Ascorbic acid	Corn silk, potassium	Kelp	Pineapple enzymes	Uva ursi-potassium
Bearberry	extract	Lactose	Plantago seed	extract
Biotin	Cupric sulfate	Lecithin	Potassium citrate	Valine
Bone marrow, red	Cyanocobalamin	Leucine	Pyridoxine hydrochloride	Vegetable
Buchu	(vitamin B$_{12}$)	Liver concentrate	(vitamin B$_6$)	Vitamin A
Buchu, potassium	Cystine	Lysine	Riboflavin	Vitamin A acetate
extract	Dextrose	Lysine hydrochloride	Rice polishings	Vitamin A palmi-
Caffeine	Docusate sodium	Magnesium	Saccharin	tate
Caffeine citrate	Ergocalciferol	Magnesium oxide	Sea minerals	Vitamin E
Calcium	Ferric ammonium	Malt	Sesame seed	Wheat germ
Calcium carbonate	citrate	Maltodextrin	Sodium	Xanthan gum
Calcium caseinate	Ferric pyrophoshate	Manganese citrate	Sodium bicarbonate	Yeast
Calcium lactate	Ferrous fumarate	Mannitol	Sodium caseinate	
Calcium pantothe-	Ferrous gluconate	Methionine	Sodium chloride (salt)	
nate	Ferrous sulfate (iron)	Methylcellulose	Soybean protein	
Carboxymethylcellu-	Flax seed	Mono- and di-glycerides	Soy meal	
lose sodium	Folic acid	Niacinamide	Sucrose	
Carrageenan	Fructose	Organic vegetables	Thiamine hydrochloride	
Cholecalciferol	Guar gum	Pancreatin	(vitamin B$_1$)	
Choline	Histidine	Pantothenic acid	Thiamine mononitrate	
Chondrus	Hydrastis canadensis	Papain	(vitamin B$_1$	
Citric acid	Inositol	Papaya enzymes	mononitrate)	

OBESITY & HEALTH;
FEDERAL REGISTER,
Aug 8, 1991, 56:153:37792-37797

gredients are allowable and bans *all* others.

The delay of a monograph on such an abused category of drugs is shocking, says Rep. Ron Wyden (D, Ore.). "But given the chaotic state of research on obesity and weight control this lapse was predictable."

Regional FDA director Don Aird, Minneapolis, is disappointed: "The most straight-forward way to handle this would be to say, 'There are only two ingredients which are acceptable – anything else is not.' That's what a monograph is all about."

However, FDA says this is a step in moving toward a monograph.

With a new chief at the helm of FDA there have been encouraging signs of the agency becoming more active in fighting fraud. David A. Kessler, MD, who took over as commissioner last No-

vember says, "People are being ripped off. We can't have an FDA inspector on every corner, but as an agency we'll

---

New chief at FDA says he'll crack down on quack products

---

do our part."

Kessler says he plans to crack down on purveyors of quack remedies.

PPA: safe and effective?

The ban does not include two other weight control ingredients, phenylpropanolamine (PPA) and benzocaine, which were listed as safe and effective by FDA in 1982. These are listed as ingredients in most weight control pills found on grocery and drug

store shelves. For example, of 27 products listed in an "appetite suppressant product table" in the latest edition of the *Handbook of Nonprescription Drugs,* all contain either PPA or benzocaine. FDA has reopened its investigation of PPA and benzocaine as nonprescription drugs for weight control. The agency is still accepting comments and reviewing information in regard to the safety, effectiveness and abuse of these two drugs.

Hearings on PPA were held May 9, with much testimony given both for and against its use by drug manufacturers and public health personnel.

(See O&H Jan/Feb 1991, page 9-12, for the case against PPA from the Wyden hearings.)

FRANCES M. BERG

Nutritional Supplements for Athletes?

Calories, Not Capsules, Enhance Performance

Kristine Napier

Kristine Napier, M.P.H., R.D., is a Cleveland-based freelance medical and science writer.

The 6th Century B.C. Greek Olympian wrestler, Milo of Crotona, was the first purported athlete to utilize unusual nutritional practices in his quest for greater physical prowess. Legend has it that daily he ate 20 pounds of meat and lifted a growing calf, essentially practicing progressive resistance training. When the calf reached four years of age, he supposedly carried her the length of the Olympia stadium, killed, roasted and ate her.

With a passion for victory, today's athletes also experiment with radical nutrition habits akin to Milo's daily 20 pounds of meat. They take preposterous quantities of protein, vitamin and mineral supplements hoping to enhance their performance, despite the lack of any evidence confirming the effectiveness of such practices.

Although some nutritional poppycock from magazine ads and on health food store shelves advises people to take supplements that are at most an innocuous placebo, other such advice catapults athletes into jeopardy. Indeed, these habits are as short-sighted as they are extreme. Athletes who engage in such activities, according to high performance nutritionist Susan Kleiner, Ph.D., R.D., are bartering tomorrow's health for today's glory.

Faulty Assumptions on Which Athletes Are Acting

The Protein Panacea—The overwhelming majority of athletes since Milo's days are under the mistaken assumption that extra animal muscle—protein—will augment their own musculature.* The great majority of Americans, however, consume at least as much protein as power-sport athletes need, and most athletes eat at least 300 percent of their recommended daily allowance (RDA) for protein *before* they beef up their diets with protein and/or amino acid supplements. In a word, protein is the nutrient most Americans, including athletes, get in the greatest excess.

Amino acid supplements (amino acids are the building blocks of protein) are one of the most popular ergogenic (work-enhancing) aids for endurance athletes and bodybuilders. Promoters claim that the supplements can do what anabolic-androgenic

*The RDA for protein is 0.8 grams per kilogram of body weight; athletes in power sports require slightly more, or 1.2 to 1.5 grams per kilogram. Three ounces of lean ground beef or white meat chicken without skin contain about 25 grams of protein, almost 40 percent of the daily requirement (64 grams) for a normally active 175 pound person.

steroids can, including build muscle, aid fat loss, provide energy and speed muscle repair. They're even superior, boast their manufacturers, because they're legal.

The great majority of Americans consume at least as much protein as power-sport athletes need, and most athletes eat at least 300 percent of their RDA for protein before *they beef up their diets with protein and/or amino acid supplements.*

Certain amino acids are even touted to have very specific, almost magical powers. Manufacturers promise athletes that the amino acids leucine, isoleucine and valine, called branched chain amino acids, are the body's preferred energy source during endurance exercise. There is absolutely no evidence to substantiate this claim. Extensive research confirms that carbohydrates are the body's most efficient energy source. When carbohydrate fuel sources are low, the body preferentially relies for fuel on branched chain amino aids stored in the liver (supplied in abundance from regular food), but only as the body's second choice.

From *Priorities*, Fall 1992, pp. 36-38. Reprinted with permission from *Priorities*, a publication of the American Council on Science and Health, New York, NY.

"SUPPLEMENTS" PROMOTED TO ATHLETES, ALL WITH NO KNOWN BENEFIT:

BIOFAVONOIDS: substances in foods that meet no nutritional need. Some are called vitamin P (erroneously) by faddists.

CELL SALTS: a mineral preparation supposedly prepared from living cells.

DNA (deoxyribonucleic acid): one of the genetic materials of cells.

GELATIN: a soluble form of the protein collagen, used to thicken foods.

GLYCINE: a nonessential amino acid, promoted as an ergogenic aid because it is a precursor of the high-energy compound phosphocreatine.

HERBAL STEROIDS: a mixture of herbs, falsely referred to as "adaptogens" or "aphrodisiacs," marketed with false claims that they contain hormones or enhance hormonal activity.

PHOSPHATE PILLS: pills of a salt that has been demonstrated to increase the levels in red blood cells of a metabolically important phosphate-compound (diphosphoglycerate) and increase the potential of the cells to deliver oxygen to the body's muscle cells.

RNA (ribonucleic acid): one of the genetic materials of cells, necessary in protein synthesis.

ROYAL JELLY: a substance produced by worker bees and fed to the queen bee.

SUPEROXIDE DISMUTASE (SOD): an enzyme made in cells that protects them from oxidative damage. When taken orally, the body digests and inactivates this protein enzyme.

WHEAT GERM OIL: oil extracted from wheat kernels, often falsely promoted as an energy booster.

Source: Whitney, Eleanor Noss. Nutrition Concepts and Controversies, *5th edition. New York: West Publishing, 1991.*

Other amino acids, especially arginine and ornithine, are marketed as growth hormone stimulators. The rationale is that growth hormone, naturally present in the body, causes muscle to grow larger. It does not, however, cause muscle strength to increase. Excess growth hormone, in fact, causes a condition called acromegaly, in which muscles become larger but weaker.

Athletes use the amino acid tryptophan and other B complex vitamins to stimulate brain chemicals that act as natural tranquilizers, believing this may calm their jitters and improve their performance. After April 1990, when more than 1,000 cases and about 20 deaths from ensinophilia myalgia, a serious muscle disorder, were reported among users of L-tryptophan, it should be clear that this, too, is dangerous. Even though products containing tryptophan were recalled at the request of the FDA in 1989, such products are still available.

Extra protein will not build muscle, stimulate production of growth hormone, calm jitters or provide a superior fuel for exercising muscles. There is simply no evidence that a well-nourished athlete needs protein or amino acid supplements, which are not only outrageously expensive but may be downright dangerous. Whether as amino acids or complete protein powders, excess protein can cause calcium loss, excessive weight gain, dehydration, gout and even liver and kidney damage. Furthermore, explains Joanne L. Slavin, Ph.D., R.D., professor of nutrition at the University of Minnesota, "Athletes should realize that single amino acid supplements in large doses have not been tested in humans, and therefore no margin for safety is available. Amino acids taken in large doses are essentially drugs with unknown physiological effects."

Vitamythology—Surveys indicate that nearly 100 percent of female and 90 percent of male athletes take vitamin/mineral supplements, believing them necessary for maximum performance. Extensive research verifies, however, that athletes consuming a well-balanced diet do not require vitamin/mineral supplements and, according to the American Dietetic Association, "There is no conclusive evidence of performance enhancement with intakes of any single nutrient or nutrient combination in excess of the RDA."

Because athletes consume so many calories—male football players and bodybuilders typically consume around 6,000 calories per day and female swimmers around 4,000—they generally consume at least 400 percent of the RDA before supplementation. Adding supplements may push athletes over the toxicity barrier and into the danger zone, especially for fat-soluble vitamins. (The exception may be female athletes or non-athletes who don't get enough iron and/or calcium, because of their dietary patterns.)

There is simply no evidence that a well-nourished athlete needs protein or amino acid supplements, which are not only outrageously expensive but may be downright dangerous.

Athletes are also lured by unscrupulous manufacturers into taking substances erroneously labeled as "vitamins" with promises of enhanced performance. Carnitine is promised to help burn fatty acids during a workout; wheat germ, especially its component octacosanol, is pushed as an overall performance enhancer; vitamin E is supposed to improve oxygen utilization at high altitudes; and vitamin B-15, marketed under a variety of names including calcium pangamate, is supposed to improve cardiovascular or metabolic responses during a workout. Runners are promised that bee pollen will help them recover faster after a workout, and spirulina, a microscopic blue-green alga, is promoted as a performance-enhancing supplement.

There is, however, no indication that any of these claims are true, and while the supplements are useless, they may not be harmless. Because vitamin E is stored in body fat, levels accumulate that could be toxic. Bee pollen may cause an allergic reaction in people who are sensitive to it, and spirulina is potentially toxic. Finally, there is little, if any, quality control on these products, and certainly no industrial or scientific standards for their production.

Why Does the Government Allow these Products?

Unfortunately, a 1975 Federal court ruling stripped FDA of its power to regulate nutritional supplements, except those for pregnant and lactating women and children under 12. The Federal Trade Commission does prohibit manufacturers from making claims about the purported benefit of products on their labels. But, manufacturers have weaseled around this by placing product pamphlets—which make all the false promises—in close proximity to the product. Another classic ploy is to position a feature article on a particular nutrient adjacent to an advertisement for that product. A close look would often reveal that the product is sold by the publisher of the magazine, who also wrote the "scientific" review of the product.

Healthy Alternatives

According to Dr. Kleiner, there are healthy alternatives. "For body builders, calories are by far the most important factor, and most people who want to build muscle simply don't get enough. Athletes continue to take excess protein, and often excess fat because of their exceptionally high meat intake, but still fall short of their calorie requirements. Not only do they not build muscle, but they wind up with unhealthy blood fat profiles because of their unhealthy eating practices."

Dr. Kleiner advises body builders to limit their protein intake to 1.2 to 1.6 grams of protein per kilogram of body weight, their fat to 20 percent of total calories, and to achieve a daily caloric intake of 4,500–5,000 for 155 pound males, 2,500–3,000 for the average 5' 4" female, making up the balance with complex carbohydrates such as whole grains, juices and pasta.

Sports medicine experts agree that all types of athletes, not just body builders, fail to appreciate the number of calories needed to support their athletic activity. Because they simply run out of energy, they don't perform as well as they might.

Jim Long, M.A., P.T., Director of Sports Medicine Rehabilitation at the Cleveland Clinic Foundation, reiterates the wisdom of getting enough calories in a healthy diet: "Instead of using supplements, be an improved eater. You need to spend only a fraction of the money you'd spend on supplements to have a nutritionally sound diet, and you'll have a far better outcome."

Hunger and Global Issues

The difference between a rich man and a poor man, is this—the former eats when he pleases, and the latter when he can get it.

—Sir Walter Raleigh

Not enough to eat! One in nine children goes hungry! Two hundred thousand face death in Ethiopia! Such are the headlines that greet us with the morning newspaper or the six o'clock news. Today's world is a paradox. On the one hand it is richer, more technologically advanced, and able to produce enough food for everyone and still have a surplus. Yet nearly 800 million people are always hungry and approximately 60 thousand die daily of hunger and its effects. Fifteen thousand of them are children.

Hunger hurts, but by the time one can see it in a child's eyes, he or she may no longer feel it. The damage done will depend upon the length and severity of the malnutrition and on when it occurs in the growth period. The effects may be found in behavior, physical growth, or mental development. It is impossible to determine the extent to which the child's recovery might be accomplished with appropriate intervention.

Death certificates of millions of children in the developing world list dysentery, measles, or other communicable diseases as the cause of death. But the same child living in the Western countries with adequate nutrition would have recovered quickly. Other countless millions suffer blindness, die from lack of vitamin A, get scurvy and pellagra, or are victims of protein-calorie deficiencies. Still others are cretins or will develop goiters like their parents.

A mother's nutritional status before and during pregnancy dramatically affects the outcome of that pregnancy. One good indicator of this is the infant mortality rate (IMR). An IMR greater than 50 is said to show that hunger exists as a chronic, society-wide condition. Worldwide the IMR is 68 infant deaths for every 1,000 live births. In Africa, where the average IMR is 99, only 6 of the 54 countries have IMRs less than 50. The rate in the United States has dropped to 9.0, while in Japan it is 4.6.

Other consequences of hunger and malnutrition can be found. An experimental study to determine the effects of starvation (article 64) produced dramatic changes in energy levels, work capabilities, and behaviors and is an eye-opener to the changes that take place. Also wide variances in life expectancies around the world can be partially explained by inadequate calories and nutrients. A person born in the United States can now expect to reach 75 years of age, 79 years in Japan. The global average is 65 years, but in Africa it is 53 years, and in Afghanistan it is only 41 years.

World food relief efforts are not sufficient, although many have been heroic. In fact, some critics argue that foreign food aid is part of the problem rather than the solution. It is commonly agreed that major problems of buying power, distribution, political decisions and policies, and environmental issues all contribute to defy a solution. Still, not all people have lost hope. In December 1992 the International Conference on Nutrition was held in Rome. A unique event, it grappled with ways to focus awareness and enthusiasm on realistic goals based in solid science, to establish an ongoing forum for discussion, and to create a collaborative effort in nutrition education (article 61).

Hunger has no geographical boundaries. It is not confined to Africa or Asia; it is also increasingly visible at home. Nor has it remained within class boundaries. With the recent economic recession people have lost jobs, and evidence of hunger has spread to the middle classes as well. In our country, 30 million are said to go to bed hungry, 50 percent higher than in the mid-1980s. In the average classroom, 4 children out of 30 do not have enough to eat. But, experts say, U.S. hunger differs from that in developing countries in that its cause is poverty uncomplicated by natural disasters, war, or an undeveloped economy. During the last decade, average incomes dropped for the very poor, those workers earning the lowest incomes increased by 50 percent, and the total number living below the official poverty line reached nearly 36 million. Furthermore, minorities represent a disproportionate number of the poor, equaling one-third of all African-American families and one-quarter of all Hispanics.

Many efforts have been made by the federal government (articles 62 and 63) to feed the needy. In 1992, $22 billion was spent on the Food Stamp Program to help feed 26 million Americans, nearly 10 percent of the population, but only half of those eligible. The intent of the Food Stamp Program is to supplement the family's food budget; instead it has become the only source of food for many. An additional $10.7 billion was spent on other antihunger programs such as school meals and the program for women, infants, and children (WIC). Total costs exceeded 1991 figures by $5 billion.

And still that is not enough. Congressional figures indicate that more than 20 million Americans rely on soup kitchens and food banks for food. Such private sector programs have multiplied all over the country, but the need sometimes exceeds the supply. Soup kitchens and emergency food ministries report turning people away or closing temporarily due to lack of supplies.

A disproportionate portion of our poor are also children. One Baltimore soup kitchen served 911 children in August 1992, nearly five times the number served in 1991. In Georgia, a Kids Kitchen has opened, and 5 more are slated to open in other parts of the country by year's end. Children line up each afternoon, 4-year-olds who arrive alone, 7-year-olds who bring their toddler siblings. It may be the only meal they eat. When summer arrives and there is no longer access to meals at school, the situation becomes even more serious.

Surveys show that voters are concerned. More than 60 percent of Americans surveyed agree that hunger is a serious and growing problem. Over one-third reported knowing someone who in the past year had not had enough to eat. More than 70 percent volunteer time or contribute money to feed hungry people. Half or more see hunger as a solvable problem and would be willing to pay $100 more in taxes to end hunger. This resolve can be seen in the Medford Declaration to End Hunger in the United States, which asserts that hunger in America can be virtually eliminated by 1995. More than 1,500 community and business organizations have supported this declaration, which focuses on the expansion of existing programs and efforts to improve purchasing power for the poor.

Mark Twain said that hunger is the handmaid of genius. Certainly the hunger felt or vicariously experienced by millions has aroused intense emotions of survival and compassion. Experts and ordinary citizens have been challenged to find solutions. Their tireless courage and successful efforts will provide the energy from which more victories will come.

Looking Ahead: Challenge Questions

What should be done to end hunger in the United States? Should the federal government spend more money to eradicate hunger?

What should be the roles of the United States and other developed countries in solving world hunger? To what extent should countries be expected to solve their own problems?

What criteria would you use to decide when to help another country and how much?

Some argue that we should all become vegetarians. Would this solve the hunger problem at home or abroad? What are the implications of changing the Western diet to one based on plants?

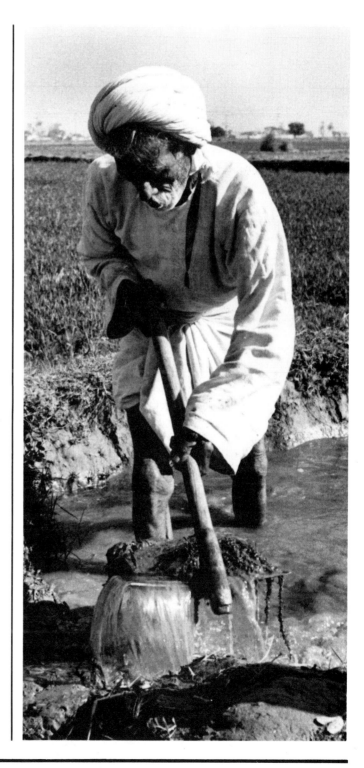

NUTRITION
WORLD HUNGER

Every day, hundreds of millions of people in the world go hungry, an appalling reality brought home to all of us most recently in the television images of Ethiopia and drought-stricken Africa. Hunger today is not, for the most part, caused by any shortfall in the earth's resources, but rather by a cycle of poverty, malnutrition, environmental degradation and poor agricultural policies that intensify traditional problems of harsh climates and low rainfall. In addition, in some areas of relative plenty, malnutrition can exist because of ignorance of basic nutritional needs.

These factors are partially the cause and partially the result of poverty. For example, people who cannot afford fuel cut down trees for firewood, which in turn contributes to environmental degradation, which in turn leads to reduced crop yields, which in turn increases both poverty and malnutrition.

There is no doubt that the technical, economic and financial resources to eliminate hunger in the world *do* exist today. But since the causes are various and complex, a comprehensive strategy will be necessary to end this scourge of mankind. The first step is learning to develop an awareness and an understanding of what human needs are, what resources are available to meet these needs and how best to use these resources.

Without nutritionally-satisfied bodies and minds, millions of people will continue to lead lives of hunger, want and pain. Those who survive may be crippled for life. The challenge now is to grasp the alternative, to use the great resources the world has available to conquer hunger and malnutrition.

THE SINISTER ALLIANCE:
Malnutrition and Infection

On a worldwide scale, almost half a billion people suffer from malnutrition. Nearly one child out of every ten children in the developing world dies before it reaches the age of five, and inadequate diet is a significant factor contributing to its death. But for this child . . . and the children of almost every poor village and neighborhood anywhere in the developing world . . . life and health are threatened by a common enemy. That enemy is the alliance of infection and malnutrition that strikes at the growth of both body and mind. Anemia, diarrhea, measles, chicken pox, pneumonia, whooping cough—minor, or at least controllable diseases in the United States—are routine causes of death for children already weakened by malnutrition.

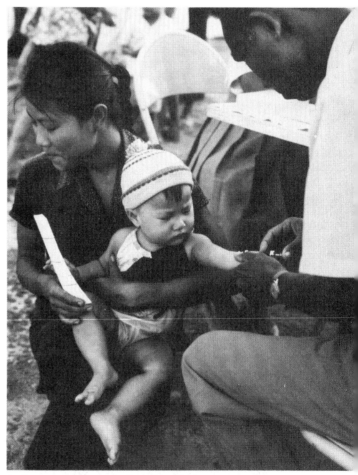

An important component of UNICEF's Child Survival and Development Revolution is immunization against polio, tetanus, diphtheria, measles, tuberculosis and whooping cough—the six major killers of children and a major cause of malnutrition. With other agencies, UNICEF is working toward the goal of Universal Immunization by 1990.   ICEF/4625/Jack Ling

The Struggle to Survive

Most of the 40,000 children who are now dying *each day* are dying not because they lost a battle, but because they lost a war—a long, losing war against the sheer frequency of assaults on their growth during their most vulnerable years. Each infection, whether it be measles or diarrhea

Reprinted by courtesy from *UNICEF*, 1993, pp. 1-5. *UNICEF*, U.S. Committee for UNICEF, 331 East 38th Street, New York, NY 10016.

or whooping cough, lowers the child's nutritional status and leaves the child weaker and more susceptible to further infection.

In the industrialized world, too, infection weakens children, burns up calories, reduces the absorption of nutrients, depresses the appetite and slows growth. But when the infection itself passes and appetite is regained, the child usually "catches up" the growth that has been lost. In other words, the part that illness plays in the story of the child's development is that of a temporary setback from which a full recovery is normally made.

In a poor community of the developing world, however, the whole relationship between illness, nutrition and a child's development is fundamentally different. Instead of being a temporary setback, an illness is often the first step towards an early death or, for the survivors, permanently-retarded growth.

The Downward Spiral

The self-perpetuating cycle of malnutrition and infection means that one setback follows another with a frequency that disrupts normal growth during the vital early years. The consequence, for hundreds of millions of children, is that never in their lives will they fulfill their own potential. And the result of that, in turn, is to set up another self-perpetuating cycle of poverty, whereby children who do not fulfill their potential for either mental or physical achievement are thereby condemned to remain in poverty and bring up their own children in circumstances where the cycle may well begin all over again. . . .

A UNICEF PRIORITY:
Preventing Malnutrition

UNICEF participates in programs to improve the lives of children in over 100 countries. Adequate nutrition is vital to the effectiveness of all these programs. The over-riding objective of UNICEF's efforts is to help nations use their own resources to combat dietary deficiencies and improve the health of their people, especially vulnerable children and mothers.

UNICEF's direct investment in nutrition programs is multiplied by many other health, clean water, educational and emergency relief operations, which contribute significantly to child nutrition. UNICEF assistance to nutrition programs includes:

• **Promoting growth monitoring, oral rehydration therapy, breast-feeding and immunization**, and providing food supplements for children and pregnant women;

• **Providing tools and seeds** in villages, for school and family orchards and vegetable gardens. Vegetables, soybeans and fruits are effective malnutrition fighters. Small gardens can mean the difference between adequate and inadequate diets for both rural and urban families;

• **Teaching practical nutritional information and hygienic food preparation at rural health centers and schools.** UNICEF's challenge is to show teachers and mothers how to improve the diet with inexpensive, locally-cultivated food. UNICEF-trained community nutrition workers and government nutrition personnel can now teach disadvantaged families how to prepare simple diet supplements that are within reach and can make a vital difference in their children's health;

• **Teaching practical farming methods;**

• **Stimulating village technology.** In many African countries, rural people are being introduced to easier work and cooking techniques. They are learning how to apply simple scientific methods, within their local cultures, to store and protect water and harvested crops. These improvements can prevent substantial food loss and the malnourishment it causes;

• **Stocking community fish and poultry farms;**

• **Combating specific nutritional diseases**, such as blindness, with vitamin A; goiter, with iodated salts; anemia, with iron supplements; and rickets, with vitamin D;

• **Distributing high-protein foods**, such as wheat flour, oats, skim milk and such special UNICEF food mixtures as CSM, a nutritious blend of corn meal, soy flour, minerals and non-fat dry milk; and K-Mix-II, consisting of casein, skim milk powder and sucrose, valuable in therapeutic feeding programs;

• **Coordinating the delivery of food supplies in emergencies.** In cooperation with other relief organizations, UNICEF provides food, transport and humanitarian assistance to children and mothers suffering from the effects of natural and/or man-made disasters;

• **Encouraging, with other international agencies, the establishment of national and global early warning systems against malnutrition and famine.** These surveillance systems could identify the major locations where additional help and information is needed to make nutrition policies and actions more effective. When

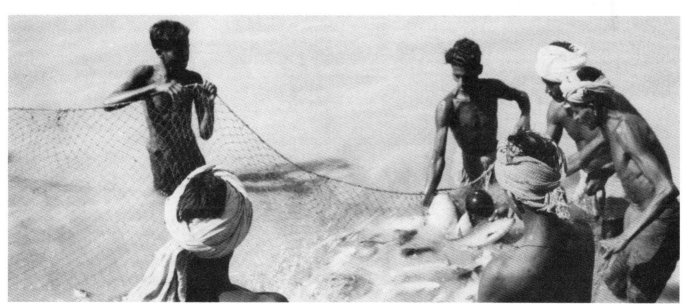

Villagers netting fish on a government fish farm in India. UNICEF assistance provides villagers with training in fish breeding in government programs designed to compensate the lack of animal protein and combat protein malnutrition.
ICEF/4308/Jack Ling

famine appears inevitable, these systems, signaling impending shortages, can use trained personnel to manage relief efforts and reduce the suffering and death of children.

Combating Child Malnutrition

• Most malnutrition is invisible and most parents of malnourished children do not know that there is anything wrong;

• Most malnourished children live in homes where there is no absolute shortage of sufficient food to provide an adequate diet for a small child;

• Most malnutrition is caused not so much by lack of food as by repeated infections that burn up calories, depress the appetite, drain away nutrients in vomiting or diarrhea and often induce mothers to stop feeding while the illness lasts.

In this context, the two most common failings of present efforts to combat child malnutrition are that they focus on the treatment of malnutrition rather than on its prevention, and that they do not sufficiently involve the mother in learning how to prevent malnutrition from recurring.

If the early signs of faltering growth could be made visible to the mother, and if at the same time she could be made aware of the special food needs of the very young child, then it would be possible to prevent perhaps half or more of all the child malnutrition in the developing world even within existing family incomes.

The Crisis in Africa

In many parts of Africa, the ravages of drought, famine and political conflict serve as dramatic reminders of how tragically vulnerable the poorest countries are. Worldwide media reports, focused on the nightmare of hunger and starvation that has besieged the people of Africa, have brought home all too painfully the extent of that vulnerability.

The crisis in Africa has been shaped by a number of factors. Chief among them are the global recession (which has hit Africa harder than any other continental area), widespread and protracted civil strife and a combination of local mismanagement and poor policies related to food production.

In good seasons today, Africa grows barely half its food needs. Population has been growing faster than domestic food production for at least a decade. More people raising ever-larger herds of cattle, goats and camels on marginal dry lands, destructive farming practices and the systematic cutting of wood for fuel have exposed millions of acres of otherwise productive land to erosion, making it vulnerable to the spreading northern deserts. Ecologists report that the Sahara has been expanding southwards at a rate of six to twelve miles a year for more than a decade.

When drought and famine reached alarming proportions in the Sahel in 1983 and 1984, victims, donors and agencies were ill-prepared. Obstacles ranged from the mobilization of aid to the transportation, storage and delivery of emergency supplies inland.

By the time help arrived, thousands already had perished, and millions more were abandoning their fields and villages for relief shelters and swelling shantytowns.

While substantial relief efforts helped millions survive in more than a dozen countries in 1984, African nations will not recover from their present plight and achieve some measure of self-sufficiency unless these efforts are accompanied by long-term commitments to domestic food production, self-sustaining, community-based services and development of human resources.

Perhaps somewhere between a half million and a million people will die in Africa in a 12-month period as a result of the current difficulties.

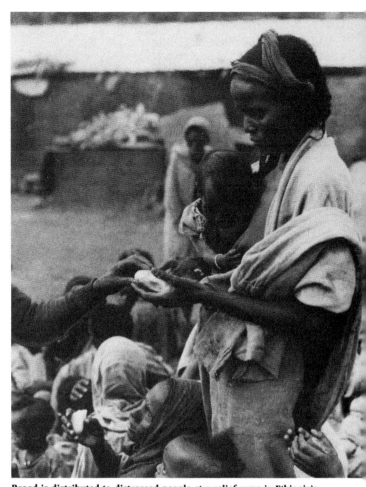

Bread is distributed to distressed people at a relief camp in Ethiopia's **Wollo Province. UNICEF assistance to governments of Africa's drought-stricken countries is aimed both at life-saving relief efforts and longer-term rehabilitation of the affected populations.   ICEF/7177/Adrian Clark**

That is a serious problem about which the world should rightly be concerned. But not many people are aware that *even if there were no drought* there would be some four to five million small children dying in Africa annually, largely from *quite readily avoidable, malnutrition-related problems.*

Thus, despite UNICEF's very deep involvement in a wide range of actions addressing many aspects of the current crisis in Africa, its primary task remains the implementation of developmental measures—rural water supply, primary health care, basic education, better food crops—that, coupled with its Child Survival strategies, are the only really effective antidote for saving children's lives in the long run.

Causes of Widespread World Hunger

• **Differing soils and climates.** The earth is not uniform. Many areas are incapable of sufficient food production because of poor soil, extremes of heat or cold and inadequate rainfall.

• **Population growth.** As the number of people living on earth increases, the demands on global food resources also rise. While these resources are limited, the current world population of 4.5 billion people is expected to double in 30 to 40 years.

• **Unsafe water.** Lack of clean water and proper sanitation affects over one billion people, who may suffer from diseases either contracted through or worsened by malnutrition.

• **Infestation and waste.** Plant diseases, rodents, insects and birds prey upon crops, leaving less for human consumption. Billions of tons of agricultural waste, most of which could be recycled for food production, pollute the environment each year.

• **Inadequate food production and distribution.** Lack of modern agricultural equipment and supplies, improper use of available resources and poor means of distribution prevent maximum growth and distribution of indigenous foods.

• **Lack of knowledge.** Many people simply do not understand the connection between proper nutrition and good health.

• **Natural and man-made disasters.** Drought, flood, misuse of land, deforestation, overgrazing and climate changes due to atmospheric pollution all produce food calamities. An ongoing calamity is desertification: 43 percent of the earth's total land surface is either desert or faced with desertification, and this figure increases every day.

• **Recession.** The worst effects of the recession in the industrialized world are being passed on, often multiplied many times over, to the poorest nations, where economic advance has been slowed, halted or even severely set back. And within these nations, it is the poor, and especially their children, who are the hardest hit.

• **Military spending.** In less than one day, the world spends more on armaments and military equipment than UNICEF has at its disposal for an entire year.

• **Export crops.** Many developing countries produce cash crops such as coffee and tea for export rather than grow food needed for their own populations.

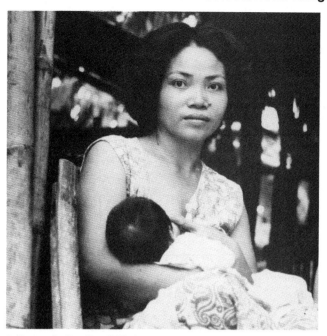

By breast-feeding her child, this young mother in the Philippines is providing her baby with the most nutritious and hygienic infant food. Breast-feeding offers a degree of immunity from infection and fosters the bonds of love between mother and child, as well as the baby's socio-psychological development.   **UNICEF Photo**

BREAST-FEEDING:
The Key to Infant Nutrition

Breast-feeding is the natural way to nourish infants. This simple fact has become blurred in the age of processed foods and reliance on infant formula, but the obvious nutritional and emotional link between mother's milk and children is regaining its once unchallenged position.

The exceptional nutritional quality of human milk has long been recognized. It is designed for easy digestion and has inherent anti-infective properties. The protective function of mother's milk is especially important in developing countries, where there is a high exposure to infection and where facilities for proper and sanitary preparation of infant formula are lacking or nonexistent.

The advantages of breast-feeding are many. It is economical; it is convenient—breast milk needs no preparation, is always ready at the right temperature; and it fosters the bonds of love between mother and baby as well as the baby's socio-psychological development.

Unfortunately, there was a significant worldwide decline in breast-feeding over the past few decades in both developed and developing countries. Apart from the nutritional and emotional inadequacies born out of this shift, ignorance of disease transmission through unsterile bottles or improperly prepared formulas can cause serious health problems among non-breast-feeding populations, especially in the developing world.

In 1981, the WHO/UNICEF "International Code of Marketing of Breast Milk Substitutes" was unanimously adopted by the World Health Assembly in recommendation form. The Code, which is designed to support breast-feeding and to regulate the marketing of artificial baby foods, was subsequently approved, and its implementation will mean that infants in many countries will not fall victim to the fashion for bottle-feeding.

Reversing the bottle-feeding trend is not an easy task. It means re-education not only of the general public, but of medical and health personnel. Programs to promote breast-feeding need the commitment of governments, with support from health, education, labor, judiciary and community development ministries.

In the past few years, there has been a noticeable revival of interest in breast-feeding and a growing awareness of its importance to the well-being of infants (and of mothers). This is an encouraging development that must be continued. . . .

World Declaration on Nutrition

Rome, December 1992

Editor's Note: From December 5 to 11, 1992, the International Conference on Nutrition was held in Rome, Italy, under the joint auspices of the Food and Agriculture Organization (FAO) and the World Health Organization (WHO). Official delegations from all the countries of the world met to consider, and eventually ratify, a Declaration and a Plan of Action for world nutrition that was meant to be a blueprint for eradicating hunger and malnutrition in the future. The conference was the culmination of more than two years of effort by international agencies and nongovernmental organizations. Such an event, with high-level participation of Ministers of Foreign Affairs, Health, and Agriculture from essentially all countries, occurs only once in a generation.

1. We, the ministers and the plenipotentiaries representing States and the EEC at the International Conference on Nutrition declare our determination to eliminate hunger and to reduce all forms of malnutrition. Hunger and malnutrition are unacceptable in a world that has both the knowledge and the resources to end this human catastrophe. We recognize that access to nutritionally adequate and safe food is a right of each individual. We recognize that globally there is enough food for all; inequitable access is the main problem. Bearing in mind the right to an adequate standard of living, including food, contained in the Universal Declaration of Human Rights, we pledge to act in solidarity to ensure that freedom from hunger becomes a reality. We also declare our firm commitment to work together to ensure sustained nutritional well-being for all people in a peaceful, just and environmentally safe world.

2. Despite appreciable worldwide improvements in life expectancy, adult literacy and nutritional status, we all view with the deepest concern the unacceptable fact that about 780 million people in developing countries—20 percent of their population—still do not have access to enough food to meet their basic needs for nutritional well-being.

3. We are especially distressed by the high prevalence and increasing numbers of malnourished children under five years in parts of Africa, Asia, and Latin America. Moreover more than 2000 million people, mostly women and children, are deficient in one or more micronutrients; babies continue to be born mentally retarded as a result of iodine deficiency; children go blind and die of vitamin A deficiency; and enormous numbers of women and children are adversely affected by iron deficiency. Hundreds of millions of women and children are adversely affected by iron deficiency. Hundreds of millions of people also suffer from communicable and non-communicable diseases caused by contaminated food and water. At the same time, chronic non-communicable diseases related to excessive or unbalanced dietary intakes often lead to premature deaths in both developed and developing countries.

4. We call on the United Nations to consider urgently the issue of declaring an International Decade of Food and Nutrition, within existing structures and available resources, in order to give additional emphasis towards achieving the objectives of this World Declaration on Nutrition. Such consideration should give particular emphasis to the food and nutrition problems of Africa, and of Asia, Latin America and the Caribbean.

5. We recognize that poverty and lack of education, which are often the effects of underdevelopment, are the primary causes of hunger and under-

Reprinted from *Nutrition Reviews*, Vol. 51, No. 2, February 1993, pp. 41-43. Copyright © 1993 by ILSI North America.

nutrition. There are poor people in most societies who do not have adequate access to food, safe water and sanitation, health services and education, which are the basic requirements for nutritional well-being.

6. We commit ourselves to ensure that development programmes and policies lead to a sustainable improvement in human welfare, are mindful of the environment and are conducive to better nutrition and health for present and future generations. The multifunctional roles of agriculture, particularly with regard to food security, nutrition, sustainable agriculture, and conservation of natural resources are of particular importance in this context. We must implement at family, household, community, national and international levels, coherent agriculture, animal husbandry, fisheries, food, nutrition, health, education, population, environmental, economic and social policies and programmes to achieve and maintain balance between the population and available resources and between rural and urban areas.

7. Slow progress in solving nutrition problems reflects the lack of human and financial resources, institutional capacity and policy commitment in many countries needed to assess the nature, magnitude, and causes of nutrition problems and to implement concerted programmes to overcome them. Basic and applied scientific research, as well as food and nutrition surveillance systems, are needed to more clearly identify factors that contribute to the problems of malnutrition and to identify the ways and means to eliminate these problems particularly for women, children and aged persons.

8. In addition, nutritional well-being is hindered by the continuation of social, economic and gender disparities; discriminatory practices and laws; floods, cyclones, drought, desertification and other natural calamities; and many countries' inadequate budgetary allocations for agriculture, health, education and other social services.

9. Wars, occupation, civil disturbances, natural disasters, as well as human rights violation and inappropriate socioeconomic policies, have led to tens of millions of refugees, displaced persons, war-affected non-combatant civilian populations, and migrants who are among the most nutritionally vulnerable groups. Resources for rehabilitating and caring for these groups are often extremely inadequate and nutritional deficiencies are common. All responsible parties should cooperate to ensure the safe and timely passage and distribution of appropriate food and medical supplies to those in need, in accordance with the charter of the United Nations.

10. Changing world conditions and reduction of international tensions improve the prospects for the peaceful solution of conflicts and give us an opportunity as never before to redirect our resources increasingly towards productive and socially useful purposes for ensuring the nutritional well-being of all people, especially the poor, deprived and vulnerable.

11. We recognize that nutritional well-being of all people is a pre-condition for the development of societies and that it should be a key objective of progress in human development. It must be at the centre of our socio-economic development plans and strategies. Success is dependent on fostering participation of the people and the community and multisectoral actions at all levels taking into account their long-term effects. Shorter-term measures to improve nutritional well-being may need to be initiated or strengthened to complement the benefits arising from longer-term development efforts.

12. Policies and programmes must be targeted toward those most in need. Our priority should be to implement people-oriented policies and programs that increase access to and control of resources by the rural and urban poor, raise their productive capacity and incomes, and strengthen their capacities to care for themselves. We must support and promote initiatives by people and communities, and ensure that the poor participate in decisions that affect their lives. We fully recognize the importance of the family unit in providing adequate food, nutrition and a proper caring environment for meeting the physical, mental, emotional and social needs of children and other vulnerable groups, including the elderly. In circumstances where the family unit can no longer undertake these responsibilities adequately the community and/or government should offer a support network to the vulnerable. We, therefore, undertake to strengthen and promote the family unit as the basic unit of society.

13. The right of women and adolescent girls to adequate nutrition is crucial. Their health and education must be improved. Women should be given the opportunity to participate in the decision-making process and to have increased access to and control of resources. It is particularly important to provide family planning services to both men and women and to provide support for women, especially working women, whether paid or unpaid, throughout pregnancy, breast-feeding and during the early childhood period. Men should also be motivated through appropriate education to assume an active role in promoting nutritional well-being.

14. Food aid may be used to assist in emergencies and provide relief to refugees and displaced persons, to support household food security and community and economic development. Countries receiving emergency food aid should be provided with sufficient resources to enable them to move on from the rehabilitation phase to development, so

7. HUNGER AND GLOBAL ISSUES

that they will be in a position to cope with future emergencies. Care must be taken to avoid creating dependency and to avoid negative impacts on food habits and on local food production and marketing. Before food aid is reduced or discontinued, steps should be taken to alert recipient countries as much in advance as possible so that they can identify alternative sources and implement other approaches. Where appropriate, food aid may be channeled through non-governmental organizations with local and popular participation, in accordance with domestic legislation of each country.

15. We affirm our obligations as nations and as an international community to protect and respect the needs for nutritionally adequate food and medical supplies for civilian populations situated in zones of conflict. We affirm in the context of international humanitarian law that food must not be used as a tool for political pressure. Food aid must not be denied because of political affiliation, geographic location, gender, age, ethnic, tribal or religious identity.

16. We recognize the fact that each government has the prime responsibility to protect and promote food security and nutritional well-being for its people, and especially to protect vulnerable groups. However, we also stress that such efforts of low-income countries should be supported by actions of the international community as a whole. Such actions should include an increase in official development assistance in order to reach the accepted United Nations target of 0.7 percent of the GNP of developed countries as reiterated at the 1992 United Nations Conference on Environment and Development.* Also, further renegotiation or alleviation of external debt could contribute in a substantive manner to the nutritional well-being in medium- as well as in low-income countries.

17. We acknowledge the importance of further liberalization and expansion of world trade, which would increase foreign exchange earnings and employment in developing countries. Compensatory measures will continue to be needed to protect adversely affected developing countries and vulnerable groups in medium- and low-income countries from negative effects of structural adjustment programmes.

18. We reaffirm the objectives for human development, food security, agriculture, rural development, health, nutrition and environment and sustainable development, enunciated in a number of international conferences and documents.** We reiterate our commitment to the nutritional goals of the Fourth United Nations Development Decade and the World Summit for Children.

19. As a basis for the Plan of Action and guidance for formulation of national plans of action, including the development of measurable goals and objectives within time-frames, we pledge to make all efforts to eliminate before the end of this decade:

• Famine and famine-related deaths;
• Starvation and nutritional deficiency diseases in communities affected by natural and man-made disasters;
• Iodine and vitamin A deficiencies.

We also pledge to reduce substantially within this decade:

• Starvation and widespread chronic hunger;
• Undernutrition, especially among children, women and the aged;
• Other important micronutrient deficiencies, including iron;
• Diet-related communicable and non-communicable diseases;
• Social and other impediments to optimal breast feeding;
• Inadequate sanitation and poor hygiene, including unsafe drinking water.

20. We resolve to promote active cooperation among governments, multilateral, bilateral, and non-governmental organizations, the private sector, communities and individuals to eliminate progressively the causes that lead to the scandal of hunger and all forms of malnutrition in the midst of abundance.

21. With a clear appreciation of the intrinsic value of human life and the dignity it commands, we adopt the attached Plan of Action and affirm our determination to revise or prepare, before the end of 1994, our national plans of action, including attainable goals and measurable targets, based on the principles and relevant strategies in the attached Plan of Action. We pledge to implement it.

---

* The developed countries reiterate their commitment to earmark 0.7 percent of their GNP to ODA—the figure set by the UN and approved by these countries, and, where this has not already been done, agree to reinforce their aid programmes so as to attain this target at the earliest possible date, and to follow up Agenda 21 as quickly and effectively as possible. Some countries have agreed to reach this target figure before the year 2000.

** The World Food Conference, 1974; the Alma Ata Conference on Primary Health Care, 1978; the World Conference on Agrarian Reform and Rural Development, 1979; the Convention on the Elimination of All Forms of Discrimination Against Women 1979, especially articles 12 and 13; the Innocenti Declaration on the Protection, Promotion and Support of Breastfeeding, 1990; the Montreal Policy Conference on Micronutrient Malnutrition, 1991; the Rio Declaration on Environment and Development, 1992.

HUNGER AND UNDERNUTRITION IN AMERICA

Visible signs of widespread hunger include the nationwide demand for emergency food distributed by soup kitchens, food pantries, and other charitable organizations, and the rise in the homeless population, especially families with children (3,4).

HUNGER

Attention to hunger as a major social problem in the United States is not new (1,2). In the 1960s, problems of hunger led the federal government to create new and expand existing programs to alleviate hunger such as the Food Stamp Program, the School Lunch and Breakfast programs, and the Special Supplemental Food Program for Women, Infants, and Children (WIC) (3,4).

These programs were successful in significantly reducing hunger and malnutrition by 1980. However, during the 1980s, cutbacks in federal spending for many food assistance programs and other programs for the poor and unemployed, increases in food prices, and inflationary economics contributed to a resurgence of hunger (3,4).

This *Digest* focuses on the prevalence and ramifications of hunger in the U.S., especially among children. This issue also addresses the role of federal food assistance programs in alleviating this preventable, tragic problem.

Recent surveys provide more quantitative evidence of the hunger epidemic in America. These surveys include ones carried out by the Food Research and Action Center (FRAC), a Washington, DC-based anti-hunger advocacy group (2), the Physician Task Force on Hunger in America (5), and the U.S. Conference of Mayors (1). Today, hunger is recognized as a serious national health problem (1,2,5,6). Health professionals, policy makers, and the general public are particularly concerned about the rise in hunger among children (6,7).

How Is Hunger Defined? Lack of a universal definition of hunger can pose a problem when identifying and determining the prevalence of hunger (4). A joint Task Force on Hunger and Malnutrition initiated by the American Institute of Nutrition and the American Society for Clinical Nutrition in 1988 defined hunger as "...a recurrent, involuntary lack of access to food" (8). If prolonged, hunger may produce malnutrition (8). According to The American Dietetic Association (6), hunger is "...discomfort, weakness, or pain caused by lack of food."

Medical experts generally agree that hunger is the mental and physical condition that results from insufficient food (and nutrients) necessary for growth and health (2,4,9,10). Hunger can be relieved quickly with food. However, if prolonged, it can increase risk of undernutrition (10).

What Causes Hunger? The cause of hunger is more complex than simply insufficient food. Many diverse, interrelated factors contribute to this condition. According to the 1991 U.S. Conference of Mayors Survey (1), employment-related problems such as layoffs, low wages, and lack of skills are leading causes of hunger. Other contributing factors include:
- Poverty or inadequate income. The recent recession has led to the growing number of "suddenly poor" and maintained the number of individuals who are "chronically poor" (1,6). Over 13 million children under 18 years of age live in poverty (11). Poverty is a root cause of hunger (4,6).
- Lack of affordable housing. Many poor families spend a huge proportion of their income on housing, leaving insufficient

Reprinted from *Dairy Council Digest,* Vol. 63, No. 2, March/April 1992, pp. 8-12. Copyright © 1992 by the National Dairy Council, Rosemont, IL.

money for food. The U.S. Department of Housing and Urban Development defines affordable housing as costing less than 30 percent of income. Fifty-six percent of all poor renters spend at least half of their income on shelter, and 81 percent are paying 30 percent or more (12).

- A social-welfare system that provides insufficient help (1,4). For example, benefits in the Aid to Families with Dependents' Program, the nation's primary public assistance program, declined 36 percent from 1972 to 1990, after adjusting for inflation (13).
- Mental illness and inadequate mental health services.
- Substance abuse and limited substance abuse services.
- Federal, state, and local budget cuts.

How Prevalent Is Hunger? The 1985 Physician Task Force estimated that hunger affects 20 million Americans, or one in twelve (5). The prevalence of hunger among Americans has increased dramatically during the past year (1,2). The demand for emergency food assistance increased by an average of 26 percent between 1990 and 1991, according to a recent U.S. Conference of Mayors survey on hunger in 28 major cities (1). Children and their parents account for more than two-thirds of those requesting emergency food assistance (1). Unfortunately, available resources (food, funds, volunteers) are insufficient to meet the needs of these hungry people (1).

Startling high levels of hunger were identified in FRAC's Community Childhood Hunger Identification Project (CCHIPS) (2). One in eight American children under 12 years of age is hungry and millions more are at risk of going hungry, according to findings of this survey (2).

CCHIP researchers interviewed members of 2,335 low-income families (incomes at or below 185% of federally defined poverty guidelines) with children under 12 years of age in seven sites across the country (2). Families were asked whether lack of money in the previous year caused them to cut food portions, skip meals, limit the number of foods served, or send children to bed hungry (2). Respondents who answered "yes" to five out of eight questions were defined

as "hungry," while those who answered "yes" to any one question were defined as "at risk" of hunger (2). This door-to-door survey documented both chronic food shortages and associations between hunger and child health problems.

The homeless are at high risk of hunger (14-16). Nearly six times as many homeless children as housed poor children said that they were "fairly often" or "always" hungry because their families ran out of food, according to a recent study conducted in Los Angeles, California (14). Children comprise the fastest growing segment of the homeless population (17). In the cities surveyed by the U.S. Conference of Mayors (1), children accounted for 24 percent of the homeless population. Homeless children from large families and from families with single mothers are particularly at high risk of hunger and its long-term consequences such as growth stunting (16).

Lack of food, inadequate diets, poor nutritional status, and infections are common among homeless people (15). This situation has led to efforts to increase the availability of health and nutrition services to the homeless, especially families with children (15).

Manifestations of Hunger. Although hunger can affect everyone, pregnant women, infants, children, and the elderly are most vulnerable to the adverse effects of hunger (6). Hunger can exert both short-term and long-term negative effects on health and behavior (1,2,4,6,8,9,18,19).

Studies in the 1970s and 1980s concluded that short-term hunger due to lack of breakfast adversely affects emotional behavior, arithmetic and reading ability, and physical work output (9,18-20). Hunger resulting from missing a meal such as breakfast can reduce a child's ability to respond to the environment and to acquire information (9). As a result, a hungry child does not pay as much attention or learn as rapidly as a well-fed child (9,21,22). Apathy, disinterest, irritability, and a low tolerance for frustration are behaviors common in hungry children (6,8).

Hungry children who receive food supplements are better able to learn (9). In the National Evaluation of the Special Supplemental Food Program for Women, Infants,

In all, 11.5 million children under 12 years of age in the U.S. are hungry or at risk of hunger (2). Hunger interferes with children's ability to learn.

and Children (WIC) (23), children who received the WIC food supplement exhibited an increased attention span and were less irritable, and more creative (all characteristics conducive to learning).

If prolonged, hunger can increase the risk of undernutrition and contribute to low birth weight in infants, reduced rate of growth in height in children, and a low resistance to infection (reduced immune response) (2, 4,6). In addition to growth impairment and increased morbidity, chronic hunger may adversely affect social-emotional performance and cognitive function (1,2,8).

FRAC's CCHIP survey found that hungry children experienced more health problems such as unwanted weight loss, fatigue, irritability, dizziness, frequent headaches, colds, ear infections, and concentration problems than children who were not hungry (2). These problems in turn affected school attendance. Hungry children missed an average of one and a half more days of school a year than other children (2).

FEDERAL FOOD ASSISTANCE PROGRAMS

Food assistance programs, administered by USDA's Food and Nutrition Service in cooperation with State and local governments, are responding to the resurgence of hunger in America (10,24). These programs are designed to improve the health and nutritional well-being of all participants.

Included among these programs are the Food Stamp Program, WIC, the National School Lunch Program, and the School Breakfast Program (10,24).

Other important programs include the Child and Adult Care Food Program which provides financial and commodity assistance for meals served in child care centers and group day care homes; the Special Milk Program which encourages consumption of milk by school children; the Summer Food Service Program for Children which targets children from low-income areas; and the Commodity Supplemental Food Program, a companion program to WIC that also serves a limited number of elderly participants (10).

The Food Stamp Program. The Food Stamp Program is the largest of the federal food assistance programs, both in terms of the amount of money spent and people served. Between 1990 and 1991, federal expenditures for, and participation in, this program increased 23 and 15 percent, respectively (25). In October 1991, 24.16 million people participated in the program, up 400,000 from a month earlier, and up 3.23 million from a year earlier (Fig., 25). More than half of all food stamp recipients are children and over 80 percent of the benefits go to families with children (2).

Started in the early 1960s, the Food Stamp Program issues coupons to eligible low-income households to purchase food at retail stores (24). Food stamp benefits, which are received on a monthly basis, are adjusted annually, based on the cost of USDA's Thrifty Food Plan for a family of four (24). The Food Stamp Program is available to most of the nation's poor. However, many eligible people fail to participate because of bureaucratic barriers, ignorance about eligibility, and embarrassment to use food stamps (2).

The Special Supplemental Food Program for Women, Infants, and Children (WIC). Similar to the Food Stamp Program, WIC funding and participation have grown rapidly. Between October 1990 and 1991, federal expenditures for WIC increased 12.5 percent (25). And WIC participation averaged 5.3 million in October 1991, compared to 4.6 million a year earlier (Fig.,25). Launched in 1974, WIC is designed to improve the health and nutritional status of low-income, nutritionally at-risk pregnant women, infants, and children up to five years of age (10). Participants receive monthly vouchers to be exchanged for foods such as iron-fortified infant formula, eggs, fruit juices with vitamin C, milk, cheese, and cereal. The program also offers nutrition education and referrals to health services (10). As part of the Hunger Prevention Act of 1988, WIC services have been expanded to reach eligible homeless mothers, infants, and children (10).

WIC is effective in improving maternal

In the last year alone, federal expenditures for food assistance programs increased dramatically in an effort to alleviate hunger (24,25).

health, pregnancy outcome, and the health and nutritional intake of preschool children (23). Although the program has grown over the years, not all eligible persons receive WIC benefits (10). At present, WIC serves just over one-half of those who are eligible.

The National School Lunch Program (NSLP).
In October 1991, 24.9 million children participated in the NSLP (Fig.,25). Not only does this number exceed the level of participation in 1990, but it also is greater than the average daily participation for any year since 1981. Over one-half or 51 percent (12.7 million) of all children who ate school lunches in October 1991 received these meals at no cost or at a substantially reduced price (25).

The NSLP, established in 1946, is available to all school districts which choose to participate. Food served under the NSLP must meet federal "meal pattern" requirements regarding specific amounts of foods (i.e., milk, meat/meat alternate, vegetable/fruit, bread/bread alternate) (10). The goal of the NSLP is to provide approximately one-third of children's Recommended Dietary Allowances for nutrients and calories (10,26). Eligibility for free and reduced-price meals is determined by household size and income (10).

The School Breakfast Program (SBP).
The SBP has grown steadily since the early 1980s (24). In October 1991, the program served daily breakfasts to 4.9 million students in 46,000 schools (Fig.,25). Nearly 90 percent (87.2 percent) of the breakfasts served were free or at a reduced price (25). Although the SBP recently has grown in participation, less than half of the schools nationwide offer this program (2).

Studies indicate that eating breakfast improves academic performance (18-22, 27). A 1987 study of over 1,000 low-income children in grades three through six linked participation in the SBP over a semester with improvements in standardized achievement test scores, fewer school absences, and reduced tardiness (21).

The effect of breakfast on cognitive functions appears to be influenced by

children's nutritional status (27), the size and composition of the breakfast (28,29), the length of participation in the breakfast program (21,29), and the cognitive function studied (28). One study found that increasing the size of adolescents' breakfast enhanced short-term memory but decreased concentration (28). The authors emphasize the need to measure several aspects of behavior (28).

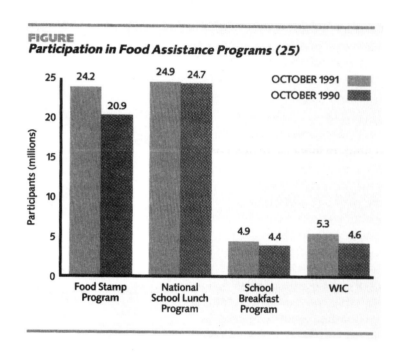

FIGURE
Participation in Food Assistance Programs (25)

In addition to breakfast's positive effect on learning, findings of a preliminary study suggest that children who consume breakfast, particularly a ready-to-eat cereal with fiber, have lower blood cholesterol levels than children who regularly skip breakfast (30).

SOLVING THE HUNGER PROBLEM

A number of measures are being taken to increase benefit levels and remove barriers to participation in existing federal programs (1,6,31). For example, a universal school lunch and breakfast program is being experimentally operated in selected sites nationwide. Congress could make lunch and breakfast available to all elementary schools nationwide without charge, provided that the schools participate in the program (31). Among its advantages, this program would fight childhood hunger without the welfare stigma attached to current programs.

FRAC, in partnership with other local and national organizations, has initiated a Campaign to End Childhood Hunger. Goals of this campaign focus on increasing participation in the Food Stamp Program, WIC, NSLP, and SBP. For example, FRAC is urging more schools that offer the school lunch program to also offer breakfast. The SBP is one of the most beneficial, but underused federal nutrition programs. Fewer than half (48.8 percent) of the schools that offer lunch also offer breakfast (32). And although almost 12 million school children receive free or reduced price school lunches, less than one-third of them receive school breakfast. Many schools are reluctant to adopt the SBP, citing financial barriers, problems with transportation, and the belief that breakfast is a family meal.

The federal government also is committed to expanding the SBP. The USDA has provided Congressionally-mandated grants to a number of school districts to help start school breakfast programs ($3 million for 1990 and $5 million for each year through 1994) (33). Partly as a result of these grants, participation in the SBP increased 15 percent between 1989 and 1991 (33).

REFERENCES

1. The United States Conference of Mayors. *A Status Report On Hunger And Homelessness In America's Cities: 1991. A 28-city survey.* December, 1991. Washington, DC: The U.S. Conference of Mayors, 1991.

2. Food Research and Action Center. *Community Childhood Hunger Identification Project. A Survey of Childhood Hunger in the United States.* Executive Summary. Washington, DC: Food Research and Action Center, March 1991.

3. Mayer, J. J. Nutr. *120:* 919, 1990.

4. Brown, J.L. Sci. Am. *256:* 37, 1987.

5. Physician Task Force on Hunger in America. *Hunger in America: The Growing Epidemic.* Boston, MA: Harvard University School of Public Health, 1985.

6. The American Dietetic Association. J. Am. Diet. Assoc. *90:* 1437, 1990.

7. Anonymous. Survey shows public concern for child hunger. CNI *21(49)* Dec. 13: 3, 1991.

8. Dietz, W.H., and F.L. Trowbridge. J. Nutr. *120:* 917, 1990.

9. Allen, L.H. J. Nutr. *120:* 924, 1990.

10. Child Nutrition Programs: Issues of the 101st Congress. School Food Service Research Rev. *131(1):* 3, 1989.

11. U.S. Department of Health & Human Services, Public Health Service, Health Resources and Services Administration, Office of Maternal and Child Health. *Child Health USA '90.* HRS-M-CH 90-1. October 1990.

12. *A Place to Call Home: The Low Income Housing Crisis Continues.* Center on Budget and Policy Priorities and Low Income Housing Coalition. Washington, DC, December 1991.

13. Committee on Ways and Means. U.S. House of Representatives. *Overview of Entitlement Programs.* May 7, 1991.

14. Wood, D.L., R.B. Valdez, T. Hayashi, et. al. Pediatrics *86:* 858, 1990.

15. Wiecha, J.L., J.T. Dwyer, and M. Dunn-Strohecker. Public Health Reports *106(4):* 364, 1991.

16. Fierman, A.H., B.P. Dreyer, L. Quinn, et. al. Pediatrics *88:* 918, 1991.

17. Anonymous. CNI *21(47)* Nov. 29: 6, 1991.

18. Pollitt, E., R.L. Liebel, and D. Greenfield. Am. J. Clin. Nutr. *34:* 1526, 1981.

19. Pollitt, E., N.L. Lewis, C. Garza, et. al. J. Psychiatr. Res. *17:* 169, 1982-1983.

20. Radzikowski, J., and S. Gale. Am. J. Clin. Nutr. *40:* 454, 1984.

21. Meyers, A.F., A.E. Sampson, M. Weitzman, et. al. Am. J. Dis. Child. *143:* 1234, 1989.

22. Meyers, A.F., A.E. Sampson, and M. Weitzman. Clin. Appl. Nutr. *1(2):* 13, 1991.

23. The National WIC Evaluation: Evaluation of the Special Supplemental Food Program for Women, Infants, and Children. Am. J. Clin. Nutr. *48 (Suppl):* 389, 1988.

24. Matsumoto, M. Food Rev. *14(3):* 43, 1991.

25. USDA, Food and Nutrition Service, Program Information Division, Data Base Monitoring Branch. Preliminary summary of food assistance program results for October 1991. December 23, 1991.

26. Committee on Dietary Allowances, Food and Nutrition Board, National Research Council. *Recommended Dietary Allowances,* 10th ed. Washington, DC: National Academy Press, 1989.

27. Simeon, D.T., and S. Grantham-McGregor. Am. J. Clin. Nutr. *49:* 646, 1989.

28. Michaud, C., N. Musse, J.P. Nicolas, et. al. J. Adol. Health *12:* 53, 1991.

29. Cromer, B.A., K.J. Tarnowski, A.M. Stein, et. al. Developmental & Behavioral Pediatr. *11(6):* 295, 1990.

30. Resnicow, K. J. Sch. Health *61(2):* 81, 1991.

31. American School Food Service Association. Universal vision: preparing the nation's children for school. October 16, 1991.

32. Food Research and Action Center. *School Breakfast Score Card.* Washington, DC: Food Research and Action Center, February 1992.

33. U.S. Department of Agriculture. USDA awards grants for school breakfast programs in 30 states. Ag New Fax July 17, 1991.

ACKNOWLEDGMENTS

National Dairy Council® assumes the responsibility for this publication. However, we would like to acknowledge the help and suggestions of the following reviewers in its preparation:

■ D. Derelian, M.S., R.D.
Educator-Consultant
Health Professions Training
Fallbrook, California

■ R.J. Fersh
Executive Director, and
L. Parker
Director of Nutrition Policy & Research
Food Research and Action Center
Washington, DC

The *Dairy Council Digest*® is written and edited by Lois D. McBean, M.S., R.D.

"Aggressive action is needed to bring an end to domestic hunger and to achieve food security for all citizens," says The American Dietetic Association in its recent position statement on hunger (6).

Hunger in the United States: Policy Implications

Marion Nestle, Ph.D., M.P.H. and
Sally Guttmacher, Ph.D.

Dr. Nestle is Professor and Chair, Department of Nutrition, Food and Hotel Management; Dr. Guttmacher is Associate Professor, Department of Health Studies, New York University, New York, NY 10003.

U.S. Hunger Policies

The Beginnings of U.S. Food Policies

The roots of present hunger policies in the United States reach back to the Great Depression of the 1930s, when unemployment, soup kitchens, and breadlines abounded and large quantities of surplus food were destroyed because the poor could not afford to buy it. In 1930, acting on legislation passed by Congress, the U.S. Department of Agriculture and the newly created Federal Emergency Relief Administration began distributing surplus farm products as food relief, thus helping farmers while feeding the poor.[1] A more formal oversight of farm prices and production was authorized in 1933, and a food-distribution program was instituted in 1935. In 1936 the first school lunch program utilized surplus commodities donated to state-supported schools, and from 1939 to 1943 an experimental food stamp program permitted exchange of vouchers for surplus commodities and other foods. With the rise in war-stimulated employment and the decline in surplus foods as U.S. production was shipped abroad to the armed forces and the Allies, the 1946 National School Lunch Act stipulated that a consider-

able portion of its food aid be cash instead of commodities. Through the 1930s and early 1940s, the major aim of food distribution programs was to dispose of surplus agricultural products rather than to feed the poor.[2]

The War on Hunger

During the 1950s and early 1960s, the majority of U.S. citizens paid little attention to growing reports of poverty and hunger in America. The nation had become prosperous, a national food-distribution system had been established with the highway network begun in the Eisenhower administration and the growth of supermarkets, and it was generally assumed that every American was well fed. In 1961, however, President Kennedy outlined a program to expand food distribution and to establish eight pilot food stamp programs in selected "poverty" areas. In 1964 the program became available nationally; in 1966 the School Breakfast Program was instituted.

Nevertheless, it was not until 1968 that a written report from the Field Foundation, *Hunger U.S.A.,*[3] and the release of a nationwide television documentary, *Hunger in America,* based on its findings, brought the issue of hunger to national attention and action. The foundation had sent a team of physicians, legislators, and other concerned citizens to more than 250 "hunger counties" in 23 states. Their report described widespread malnutrition and poverty and called for immediate expansion of federal efforts to improve food assistance to the poor. The U.S. Senate appointed a bipartisan Select committee on Nutrition and Human Needs to lead its anti-hunger efforts. From 1968 to 1977, the Committee initiated legislation that expanded food assistance for families, children, and the elderly.[4] In 1969,

Reprinted from *Nutrition Reviews,* Vol. 50, No. 8, August 1992, pp. 242-245. Originally from *Journal of Nutrition,* 1992, 24:18S-22S. Copyright © 1992 by the Society for Nutrition Education.

President Richard M. Nixon announced a "war on hunger," and called a White House Conference on Food, Nutrition, and Health to advise on national policies to eliminate hunger and malnutrition caused by poverty.[5]

During the 1970s, cash subsidies and vouchers gradually replaced commodities in federal food programs as part of an evolving strategy to increase the purchasing power of the poor. The food stamp program was expanded, the Women, Infants, and Children Program (WIC)—of which the Special Supplemental Food Program was a part—and other child food assistance programs were created, and nutrition programs were developed for the elderly. Between 1969 and 1977, annual federal expenditures for food assistance increased from $1.2 to $8.3 billion,[4] and by 1979 donated farm products accounted for less than 10% of total federal expenditures on food programs.[2] In 1977, the Field Foundation sent a team (with some of the same members of the earlier team) back to the "hunger counties" surveyed a decade before. The team found fewer cases of overt malnutrition, and concluded that although some hunger remained evident, its manifestations had become more subtle and, therefore, more difficult to identify.[6]

Hunger Studies

At the beginning of the 1980s, new national policies shifted a greater degree of responsibility for social programs from the federal government to the states and the private sector. A series of legislative acts passed in 1981 and 1982 led to significant reductions in the benefits that had, at least in part, sheltered vulnerable groups from fluctuations in the business cycle. Because these reductions occurred at the same time as an economic recession, their impact was especially severe. Emergency food and shelter providers began to report an increasing use of their services by the "new poor": children, unskilled and unemployed youths, families with insufficient resources, and the deinstitutionalized mentally ill.

In response, agencies and organizations in the public and private sectors began to document the increasing demands for food assistance through studies of hunger prevalence. Many of these reports are available only as unpublished manuscripts of limited distribution. The largest hunger study collection of which the authors are aware is that of the Food Research and Action Center (FRAC) in Washington, D.C. Although incomplete, it lists nearly 250 reports released since the early 1970s from 40 states, the District of Columbia, and Canada.[7] The index to this collection reflects the rapid impact of the reductions in welfare spending initiated early in the decade. It lists three studies in

1981, 19 in 1982, 31 in 1983, 40 in 1984, and an additional 30 or so for each of the three subsequent years. The most recent studies were published in 1991.

The most widely publicized of these reports is a study issued in 1985 by the Physician Task Force on Hunger in America. The report defined hunger in economic terms: individuals were at risk if their income fell below the poverty line or if their food stamp benefits were inadequate.[8] By these criteria, 20 million people in the U.S. were said to be suffering from hunger.*

Methodologic Issues

Hunger studies have been ignored or greeted with skepticism by local and federal policymakers, who argue that signs of malnutrition occur only rarely in the U.S. population and that federal funding for assistance to the poor has increased greatly over the years.[9] Critics point out that federal expenditures for Department of Agriculture food assistance alone exceeded $21 billion and provided benefits to more than 40 million individuals in 1989.[10]

More important for this discussion is the claim by critics that the methods used to define and identify hunger rarely meet accepted standards of scientific proof, are anecdotal, and therefore greatly exaggerate the prevalence of this condition.[11] This charge is not easy to address directly. Federal nutrition monitoring surveys do not yet measure the prevalence of hunger in the U.S. population, nor do they sample homeless people, migrant families, or certain other groups that might be expected to have limited access to food.[12] The national surveys listed in the FRAC Index provide only limited data on participation rates in food assistance programs or on poverty rates in selected cities. Although the development of standards and means of measurement that more accurately portray hunger and poverty has long been recommended,[9] the response has been slow. Because most hunger studies were conducted by advocates rather than by scientists, they often lack the systematic documentation, precise definitions, consistent study methods, and appropriate sampling techniques necessary for a determination of their reliability or applicability to large populations.

Measuring the extent of hunger is exceedingly difficult. No easily defined line of causality exists between hunger, biochemical indices of malnutrition, poor health, and disease. Chronic hunger over a substantial time may lead to undernutrition and disease, but the health effects of episodic hunger remain uncertain. Because it is difficult—and very

---

*12 million children and 8 million adults.

expensive—to measure clinical or biochemical indices of malnutrition in population surveys, few hunger studies have done so. Instead, researchers and advocates have identified a range of indirect measures of food insecurity, such as the level of poverty or unmet needs for food assistance, that can be used as indicators of hunger and malnutrition. Although each of these measures is imperfect, any one of them can be used to estimate the extent of hunger in a population. Furthermore, the use of multiple indicators should increase the reliability of such estimates.[13]

State Hunger Surveys

The lack of a coherent federal policy to deal with hunger is, in part, a result of the paucity of national prevalence data. Thus, to develop policy recommendations based on the largest population surveys, the authors selected for analysis hunger studies that had been sponsored by state governments, identified from the FRAC Index and from private collections. These studies included 28 hunger surveys that had been authorized by the governors or legislatures of 18 states. Excluded from the analysis were studies restricted to specific age groups (e.g., children), or populations (e.g., users of soup kitchens). When a state had conducted more than one study, either the most recent or the one that had employed the broadest range of hunger indicators was selected. The final sample consisted of studies authorized by 11 states between 1984 and 1988.[14–24]

Analysis of these studies provides a broader perspective on hunger issues than can be obtained from local community surveys and as much of a national perspective as is available at the present time. The studies employed a variety of methods to estimate the extent of hunger and food insecurity in their populations. All had collected subjective information on professional or personal experience with the hunger problem[16–18,20,21,23] or responses to questionnaires or interviews.[14,15,19–22,24] Some had conducted secondary analyses of state data on poverty levels,[16,18] the prevalence of conditions related to undernutrition,[16,18,22] or the use of public and private food and income assistance programs.[14,16,19,23] One study[24] had used the standardized sampling and survey methods of the Community Childhood Hunger Identification Project.[25]

Despite these diverse methods, the findings were similar. Without exception, the state studies found hunger and food insecurity to be problems affecting large numbers of their people. All reported increasing demands for food assistance and the inadequacy of federal, state, and private resources.[14–24] They found the individuals most at risk of hunger to include women, children, and the elderly,[14,16–18,20,21,23,24] many of them members of minority groups.[14–16,18,24] They attributed the cause of food insufficiency to poverty,[14,15,18,20,21,23] and the poverty to unemployment or underemployment,[14,15,17–19,22,24] the high costs of housing and other basic needs,[14,15,18,23,24] and inadequate welfare and food assistance benefits.[14,16–19,23,24]

The studies' recommendations were also remarkably similar. They suggested strategies to increase the federal contribution to state food and welfare assistance programs and client access to their benefits.[14–21,23,24] Some studies also addressed more fundamental issues, such as the need for increased employment opportunities,[14,17–19,23] higher wages,[24] improved access to low-cost housing,[14,18,24] and other forms of income redistribution.[24]

Conclusions

The findings and recommendations of state hunger studies are indistinguishable from those of county, city, and community studies conducted during the past decade[26,27] and more recent studies using improved survey methods.[25] The striking consistency of the results of virtually all hunger studies, no matter how they were conducted, provides ample—and sufficient—evidence for several broad conclusions:

- Food insufficiency has become a chronic problem in the United States.[11,14–24]
- Food insufficiency is not due to food shortages.[14,15,20,21,23]
- People who lack access to a variety of resources—not just food—are most at risk of hunger.[14–19,23,24]
- The federal poverty level is an inappropriate index of hunger, since it is based on a formula that fails to account for changes in the cost of living, regional variations in costs, or unusual expenses that may be required.[28]
- The U.S. social welfare system does not provide an adequate safety net.[14,16–18,20,21,23]
- Private charity cannot solve the hunger problem. Such voluntary activities are necessarily limited in expertise, time, and resources and are likely to require government support to permit them to continue.[14,16,19]
- Hunger is inextricably linked to poverty, which in turn is inextricably linked to underemployment and the costs of housing and other basic needs.[14,15,17–19,22–24]

Policy Implications

This analysis suggests little need for more methodologically sophisticated hunger studies to prove that a significant segment of the U.S. population experiences periodic food shortages. The consistency and weight of the evidence as presented by state-authorized studies, as well as those conducted by local groups, lead to this inescapable conclusion.

The inadequacies of current welfare and food assistance policies underscore the need for alternative solutions. Both liberals and conservatives are now suggesting strategies that recall policies of the 1930s.[29,30] They focus on provision of full employment that guarantees to low-income individuals and families an income that can raise them out of poverty. They also call for an increase in the minimum wage, wage supplements, and, for low-income working families, income tax credits adjusted for the number of children.[29,31]

Serious consideration of these strategies requires understanding of hunger as a chronic societal problem that no longer can be addressed in isolation from other correlates of poverty such as underemployment, inadequate housing, or poor education. Hunger studies provide overwhelming evidence to support such an understanding.

1. Poppendieck J. Breadlines knee-deep in wheat: food assistance in the great depression. New Brunswick, NJ: Rutgers University Press, 1986

2. Kerr NA. The evolution of USDA surplus disposal programs. Natl Food Rev 1988;11(3):25–30

3. Citizens' Board of Inquiry into Hunger and Malnutrition in the United States. Hunger U.S.A. Boston: Beacon Press, 1968

4. US Senate Select Committee on Nutrition and Human Needs. Final Report. Washington, DC: US Government Printing Office, December 1977

5. White House Conference on Food, Nutrition, and Health. Final report, December 24, 1969. Washington, DC: US Government Printing Office, 1970

6. Kotz N. Hunger in America: the federal response. New York: Field Foundation, 1979

7. Food Research and Action Center. Hunger survey index. FRAC, 1875 Connecticut Ave., N.W., #540, Washington, DC 20009

8. Physician Task Force on Hunger in America. Hunger in America: the growing epidemic. Middletown, CT: Wesleyan University Press, 1985, 1986, 1988

9. President's Task Force on Food Assistance. Report. Washington, DC: The White House, January 18, 1984

10. Matsumoto M. Recent trends in domestic food programs. Natl Food Rev 1989;12(4):34–6

11. US General Accounting Office. Hunger counties: methodological review of a report by the Physician Task Force on Hunger. GAO/PEMD-86-7BR. Washington, DC: General Accounting Office, March 1986

12. Nestle M. National nutrition monitoring policy: the continuing need for legislative intervention. J Nutr Ed 1990;22:141–4

13. Anderson SA, ed. Core indicators of nutritional state for difficult-to-sample populations. J Nutr 1990;120(suppl 11):1559–600

14. The Department of Health and Rehabilitative Services and the Florida Task Force on Hunger. Hunger in Florida: a report to the legislature, April 1, 1986

15. Iowa Department of Human Services and the Governor's Advisory Committee on Commodity Food and Shelter Programs. Results of the Iowa Food and Hunger Survey, March 1984

16. State of Maryland, Governor's Task Force on Food and Nutrition. Interim report, November 1984, and final report, executive summary, November 1985

17. Michigan Department of Public Health. A right to food: food assistance—the need and response. Proceedings and recommendations of the Food and Nutrition Advisory Commission Hearings, May 1984

18. New Jersey Commission on Hunger. Hunger: report and recommendations. Trenton, 1986

19. Ohio Senate Hunger Task Force. Final report, 1984

20. The Interim Study Committee on Hunger and Nutrition in South Carolina. Accounting for hunger: hunger and nutrition in South Carolina, September 1986

21. Senate Interim Committee on Hunger and Malnutrition. Faces of hunger in the shadow of plenty; 1984 report and recommendations. Austin, Texas: November 30, 1984

22. Utahns Against Hunger and Utah Department of Health. Utah nutrition monitoring project: study of low income households, Utah 1985. Salt Lake City: May 1986

23. The Governor's Task Force on Hunger. Hunger in Vermont, June 1986

24. Governor's Task Force on Hunger. Hunger in Washington State, October 1988

25. Community childhood hunger identification project: a survey of childhood hunger in the United States. Washington, DC: Food Research and Action Center, March 1991

26. Brown L. When violence has a benevolent face: the paradox of hunger in the world's wealthiest democracy. Int J Health Serv 1989;19:257–7

27. Cohen B, Burt MR. Eliminating hunger; food security policy for the 1990s. Washington, DC: The Urban Institute, 1989

28. Goodwin MY. Can the poor afford to eat? In: Wright HS, Sims LS, eds. Community nutrition; people, policies and programs. Boston: Jones Bartlett, 1981

29. Ellwood DE. Poor support: poverty in the American family. New York: Basic Books, 1988

30. Domestic Policy Council Low Income Opportunity Working Group. Up from dependency: a new national public assistance strategy. Washington, DC; The White House, December 1986

31. Shapiro I, Greenstein R. Making work pay: a new agenda for poverty policies. Washington, DC: Center on Budget and Policy Priorities, March 21, 1989

Effects of human starvation

*Physical and personality changes
documented in the Minnesota Experiment
in human starvation may be especially
relevant to facilitators of diet programs,
eating disorder specialists, health policy
makers and wrestling coaches.*

Frances M. Berg

Much critical information on the adverse effects of rapid weight loss can be found in the classic 1950 book, *The Biology of Human Starvation* by Ancel Keys and colleagues at the University of Minnesota.

In this impressive two-volume 1,385-page work, Keys documents the physical and mental effects on the 32 men who took part in the Minnesota Experiment in starvation of 1944-1945.

A well-educated and idealistic group, the volunteers were designated wartime conscientious objectors. All had at least one year of college; over half were college graduates. Personality scores were in the normal range by the Minn. Multiphasic Personality test.

Many had volunteered to serve overseas in relief operations. The study was designed to aid famine sufferers in wartorn Europe and Asia, and in participating in the research, the men hoped to make an important contribution to starving people throughout the world. They expected to assist overseas after the war.

Unfortunately, their altruism disappeared during the starvation period and they became self-serving and self-absorbed.

The study lasted one year: three months of an initial control period, six months of semi-starvation, and three months of re-feeding. Extensive testing was done at each stage and during the following year.

The semi-starvation diet, averaging 1,570 calories, was less than half the amount eaten during the control period (3,492 calories). The volunteers were required to lose 19 to 28 percent of body weight, depending on body composition (an average of 24 percent). If weekly weight loss for an individual fell short of what was expected, bread and potatoes were decreased; if weight loss was too high, these foods were increased.

Physical activity was vigorous. Each week the men walked 22 miles, participated in 30 minutes of treadmill testing, and worked 15 hours in clerical or maintenance work. They also walked a distance to the dining hall, adding another two to three miles each day. This continued throughout the study, however it is noted their work was done poorly during the final two months of semi-starvation.

As semi-starvation progressed, a great many physical and psychological changes were documented.

These may be similar to changes experienced by modern dieters, and are especially relevant to facilitators of weight loss programs, eating disorder specialists, health policy makers, and coaches of wrestling and other weight-cutting athletic teams.

The Minnesota Experiment in human starvation

Male subjects	Average
Age	25 years
Height	5 ft. 10 in.
Initial weight	153 pounds
Calorie intake	1,570 calories per day
Exercise level	22 miles hiking per week, plus treadmill/walking
After 6 months semi-starvation	
Weight	decreased 24%
Size (arms/thighs)	decreased 25%
Basal metabolism	decreased 40%, saving 600 calories/day
Strength	decreased 30%
Heart volume	reduced 20%
Heart work output	reduced 50%
Pulse rate	decreased from 56 to 37.8 beats/min.

The Minnesota Experiment in human starvation of 1944-1945 included 32 male volunteers and lasted one year (3 months initial control period, 6 months semi-semistarvation, 3 months re-feeding). OBESITY & HEALTH

Reprinted from *Obesity & Health*, Journal of Research, News and Contemporary Issues, Vol. 7, No. 1, January/February 1993, pp. 12-15. Copyright © 1993 by Health Living Institute, Hettinger, ND.

Physical changes

- Weight decreased an average of 24 percent, ranging from 18.8 to 29.3 percent (the men initially averaged 153 pounds, at 5-feet-10).
- Size decreased, especially in the diameter of upper thigh and upper arm where reduction was 25 percent; decrease in upper trunk breadth and depth, waist breadth and depth, pelvic depth, and neck breadth varied from about 9 to 15 percent.
- Heart volume decreased an average of about 20 percent; variability in heart volume was increased during starvation.
- Work output of heart per minute was reduced about 50 percent.
- Pulse rate slowed, from a mean of 56 initially to 37.8 beats per minute.
- Small decrease in body temperature.
- Veins were less prominent, and often collapsed when blood was drawn.
- Basal metabolism rate decreased by almost 40 percent by the end of 6 months of semi-starvation; metabolism was reduced per unit of tissue mass, as well as because of decreased size. This was calculated as equal to adaptive savings of 600 calories per day. (The researchers say some famine reports indicate women may have a greater decrease in metabolic rate than males, and also that women may have greater survival rates in times of starvation.)
- The men had an abnormal accumulation of fluid, which gave increased measurements for some in the ankle and wrist. (Edema is so closely related to semi-starvation that early terms linking the two were "hunger edema," "famine edema," and "war edema," writes Keys.)
- All the men felt cold and frequently complained of cold hands and feet. Even in mid-July, they wore jackets during the day and piled on blankets at night.
- The men felt weak and tired easily; voluntary movements became slower; their energy output decreased, even though regular physical activity was maintained including 22 miles of hiking per week.
- Their capacity to work decreased, especially that involving lifting, pushing and carrying loads. Also diminished was their ability to climb, walk long distances, and stand for long periods. Speed and accuracy were less impaired.
- Decrease in strength by about 30 percent in the forearm, legs and back.
- Decrease in endurance.
- Giddiness and momentary blackouts upon rising were common.
- Frequent reports of muscle cramp, soreness, and extremities that "went to sleep"; tendon reflexes were more sluggish.
- Frequency of urination.
- No increase in diarrhea, bloating, flatulence or colic such as has been observed in natural starvation areas.
- Sexual function and testes size was reduced. (It is noted that European famine reports frequently mention amenorrhea in women, impotence in men, delayed puberty in children, and decreased birth rate.)
- No impairment of visual ability was found, but there was an inability to focus, frequent eye-aches and spots before the eyes.
- Acuteness of hearing improved significantly, along with sensations of ringing in the head. Ordinary sounds were disturbing.
- Skin became pale, cold, dry, thin, scaly, rough, inelastic and marked with brownish pigmentation; skin ulcers and sores were common.
- Teeth and bones were apparently not demineralized as had been theorized; teeth were X-rayed at beginning and end, and decay was considered normal for a 6-month period. It is noted there is no evidence of teeth or bone deterioration from famine areas, and starving prisoners emerged from Japanese internment camps with teeth in remarkably good condition.
- Hair became thin, dry, and fell out.
- Senses of taste, smell and pressure seemed unaffected.
- The men appeared as if older, and behaved much older. They often said they felt old, but there were no indications of an accelerated aging process.

Personality changes

- Apathy, depression and tiredness increased.
- Irritability and moodiness increased.
- Self-discipline, mental alertness, comprehension and concentration decreased.
- Deterioration of spontaneous activity, including intellectual pursuits.
- Loss of ambition, a narrowing of interests.
- Feeling ineffective in daily living.
- The men felt distracted when they attempted to continue their cultural interests and studies. They were frustrated by the discrepancy between what they wanted to do and did do.

- They believed their judgment was impaired; however, tests showed this was unchanged, and they appeared to think clearly. (The researchers suggest this erroneous belief stemmed from feelings of apathy and narrowed interests).
- Decrease in sexual interest and loss of libido.
- Personal appearance and grooming deteriorated; the men often neglected to shave, brush their teeth, or comb their hair; they continued bathing, however, as one source of pleasure in feeling warm, and relieving aches, pain and fatigue.
- An average rise toward the neurotic end of profile.
- Six subjects reacted to semi-starvation stress with severe "character neurosis." Two cases bordering on psychosis included violence and hysteria.
- A rise in hysteria scores.
- Sensitivity to noise.
- Sometimes highly nervous, restless and anxious.
- The men carried out their chores and duties poorly.

Food preoccupation

- Increase in food interest; there was a preoccupation with food talk and food thoughts, though some subjects became annoyed by this in others.
- The men spent much time collecting recipes, studying cookbooks and menus, and fixing food saved from mealtime.
- An increased anticipation heightened their craving for food at meals.
- The men did much planning about how they would handle the day's allotment of food.
- Food dislikes disappeared. Taste appeal of the monotonous meals increased as time went on.
- The men became possessive about their food.
- They demanded food and beverages be hot.
- They toyed with their food to make it seem like more and of greater variety. Often, toward the end, they would dawdle over a meal for two hours.
- For some there appeared a conflict in whether to stall out eating or ravenously gulp their food.
- The men became angry when they saw others wasting food.
- They ate their food to the last crumb and licked their plates.
- They did not dream of food, however, as some other reports have suggested.
- Extensive gum chewing; one man increased his gum chewing to 40 packs a day.
- Increased drinking of coffee and tea.
- The men increased their smoking, and some non-smokers began smoking.

- Nail-biting, not seen in the initial control period, became common.
- The men became somewhat acquisitive in purchasing useless articles they could hardly afford and afterwards did not want; others became extremely anxious about saving money for "a rainy day."

Social activities

- Deterioration was seen in the group spirit. During initial 12-week control period a group feeling had developed which was lively, responsive, tolerant and happy, with outstanding qualities of humor and high spirits. This gradually disappeared, and the tone became sober, serious, and what humor remained tended to be sarcastic.
- The men became reluctant to make group decisions or to plan activities, even though earlier they had taken an active interest in making policies and rules.
- They were reluctant to participate in group activities, saying it was too much trouble to contend with other people; they spent more time alone, became self-centered and egocentric.
- Social interaction seemed stilted, and politeness artificial.
- Food was the central topic of conversation; the men talked of little but hunger, food, weight loss, and their "guinea pig" way of life.
- The men were aware of their hyper-irritability, but were not entirely able to control emotionally charged responses, outbursts of temper, periods of sulking, and violence. Some men became scapegoats and targets of aggression for rest.
- Occasionally, exhilaration and feelings of well-being were brought on by such things as a variation in daily routine, lasting from a few hours to several days, but these were inevitably followed by "low" periods.
- Educational programs, which the men had originally designed to prepare themselves for anticipated careers in foreign relief work, quietly collapsed.

Refeeding

For six weeks the men received varied calorie levels, from 1,877 to 4,158 calories, in four groups.

- The men's spirits continued low for six weeks, and many were more depressed and irritable than ever.
- There was a slump in morale, and the men lost all

interest in their earlier humanitarian concerns for the welfare of starving people.

- They became argumentative, and questioned the value of the experiment, as well as the competence of the researchers; they expressed feelings of being "let down." (This aggressiveness was seen by the researchers as evidence of increasing energy, and that the men were becoming less introverted and more interested in their environment.)
- Hunger pangs were reported as being more intense than ever.
- During the first 12 weeks of rehabilitation, appetites were insatiable; all the men, including those on the highest calorie diets, wanted more food even when they were physically full.
- Many found it hard to stop eating, although "stuffed to bursting."
- The men were still concerned with food and their rations, above all else.
- They continued licking their plates, playing with food, and avoiding waste. Although this was a highly educated group, the men's table manners and eating habits had deteriorated, and during refeeding several deteriorated even more.
- The urgent desire for dietary freedom was so extreme that postponing it another week produced severe emotional crisis and nearly open rebellion. All were counting the hours until they would have more food, even those who had been eating over 4,000 calories a day for two weeks.
- During week 13, when restrictions were lifted, the men ate an average of 5,218 calories per day. Their time was largely devoted to eating and sleeping, and they ate nearly continuously, eating as many as three consecutive lunches.
- By week 15, there was more social behavior at meals.
- By week 15, the table manners of 19 of 26 men were normal or normal, but the other 7 still gobbled their food, had the desire to lick their plates and licked their knives when they could.
- Of 17 who left the laboratory, 15 reported they ate from 50 to 200 percent more than before the experiment and snacked often; one said he ate immense meals and then started snacking an hour after finishing a meal.
- By week 20, all said they felt nearly normal and were less preoccupied with food.
- By week 33, 10 of the 14 who remained at the laboratory were eating normal amounts. The others ate more than before. One man, who ate 25 percent more and was gaining excess weight, tried to eat less but became so hungry he said he couldn't stand it and returned to excessive eating.
- Slowly humor, enthusiasm and sociability returned, and the men began looking forward to their plans for the future.

Physical effects in refeeding

- Physical discomforts continued, and the expected relief did not come quickly.
- The men gained fat tissue rapidly, and "soft roundness" became their dominant characteristic; in three months they had gained back an average of half their fat loss.
- Lean tissue recovered more slowly. Abdomen circumference reached 101 percent in three months for the highest calorie group, while arm, calf and thigh circumference recovered only 50 percent of initial size.
- The most rapid recovery was from dizziness, apathy and lethargy, with slower recovery from tiredness, weakness and loss of sex drive.
- Work capacity increased by week 13.
- The men had some problems with constipation, stomach pains, heartburn and gas, especially when they overate.
- Sleepiness and headaches increased for some.
- Thirst increased and edema continued to be a problem.

Source: Keys, Ancel, J Brozek, A Henschel, O Mickelsen, H Taylor. The Biology of Human Starvation. School of Public Health, 1950. University of Minnesota Press, Minneapolis, MN.

Frances M. Berg, M.S., is the editor and publisher of Obesity & Health.

Glossary

Absorption The process by which digestive products pass from the gastrointestinal tract into the blood or lymphatic systems.

Acid/base balance The relationship between acidity and alkalinity in the body fluids.

Amino acids The structural units that make up proteins.

Amylopectin A component of starch, consisting of many glucose units joined in branching patterns.

Amylase An enzyme that breaks down starches; a component of saliva.

Amylose A component of starch, consisting of many glucose units joined in a straight chain, without branching.

Anabolism The synthesis of new materials for cellular growth, maintenance, or repair in the body.

Anemia A deficiency of oxygen-carrying material in the blood.

Anorexia nervosa A disorder in which a person refuses food and loses weight to the point of emaciation and even death.

Antioxidant A substance that prevents or delays the breakdown of other substances by oxygen; often added to food to retard deterioration and rancidity.

Arachidonic acid An essential polyunsaturated fatty acid.

Arteriosclerosis Condition characterized by a thickening and hardening of the walls of the arteries and a resultant loss of elasticity.

Ascorbic Acid Vitamin C.

Atherosclerosis A type of arteriosclerosis in which lipids, especially cholesterol, accumulate in the arteries and obstruct blood flow.

Avidin A substance in raw egg white that acts as an antagonist of biotin, one of the B vitamins.

Basal metabolic rate (BMR) The rate at which the body uses energy for maintaining involuntary functions such as cellular activity, respiration, and heartbeat when at rest.

Basic Four The food plan outlining the milk, meat, fruits and vegetables, and breads and cereals needed in the daily diet to provide the necessary nutrients.

Beriberi A disease resulting from inadequate thiamin in the diet.

Betacarotene Yellow pigment that is converted to vitamin A in the body.

Biotin One of the B vitamins.

Bomb calorimeter An instrument that oxidizes food samples to measure their energy content.

Buffer A substance that can neutralize both acids and bases to minimize change in the pH of a solution.

Calorie The energy required to raise the temperature of one gram of water one degree Celsius.

Carbohydrate An organic compound composed of carbon, hydrogen, and oxygen in a ratio of 1: 2: 1.

Carcinogen A cancer-causing substance.

Catabolism The breakdown of complex substances into simpler ones.

Celiac disease A syndrome resulting from intestinal sensitivity to gluten, a protein in some cereals.

Cellulose An indigestible polysaccharide made of many glucose molecules.

Cheilosis Cracks at the corners of the mouth, due primarily to a deficiency of riboflavin in the diet.

Cholesterol A fatlike alcohol found only in animal products; important in many body functions but also implicated in heart disease.

Choline A substance that prevents the development of a fatty liver; frequently considered one of the B-complex vitamins.

Chylomicron A very small emulsified lipoprotein that transports fat in the blood.

Cobalamin One of the B vitamins (B_{12}).

Coenzyme A component of an enzyme system that facilitates the working of the enzyme.

Collagen Principal protein of connective tissue.

Colostrum The yellowish fluid that precedes breast milk, produced in the first few days of lactation.

Cretinism The physical and mental retardation of a child resulting from severe iodine or thyroid deficiency in the mother during pregnancy.

Dehydration Excessive loss of water from the body.

Dextrin Any of various small soluble polysaccharides found in the leaves of starch-forming plants and in the human alimentary canal as a product of starch digestion.

Diabetes (diabetes mellitus) A metabolic disorder characterized by excess blood sugar and urine sugar.

Digestion The breakdown of ingested foods into particles of a size and chemical composition that can be absorbed by the body.

Diglyceride A lipid containing glycerol and two fatty acids.

Disaccharide A sugar made up of two chemically combined monosaccharides, or simple sugars.

Diuretics Substances that stimulate urination.

Diverticulosis A condition in which the wall of the large intestine weakens and balloons out, forming pouches where fecal matter can be entrapped.

Edema The presence of an abnormally high amount of fluid in the tissues.

Emulsifier A substance that promotes the mixing of foods, such as oil and water in a salad dressing.

Enrichment The addition of nutrients to foods, often to restore what has been lost in processing.

Enzyme A protein that speeds up chemical reactions in the cell.

Epidemiology The study of the factors which contribute to the occurrence of a disease in a population.

Essential amino acid Any of the nine amino acids that the human body cannot manufacture and that must be supplied by the diet, as they are necessary for growth and maintenance.

Essential fatty acid A fatty acid that the human body cannot manufacture and that must be supplied by the diet, as it is necessary for growth and maintenance.

Fat An organic compound whose molecules contain glycerol and fatty acids; fat insulates the body, protects organs, carries fat-soluble vitamins, is a constituent of cell membranes, and makes food taste good.

Fatty acid A simple lipid—containing only carbon, hydrogen, and oxygen—that is a constituent of fat.

Ferritin A substance in which iron, in combination with protein, is stored in the liver, spleen, and bone marrow.

Fiber Indigestible carbohydrate found primarily in plant foods; high fiber intake is useful in regulating bowel movements, and may lower the incidence of certain types of cancer and other diseases.

Flavoprotein Protein containing riboflavin.

Folic acid (folacin) One of the B vitamins.

Fortification The addition of nutrients to foods to enhance their nutritional values.

Fructose A six-carbon monosaccharide found in many fruits as well as honey and plant saps; one of two monosaccharides forming sucrose, or table sugar.

Galactose A six-carbon monosaccharide, one of the two that make up lactose, or milk sugar.

Gallstones An abnormal formation of gravel or stones, composed of cholesterol and bile salts and sometimes bile pigments, in the gallbladder; result when substances that normally dissolve in bile precipitate out.

Gastritis Inflammation of the stomach.

Glucagon A hormone produced by the pancreas that works to increase blood glucose concentration.

Glucose A six-carbon monosaccharide found in sucrose, honey, and many fruits and vegetables; the major carbohydrate found in the body.

Glucose tolerance factor (GTF) A hormonelike substance containing chromium, niacin, and protein that helps the body use glucose.

Glyceride A simple lipid composed of fatty acids and glycerol.

Glycogen The storage form of carbohydrates in the body; composed of glucose molecules.

Goiter Enlargement of the thyroid gland as a result of iodine deficiency.

Goitrogens Substances that induce goiter, often by interfering with the body's utilization of iodine.

Heme A complex iron-containing compound that is a component of hemoglobin.

Hemicellulose Any of various indigestible plant polysaccharides.

Hemochromatosis A disorder of iron metabolism.

Hemoglobin The iron-containing protein in red blood cells which carries oxygen to the tissues.

High-density lipoprotein (HDL) A lipoprotein that acts as a cholesterol carrier in the blood; referred to as "good" cholesterol because relatively high levels of it appear to protect against atherosclerosis.

Hormones Compounds secreted by the endocrine glands that influence the functioning of various organs.

Humectants Substances added to foods to help them maintain moistness.

Hydrogenation The chemical process by which hydrogen is added to unsaturated fatty acids, which saturates them and converts them from a liquid to a solid form.

Hydrolyze To split a chemical compound into smaller molecules by adding water.

Hydroxyapatite The hard mineral portion (the major constituent) of bone, composed of calcium and phosphate.

Hypercalcemia A high level of calcium in the blood.

Hyperglycemia A high level of "sugar" (glucose) in the blood.

Hypocalcemia A low level of calcium in the blood.

Hypoglycemia A low level of "sugar" (glucose) in the blood.

Incomplete protein A protein lacking or deficient in one or more of the essential amino acids.

Inorganic Describes a substance not containing carbon.

Insensible loss Fluid loss, through the skin and from the lungs, that an individual is unaware of.

Insulin A hormone produced by the pancreas that regulates the body's use of glucose.

Intrinsic factor A protein produced by the stomach that makes absorption of B_{12} possible; lack of this protein results in pernicious anemia.

Joule A unit of energy preferred by some professionals over the heat energy measurements of the calorie system for calculating food energy; sometimes referred to as "kilojoule."

Keratinization Formation of a protein called keratin which, in vitamin A deficiency, occurs instead of mucus formation; leads to a drying and hardening of epithelial tissue.

Ketogenic Describes substances that can be converted to ketone bodies during metabolism, such as fatty acids and some amino acids.

Ketone bodies The three chemicals—acetone, acetoacetic acid, and beta-hydroxybutyrie—which are normally involved in lipid metabolism and accumulate in blood and urine in abnormal amounts in conditions of impaired metabolism (such as diabetes).

Ketosis A condition resulting when fats are the major source of energy and are incompletely oxidized, causing ketone bodies to build up in the bloodstream.

Kilocalorie One thousand calories, or the energy required to raise the temperature of one kilogram of water one degree Celsius; the preferred unit of measurement for food energy.

Kilojoule See Joule.

Kwashiorkor A form of malnutrition resulting from a severe protein deficiency and a mild to moderate lack of other essential nutrients but an adequate or even excessive calorie intake.

Lactase A digestive enzyme produced by the small intestine that breaks down lactose.

Lactation Milk production/secretion.

Lacto-ovo-vegetarian A person who does not eat meat, poultry, or fish but does eat milk products and eggs.

Lactose A disaccharide composed of glucose and galactose and found in milk.

Lactose intolerance The inability to digest lactose, due to a lack of the enzyme lactase in the intestine.

Lacto-vegetarian A person who does not eat meat, poultry, fish, or eggs but does drink milk and eat milk products.

Laxatives Food or drugs that stimulate bowel movements.

Lignins Certain forms of indigestible carbohydrate in plant foods.

Linoleic acid An essential polyunsaturated fatty acid.

Lipase An enzyme that digests fats.

Lipid Any of various substances in the body or in food that are insoluble in water; a fat or fatlike substance.

Lipoprotein Compound composed of a lipid (fat) and a protein that transports both in the bloodstream.

Low-density lipoprotein (LDL) A lipoprotein that acts as a cholesterol carrier in the blood; referred to as "bad" cholesterol because relatively high levels of it appear to enhance atherosclerosis.

Macrocytic anemia A form of anemia characterized by the presence of abnormally large blood cells.

Macroelements (also macronutrient elements) Those elements present in the body in amounts exceeding 0.005 percent of body weight and required in the diet in amounts exceeding 100 mg/day; include sodium, potassium, calcium, and phosphorus.

Malnutrition A poor state of health resulting from a lack, excess, or imbalance of the nutrients needed by the body.

Maltose A disaccharide whose units are each composed of two glucose molecules, produced by the digestion of starch.

Marasmus Condition resulting from a deficiency of calories and nearly all essential nutrients.

Melanin A dark pigment in the skin, hair, and eyes.

Metabolism The sum of all chemical reactions that take place within the body.

Microelements (also micronutrient elements; trace elements) Those elements present in the body in amounts under 0.005 percent of body weight and required in the diet in amounts under 100 mg/day.

Monoglyceride A lipid containing glycerol and only one fatty acid.

Monosaccharide A single sugar molecule, the simplest form of carbohydrate; examples are glucose, fructose, and galactose.

Monosodium glutamate (MSG) An amino acid used in flavoring foods; causes allergic reactions in some people.

Monounsaturated fatty acid A fatty acid containing one double bond.

Mutagen A mutation-causing agent.

Negative nitrogen balance Nitrogen output exceeds nitrogen intake.

Niacin (nicotinic acid) One of the B vitamins.

Nitrogen equilibrium (zero nitrogen balance) Nitrogen output equals nitrogen intake.

Nonessential amino acid Any of the 13 amino acids that the body can manufacture in adequate amounts, but which are nonetheless required in the diet in an amount relative to the amount of essential amino acids.

Nutrients Nourishing substances in food that can be digested, absorbed, and metabolized by the body; needed for growth, maintenance, and reproduction.

Nutrition (1) The sum of the processes by which an organism obtains, assimilates, and utilizes food. (2) The scientific study of these processes.

Obesity Condition of being 15 to 20 percent above one's ideal body weight.

Oleic acid A monounsaturated fatty acid.

Organic foods Those foods, especially fruits and vegetables, grown without the use of pesticides, synthetic fertilizers, etc.

Osmosis Passage of a solvent through a semipermeable membrane from an area of higher concentration to an area of lower concentration until the concentration is equal on both sides of the membrane.

Osteomalacia Condition in which a loss of bone mineral leads to a softening of the bones; adult counterpart of rickets.

Osteoporosis Disorder in which the bones degenerate due to a loss of bone mineral, producing porosity and fragility; normally found in older women.

Overweight Body weight exceeding an accepted norm by 10 or 15 percent.

Ovo-vegetarian A person who does not eat meat, poultry, fish, milk, or milk products but does eat eggs.

Oxidation The process by which a substrate takes up oxygen or loses hydrogen; the loss of electrons.

Palmitic acid A saturated fatty acid.

Pantothenic acid One of the B vitamins.

Pellagra The niacin deficiency syndrome, characterized by dementia, diarrhea, and dermatitis.

Pepsin A protein-digesting enzyme produced by the stomach.

Peptic ulcer An open sore or erosion in the lining of the digestive tract, especially in the stomach and duodenum.

Peptide A compound composed of amino acids joined together.

Peristalsis Motions of the digestive tract that propel food through the tract.

Pernicious anemia One form of anemia caused by an inability to absorb vitamin B_{12}, owing to a lack of intrinsic factor.

pH A measure of the acidity of a solution, based on a scale from 0 to 14: a pH of 7 is neutral; greater than 7 is alkaline; less than 7 is acidic.

Phenylketonuria (PKU) A genetic disease in which phenylalanine, an essential amino acid, is not properly metabolized, thus accumulating in the blood and causing early brain damage.

Phospholipid A fat containing phosphorus, glycerol, two fatty acids, and any of several other chemical substances.

Polypeptide A molecular chain of amino acids.

Polysaccharide A carbohydrate containing many monosaccharide subunits.

Polyunsaturated fatty acids A fatty acid in which two or more carbon atoms have formed double bonds, with each holding only one hydrogen atom.

Positive nitrogen balance Condition in which nitrogen intake exceeds nitrogen output in the body.

Protein Any of the organic compounds composed of amino acids and containing nitrogen; found in the cells of all living organisms.

Provitamins Precursors of vitamins that can be converted to vitamins in the body (e.g., betacarotene, from which the body can make vitamin A).

Pyridoxine One of the B vitamins (B_6).

Pull date Date after which food should no longer be sold but still may be edible for several days.

Recommended Daily Allowances (RDAs) Standards for daily intake of specific nutrients established by the Food and Nutrition Board of the National Academy of Sciences; they are the levels thought to be adequate to maintain the good health of most people.

Rhodopsin The visual pigment in the retinal rods of the eyes which allows one to see at night; its formation requires vitamin A.

Riboflavin One of the B vitamins (B_2).

Ribosome The cellular structure in which protein synthesis occurs.

Rickets The vitamin D deficiency disease in children characterized by bone softening and deformities.

Saliva Juices, produced in the mouth, that help digest foods.

Salmonella A bacterium that can cause food poisoning.

Saturated fatty acid A fatty acid in which carbon is joined with four other atoms; i.e., all carbon atoms are bound to the maximum possible number of hydrogen atoms.

Scurvy The vitamin C (ascorbic acid) deficiency disease characterized by bleeding gums, pain in joints, lethargy, and other problems.

Standard of identity A list of specifications for the manufacture of certain foods, stipulating their required contents.

Starch A polysaccharide composed of glucose molecules; the major form in which energy is stored in plants.

Stearic acid A saturated fatty acid.

Sucrose A disaccharide composed of glucose and fructose, often called "table sugar."

Sulfites Agents used as preservatives in foods, to eliminate bacteria, preserve freshness, prevent browning, and increase storage life; can cause acute asthma attacks, and even death, in people who are sensitive to them.

Teratogen An agent with the potential of causing birth defects.

Thiamin One of the B vitamins (B_1).

Thyroxine Hormone containing iodine that is secreted by the thyroid gland.

Toxemia A complication of pregnancy characterized by high blood pressure, edema, vomiting, presence of protein in the urine, and other symptoms.

Transferrin Protein compound, the form in which iron is transported in the blood.

Triglyceride A lipid containing glycerol and three fatty acids.

Trypsin A digestive enzyme, produced in the pancreas, that breaks down protein.

Underweight Body weight below an accepted norm by more than 10 percent.

United States Recommended Daily Allowance (USRDA) The highest level of recommended intakes for population groups (except pregnant and lactating women); derived from the RDAs and used in food labeling.

Urea The main nitrogenous component of urine, resulting from the breakdown of amino acids.

Uremia A disease in which urea accumulates in the blood.

Vegan A person who eats nothing derived from an animal; the strictest type of vegetarian.

Vitamin Organic substance required by the body in small amounts to perform numerous functions.

Vitamin B complex All known water-soluble vitamins except C; includes thiamin (B_1), riboflavin (B_2), pyridoxine (B_6), niacin, folic acid, cobalamin (B_{12}), pantothenic acid, and biotin.

Xerophthalmia A disease of the eye resulting from vitamin A deficiency.

Credits/ Acknowledgments

Cover design by Charles Vitelli

1. Trends Today and Tomorrow
Facing overview—The Dushkin Publishing Group, Inc., photo by Cheryl Greenleaf. 17—From *FDA Consumer,* June 1993, p. 8. Reprinted by permission from U.S. Department of Agriculture/ U.S. Department of Health and Human Services.

2. Nutrients
Facing overview—The Dushkin Publishing Group, Inc., photo.

3. Through the Life Span: Diet and Disease
Facing overview—The Dushkin Publishing Group, Inc., photo by Pamela Carley.

4. Fat and Weight Control
Facing overview—United Nations photo by F. B. Grunzweig.

5. Food Safety
Facing overview—The Dushkin Publishing Group, Inc., photo.

6. Health Claims
Facing overview—The Dushkin Publishing Group, Inc., photo.

7. Hunger and Global Issues
Facing overview—World Bank photo.

ANNUAL EDITIONS ARTICLE REVIEW FORM

■ NAME: _____ DATE: _____

■ TITLE AND NUMBER OF ARTICLE: _____

■ BRIEFLY STATE THE MAIN IDEA OF THIS ARTICLE: _____

_____

_____

_____

_____

■ LIST THREE IMPORTANT FACTS THAT THE AUTHOR USES TO SUPPORT THE MAIN IDEA:

_____

_____

_____

_____

_____

_____

■ WHAT INFORMATION OR IDEAS DISCUSSED IN THIS ARTICLE ARE ALSO DISCUSSED IN YOUR TEXTBOOK OR OTHER READING YOU HAVE DONE? LIST THE TEXTBOOK CHAPTERS AND PAGE NUMBERS:

_____

_____

_____

_____

_____

_____

_____

■ LIST ANY EXAMPLES OF BIAS OR FAULTY REASONING THAT YOU FOUND IN THE ARTICLE:

_____

_____

_____

_____

_____

■ LIST ANY NEW TERMS/CONCEPTS THAT WERE DISCUSSED IN THE ARTICLE AND WRITE A SHORT DEFINITION:

_____

_____

_____

_____

_____

*Your instructor may require you to use this Annual Editions Article Review Form in any number of ways: for articles that are assigned, for extra credit, as a tool to assist in developing assigned papers, or simply for your own reference. Even if it is not required, we encourage you to photocopy and use this page; you'll find that reflecting on the articles will greatly enhance the information from your text.